Carla

Care Planning and Delivery in Intellectual Disability Nursing

Edited by

Bob Gates
Professor and Head of Subject for Learning Disabilities
Thames Valley University, London

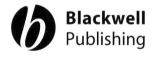

Blackwell
Publishing

© 2006 by Blackwell Publishing Ltd

Editorial offices:
Blackwell Publishing Ltd, 9600 Garsington Road, Oxford OX4 2DQ, UK
  Tel: +44 (0)1865 776868
Blackwell Publishing Inc., 350 Main Street, Malden, MA 02148-5020, USA
  Tel: +1 781 388 8250
Blackwell Publishing Asia Pty Ltd, 550 Swanston Street, Carlton, Victoria 3053, Australia
  Tel: +61 (0)3 8359 1011

First published 2006 by Blackwell Publishing Ltd

ISBN-10: 1-4051-3122-5
ISBN-13: 978-1-4051-3122-3

Library of Congress Cataloging-in-Publication Data
Care planning and delivery in intellectual disability nursing / edited by Bob Gates.
   p. ; cm.
Includes bibliographical references and index.
ISBN-13: 978-1-4051-3122-3 (pbk. : alk. paper)
ISBN-10: 1-4051-3122-5 (pbk. : alk. paper)
1. Mental retardation–Nursing. 2. Nursing–Planning. 3. Nursing care plans.
[DNLM: 1. Mental Retardation–nursing. 2. Nursing Care–methods. 3. Patient Care
Planning. 4. Quality of Health Care. WY 160 C2768 2006] I. Gates, Bob, RNT. II. Title.
RC570.C27 2006
616.85′880231–dc22
2005030637

A catalogue record for this title is available from the British Library

Set in 10/12.5pt Palatino
by Graphicraft Limited, Hong Kong
Printed and bound in Great Britain
by TJ International, Padstow

The publisher's policy is to use permanent paper from mills that operate a sustainable forestry policy, and which has been manufactured from pulp processed using acid-free and elementary chlorine-free practices. Furthermore, the publisher ensures that the text paper and cover board used have met acceptable environmental accreditation standards.

For further information on Blackwell Publishing, visit our website:
www.blackwellpublishing.com

Contents

iii

Preface

This ground-breaking text book is the first of its kind. It has been specifically written for intellectual disability nurses to assist them in care planning and delivery of care for people with intellectual disabilities. In the past little attention has been paid to care planning and delivery in intellectual disability nursing with a few notable exceptions (Aldridge, 1987, 2003). There has been, at least for the last three decades, a seemingly never-ending preoccupation with exploring the role of the intellectual disability nurse in esoteric terms, rather than articulating in operational terms what they are and should be doing. I believe it is long past the hour for apologising for the role of intellectual disability nurses in institutionalising people with intellectual disabilities in the last century. Rather they need to think of the present and the future, and it is my profound belief that what intellectual disability nurses do is of central importance to the lives of many people with intellectual disabilities, their families and carers, and that what they do has measurable impact on those individuals' quality of life (Alaszewski et al., 2001; Gates, 2002).

In Part 1 of this book the first six chapters explore: the nature of care planning and delivery, integrated care pathways, life planning, person-centred planning, legal and ethical issues of care planning and delivery and, finally, risk assessment and risk management in intellectual disability nursing. Each of these chapters contains authentic case illustrations, reader activities and is supported by contemporary research literature, as well as containing useful resources and further reading. More specifically, in Chapter 1, Zuzana Matousova-Done and Bob Gates point out that much of the care planning and delivery of intellectual nursing no longer takes place in the old long-term intellectual disability hospitals, rather it occurs in a landscape of complex service provision that includes residential care homes, independent living homes and supported living, as well as people with intellectual disabilities living in their own home or family homes. There are also larger service configurations and very specialist settings, such as treatment and assessment services and challenging behaviour units; people with intellectual disabilities may also reside in other specialist health or social care settings, such as hospices or homes for older people. Wherever people with intellectual disabilities live, if they are in receipt of nursing care, whether this comprises short intensive nursing interventions or long periods of care and support, then this care should be guided by a care plan. This chapter introduces the reader to the nature of care planning; distinctions are drawn between care planning and care management and wider caring terminology. The reader will be introduced to relevant and contemporary social policy, the Nursing and Midwifery Council's guidelines, competencies and expectations for professional practice. The use of the nursing process and nursing models and their appropriateness in care planning and delivery will be also be explored. This chapter concludes that there is a need for robust, professionally prepared care plans based on a systematic nursing assessment.

In Chapter 2, Hazel Powell and Elaine Kwiatek explore the concept of integrated care pathways. This chapter should assist readers to reflect on their practice and assist them in using integrated care pathways for people with intellectual disabilities. Promoting accessible healthcare through the use of patient passports and easier-to-read versions of patient information is also explored to enable nurses to employ these models to ensure people with intellectual disabilities obtain high quality healthcare. Integrated care pathways are defined and their application is described. The evidence base relating to integrated care pathways is also investigated along with their constraints and benefits. The use of integrated care pathways for people with intellectual disabilities is explored and suggestions are made for developing or improving their use in the area of intellectual disability nursing. The emergence of the use of communication passports both within intellectual disability services and as a means for accessing mainstream healthcare provision will be described. Finally, they review the literature concerning the communication needs of people with intellectual disabilities regarding how healthcare information is reviewed. This concludes with an overview of the use of accessible information and an exploration as to how this can be incorporated into everyday practice.

In Chapter 3, Carmel Jennings, Declan Courell and Dympna Walsh Gallagher explore life planning for individuals with intellectual disabilities. They point out that services for this group of people have witnessed fundamental changes over the last 30 years, moving from a model of care that was primarily institutional and medically focused, to one that supports community presence and inclusion. This chapter explores how we all think about and plan for our lives in different ways. The authors show that some people have very clear ideas about what they want in life, why they want it and how they can achieve it; whereas other people may only dream of what they want and dreams may never become a reality. Using person-centred approaches, the authors explain that life planning is about whom we are, what our needs, wishes and dreams are, and how we can go about achieving these needs, wishes and dreams.

In Chapter 4, Steve McNally further explores issues concerning person-centred planning (PCP). In particular the nature of PCP and its prominence in policy is reviewed. The benefits and limitations of PCP approaches are explored. The chapter also articulates some of the inherent tensions which exist between professional and personal perspectives of care planning. The implications of PCP for professionals are explored, including the need for facilitation of PCP to be acknowledged as sound professional practice. Facilitation of PCP is a role that can be integrated within the therapeutic relationship between intellectual disability nurses and people with intellectual disabilities. Finally this chapter draws on data from original research of a study on the practice of self advocacy in England. Informants from this research project express their own views on rights, choice, independence and inclusion. These are presented to provide a user perspective concerning the delivery of these principles that are central to PCP and to their lives.

In Chapter 5, Susan Harvey and Vicky Stobbart rightly point out that intellectual disability nurses are required to safeguard the interests of their clients at all times and this will require them to be clear about their scope of professional practice. They point out that intellectual disability nurses must practise in an anti-discriminatory and anti-oppressive way, remaining alert to the legal, moral and ethical implications of their practice. Additionally the authors outline how intellectual disability nurses must practise in a non-parentalistic way, recognising their duty of care. Their chapter explores all of these issues and also focuses on treatment issues, consent and the UK's Nursing Code of Professional Conduct.

In the final chapter of Part 1, Chapter 6, Phil Boulter and Alison Pointu identify ways in which nurses can support people with intellectual disabilities to live a full life whereby risk issues are recognised and managed. This chapter explores issues relating to risk and risk management, and for this purpose they focus on a number of key principles. Firstly, the chapter reflects on the historical perspective of intellectual disability practice; they then discuss a variety of frameworks available to assess and plan for risk. They raise ethical dilemmas and issues relating to individual accountability for nurses as part of the risk management process. Throughout the chapter they challenge readers to examine their practice and their organisation's approach to risk and risk management.

In Part 2 each of the chapters discuss the complexities and intricacies associated with care planning and delivery across a wide range of settings as well as exploring the wide spectrum of needs presented by people with intellectual disabilities. These chapters include: care planning for people with intellectual disabilities in forensic settings, care planning for people with intellectual disabilities in mental health settings, care planning and delivery for those requiring palliative care, care planning for people with intellectual disabilities in community settings, care planning for people with intellectual disabilities in residential settings; this is followed by chapters on health action planning for people with intellectual disabilities and, finally, care planning and delivery for people with profound intellectual disabilities and complex needs. As in Part 1, each of these chapters contains authentic case illustrations and reader activities, as well as being supported by contemporary research literature, and all contain useful resources and further reading.

In more detail for Part 2, in Chapter 7 Karina Hepworth and Mick Wolverson present a comprehensive overview of the key aspects of care planning and delivery for individuals involved with forensic services. They discuss the care pathway relating to people involved with forensic services. They point out the shift in focus of forensic provision of care from custodial to less restrictive environments, whilst placing an emphasis on individualised care plans and a care pathway that would encourage diversion from custody schemes. In particular they discuss care planning within forensic units, preventative work, holistic assessment, supporting people involved with the criminal justice system and the care programme approach. The chapter also explores forensic issues in relation to youth and adult offending perspectives. The chapter discusses care planning and delivery in relation to services and more specific assessment and care planning on inappropriate sexual behaviour and arson.

In Chapter 8, Laurence Taggart and Eamonn Slevin describe in detail care planning in mental health settings. They point out the effects of mental ill health and its potential to disintegrate personality or descend on one's life like a dark cloud and overshadow all aspects of personhood. They rightly point out that if a person also has an intellectual disability and a co-morbid mental illness or mental health problem, then this can compound the detrimental impact of these co-existing conditions. They detail a range of pertinent issues associated with planning and delivering care for people with intellectual disabilities who have mental health problems. They discuss key principles that guide the chapter, including aspects related to defining mental illness and its prevalence in the intellectually disabled population. They provide guidance on the care planning process for intellectual disability nurses and other care staff who may work with this client group.

Chapter 9 aims to achieve three things. Firstly, it identifies the challenges presented when a person with an intellectual disability is diagnosed with a palliative condition. Secondly, it integrates general palliative care principles into good practice for people with intellectual disabilities and, finally, explores concepts of care planning for people with intellectual disability that will ensure equity and parity of care delivery and accessibility. David Elliot and Sue Read next define palliative care and intellectual disabilities and clarify the contextual background of palliative care in relation to people with intellectual disabilities. They explore a holistic approach to palliative care and this is undertaken using a practical approach. Finally, they offer a model of good practice that can be used as a basis for developing an integrated, consistent, planned approach to holistic palliative care provision to people with intellectual disabilities.

In Chapter 10, Owen Barr and Maurice Devine explore the planning and delivery of nursing care in community nursing services. They point out that the majority of people with intellectual disabilities live in community settings, and many more live with family carers than live in hospitals or community-based residential accommodation. This makes effective collaboration between parents, family carers and community nurses essential. They also remind us that the range of community settings in which people with intellectual disabilities live has diversified considerably as was pointed out in Chapter 1. More opportunities now exist for people with intellectual disabilities to live in their own homes, as well as a range of supported housing options, small group homes and, for some people, larger residential or nursing home accommodation. People with intellectual disabilities also use other community-based services that include day services, further education, leisure services and employment training services, and may also be in supported or open employment. Some people with intellectual disabilities may have a complex package of day activities that combines day centres with further education, training and work in open or supported employment. These services are typically provided by statutory and independent sector providers, across a number of agencies including health, social services, education and employment. Therefore community nurses need to have effective and collaborative relationships with staff in community-based residential accommodation, and across a number of other agencies, in order to provide effective care planning and delivery to people who live in the community.

Chapter 11, by Robert Jenkins, Paul Wheeler and Neil James, explores care planning in residential settings. They identify that, central to the role of the intellectual disability nurse within residential settings, there must be a framework established that will direct the way in which services and therapeutic approaches are provided. This chapter explores issues concerning the provision of accommodation for people with intellectual disabilities. It considers the purpose of nursing, the historical development of services and the role of the intellectual disability nurse. This chapter considers how the concept of quality of life might be used as a framework for care planning.

In the penultimate chapter Helen Atherton discusses the principles of care planning in meeting the health needs of people with intellectual disabilities within the context of health facilitation and health action planning. She explores the role of the health facilitator, including those who might undertake this role. She argues that intellectual disability nurses are in a key position to lead on this role. She points out that a central feature of health facilitation is the necessity of working in a way that promotes rights, independence, choice and inclusion for people with intellectual disabilities. Throughout the chapter, best practice examples are articulated as recommended approaches to improving access to healthcare for people with intellectual disabilities.

In the final chapter Julie Clark and Bob Gates explore care planning and delivery for people with profound intellectual disabilities and complex needs. They argue that people with profound intellectual disabilities and complex needs represent one of the most marginalised groups in western society. They point out that they are at risk from social exclusion and experience poorer health than the rest of the population. This makes care planning particularly relevant for this group of people because of the high level of dependence they may have on others throughout their lives. They argue that care plans should be regarded as a way of systematically planning and documenting interventions to meet their needs to support them in all aspects of their life. In this chapter they consider the intellectual disability nurse's role in care planning and delivery for this group of people.

In the context of the recent White Paper, *Valuing People* (Department of Health, 2001), it is clear that intellectual disability nurses have much to contribute to the enormous agenda of current health and social care reforms. They have the potential to act as agents of social inclusion and assist in bringing about the inclusion of people with intellectual disabilities into their communities, away from the margins where many currently exist. For this to happen they need to continue to develop their specialist knowledge and skills, so that they are better able to offer robust care planning and delivery to people with intellectual disabilities in a range of health and social care settings.

It is hoped that this text will play some small part in this enormous agenda for all involved in the arena of intellectual disabilities, but in particular for intellectual disability nurses so that they are able to better serve people with intellectual disabilities, their families and carers, enabling them to enjoy quality lives.

Bob Gates
Head of Subject and Professor of Learning Disabilities
Thames Valley University, London

References

Aldridge, J. (1987) Initiating the use of a nursing model: the importance of systematic care planning – a ward clinician's perspective. In: *Mental Handicap: Facilitating Holistic Care* (Barber, P., ed.). London: Hodder and Stoughton.

Aldridge, J. (2003) Learning Disability nursing: a model for practice. In: *Learning Disability Nursing* (Turnbull, J., ed.). Oxford: Blackwell Publishing.

Alaszewski, A., Motherby, E., Gates, B., Ayer, S. and Manthorpe, J. (2001) *Diversity and Change: The Changing Roles and Education of Learning Disability Nurses.* London: English National Board.

Department of Health (2001) *Valuing People: A New Strategy for Learning Disability for the 21st Century.* Norwich: The Stationery Office.

Gates, B. (2002) The new learning disability nursing: agents of inclusion for the 21st Century. Guest Editorial. *Learning Disability Bulletin.* Kidderminster: British Institute of Learning Disability.

Contributors

Editor
Bob Gates MSc, BEd (Hons) RNMS, RMN, Dip Nurs (Lond), Cert Ed, RNT
Professor and Head of Subject for Learning Disabilities, Thames Valley
University, London, UK

Contributing authors
Helen Atherton PhD, BSc (Hons), RNLD
Lecturer in Learning Disability Nursing, University of Leeds, UK

Owen Barr PhD, MSc, BSc (Hons), RGN, RNMH, CNMH Cert, RNT
Senior Lecturer in Nursing, University of Ulster, Northern Ireland

Phil Boulter MA, RNMH, RMN
Consultant Nurse, Surrey and Borders Partnership NHS Trust, UK

Julie Clark BSc (Hons) Psychology, BSc (Hons) Nursing, RNLD
PhD Student/Teaching Assistant, Thames Valley University, London, UK

Declan Courell MSc, BNSc (Hons), RNID, CNMH, CPT, PGCE, RNT
Lecturer in Nursing, St Angela's College, Republic of Ireland

Maurice Devine BSc (Hons) Community Nursing, RNMH, RGN, Dip Nurs
(Lond), PG Dip, Nurse Education
Nurse Consultant, Learning Disability, Down/Lisburn Trust Northern
Ireland

David Elliott BA (Hons), MA, RNMH, Dip Grief and Ber Couns, Cert Ber
Couns
Community Nurse, Learning Disabilities, Developmental Neurosciences and
Learning Disabilities Services, South Staffordshire, UK

Susan Harvey BA Health Care Community Practice, RNMH, RN
(Psychopaedic), ENB 807
Nurse Consultant, Hounslow Primary Care Trust, and Associate Lecturer,
Thames Valley University, London, UK

Karina Hepworth MA, RGN, RNLD, Dip Behavioural Approaches
Senior Nurse Specialist, Kirklees Youth Offending Team, South West
Yorkshire Mental Health NHS Trust, UK

Neil James BSc (Hons), RNLD, PGCE
Senior Lecturer, School of Care Sciences, University of Glamorgan, UK

Robert Jenkins MSc, Dip Soc Studies, Cert Ed (FE), RNLD
Principal Lecturer, School of Care Sciences, University of Glamorgan, UK

Carmel Jennings MA (Health Education), RNID, BNT Cert Ed, RNT
Lecturer in Nursing, St Angela's College, Republic of Ireland

Elaine Kwiatek MSc, RNLD, SRN, Reg CT, Cert Ed
Lecturer and Teaching Fellow, Napier University, UK

Steve McNally PhD, MSc, Cert Ed, RNLD, RMN
Lecturer Practitioner in Learning Disabilities, Oxford Brookes University,
Oxfordshire Learning Disability NHS Trust, UK

Zuzana Matousova-Done BSc (Hons), RNLD
Teaching Assistant, Thames Valley University, London

Alison Pointu MSc (Learning Disabilities Studies), RNMH, Dip Specialist
Community Nurse
Consultant Nurse Learning Disabilities, Barnet Primary Care Trust, and
Honorary Fellow, University of Hertfordshire, UK

Hazel Powell BSc, RNLD, RMN, RNT, SPQ, PGCE
Lecturer in Learning Disabilities, Napier University, UK

Sue Read PhD, MA, RNMH, CertEd (FE), Cert in Bereavement Studies
Lecturer, School of Nursing and Midwifery, Keele University, UK

Eamonn Slevin DNSc, BSc (Hons), RNLD, RGN, RNT, PG Dip AdvNursing,
PG Dip Ed
Reader in Learning Disabilities, University of Ulster, Northern Ireland

Vicky Stobbart MSc, RNLD, Dip Nursing, ENB 807
Safer Practice Lead, National Patient Safety Agency, NHS, UK

Laurence Taggart PhD, BSc (Hons) Applied Psychology, RNLD, ENB 955
Lecturer, University of Ulster, Northern Ireland

Dympna Walsh Gallagher MSc, BNSc (Hons), RNID, DN, RGN, PGD, RNT
Lecturer in Nursing, St Angela's College, Republic of Ireland

Paul Wheeler PhD, MPhil, LLB (Hons), BSc (Hons), RNLD
Senior Lecturer, School of Care Sciences, University of Glamorgan, UK

Mick Wolverson MSc, BA (Hons), RNMH, PGCE
Lecturer in Learning Disabilities, University of York, UK

Chapter 1

The nature of care planning and delivery in intellectual disability nursing

Zuzana Matousova-Done and Bob Gates

Introduction

The practice setting for intellectual disability nursing is difficult to define because it is located in a complex landscape of service provision. This includes, for example, residential care homes, independent living homes, supported living arrangements, as well as people with intellectual disabilities living in their own homes as well as family homes. There are also larger service configurations and very specialist settings, such as treatment and assessment services and challenging behaviour units, as well as specialist health or social care settings, such as hospices or homes for older people. Therefore much of the care planning and delivery of intellectual nurses now no longer takes place in traditional settings; rather it takes place in within the context of multi-disciplinary and multi-agency settings (Alaszewski et al., 2001). However, because of professional requirements for intellectual disability nurses, regardless of where people with intellectual disabilities live, if they are in receipt of nursing care this should be guided by a care plan, whether the care comprises short intensive nursing interventions or long periods of care and support (Nursing and Midwifery Council, 2004c).

This chapter will introduce the reader to the nature of care planning, person-centred planning, care management, health action planning, life planning and the care programme approach. The reader will also be introduced to relevant and contemporary social policy, as well as the Nursing and Midwifery Council's guidelines, competencies and expectations of professional practice as they apply to nursing and their planning and delivery of care. This chapter will advocate the need for robust, professionally prepared care plans based on a systematic nursing assessment. In addition to this, reference to the nursing process and models of nursing and their appropriateness to care planning and delivery will be highlighted and explored.

The nature of care planning and its delivery

This first section describes the nature of care planning and delivery whilst simultaneously making distinctions with other 'caring' terminology. The language of human services is littered with an (un)impressive array of words, phrases and initiatives that are used in the armoury of 'caring professionals', concerning care, care planning and delivery. This terminology includes care planning, person-centred care planning, care management, health action planning, life planning and the care programme approach. Perhaps this is why it is common to find students and newly qualified practitioners in health and social care settings unclear at times about what is being referred to when such terminology is used, or what their specific role and responsibilities are; this is particularly so in the case of the intellectual disability nurse. It is hoped that this chapter will demystify some of this terminology and in this respect provide a useful foundation for the remaining chapters of this book.

In describing this caring terminology it is necessary to briefly explore each of the terms identified, and outline their specific meaning, not just for the convenience of this book but because they apply to the practice of intellectual disability nursing. This is illustrated by Fig. 1.1 which depicts the nature of the inter-relationship of care planning and delivery and caring terminology in intellectual disability nursing. This figure shows that at the heart of all that we do is the individual. Intellectual disability nurses must always remember this

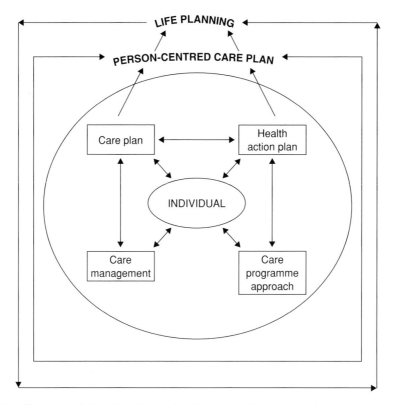

Fig. 1.1   The inter-relationship of care planning and delivery and caring terminology in intellectual disability nursing.

regardless of the environment or context of the interaction between the nurse and the person with intellectual disabilities they are supporting. It can be seen in Fig. 1.1 that some people with intellectual disabilities may have a care plan or health action plan, or be the subject of the care programme approach. These can all be seen to be located within a person-centred care plan, where all that is constructed is done so in partnership with the person with intellectual disabilities and their families or carers. It can also be seen that the process of care management is located in Fig. 1.1; this is where packages of care are constructed for some individuals with intellectual disabilities. Usually these care packages include reference to residential provision, day care provision and sometimes leisure and recreational provision. This process is usually undertaken by care managers, who typically come from a range of different professional backgrounds in intellectual disabilities, including nurses, occupational therapists and physiotherapists, but more usually, social workers. Once again good care management should put the individual at the heart of constructing a care package for an individual.

In Fig. 1.1 all of these different elements of caring terminology are shown to be first located with the broad philosophy of what has become universally known as person-centred care planning, and this is depicted within a process of life planning. This collective caring terminology is discussed more specifically below before an exploration of the nursing process and the use of nursing models to guide the planning and delivery of intellectual disability nursing care.

Care plan

Essentially this is a written document that articulates a plan of care for an individual with intellectual disabilities. This plan will typically identify what this person can and will do in their day-to-day living and what support they need to do so. This process of constructing a care plan is complex and can potentially involve a large number of people and sources of information. The use of a nursing model can help to make this process more manageable and thereby enhance care (Newton, 1991). Planning care and its delivery has different emphases depending on its purpose, function and who carries out the assessment. For example, a person with intellectual disabilities living in a community setting will require different information to be collected from health, generic and social care assessments as opposed to someone detained under the Mental Health Act in a treatment and assessment unit. It is the case that in the preceding example both of these assessments will look at different areas of need; however the overall process of care planning and its delivery should ideally take into consideration all the assessed needs/areas, and the construction of any care plan should reflect and include these. For example, an occupational therapist might assess the daily living skills of a person with intellectual disabilities living in the community, whereas a clinical psychologist might assess the behavioural needs of someone in a treatment and assessment unit; a social worker might assess someone with learning disabilities as to whether they meet eligibility criteria for services (and to identify which service is appropriate) and, finally, a nurse might assess the health needs of an individual. All of these contributions might well assist in the construction of an overall care plan for someone with intellectual disabilities.

Person-centred care planning

Person-centred care planning forms an integral part of the care planning process (Department of Health, 2001; Thompson and Cobb, 2004). Person-centred planning refers to a philosophy or set of values based on the idea that care planning should begin with the individual (Department of Health, 2001). It can also be thought of as a set of tools designed to help people with intellectual disabilities and services make plans which reflect an individual's desires and aspirations (Sanderson et al., 1997). Chapters 3 and 4 provide full and extensive discussion on person-centred care planning.

Care management

This is a system of assessing individual needs and, from this, constructing a 'package of care' to meet those needs. Care managers play a pivotal role in helping people to achieve valued, fulfilling lifestyles; they can be instrumental in commissioning new initiatives built around the needs of the person, rather than expecting them to fit into existing provision, however inappropriate. It has been observed that care managers occupy a crucial point which straddles human services and the wider community (Duffy and Sanderson, 2004). A really effective care manager is likely to practise in a person-centred way, and probably has some characteristics in common with a 'service broker' (Brandon and Towe, 1989). Intellectual disability nurses are in a strong position to carry out this role, given their specialist training and understanding of the service user's perspective based on their partnership approach. Good care management practice involves working in a person-centred way. However, one could argue that care management is still often applied as an 'administrative tool for cost management' (Walker, 1993, p. 219).

Health action planning

Health action plans are personal action plans that detail the actions needed to improve and maintain an individual's health (Department of Health, 2001). The government has introduced health action plans in an attempt to reduce some of the health inequalities that people with intellectual disabilities experience (Howells, 1986; van Schrojenstein Lantman de Valk et al., 2000; Elliott et al., 2003; Mencap, 2004). These should form part of a person-centred care plan and should be developed using the same philosophy. Nurses must recognise that they have to balance a duty of care with respect for the client's right to make choices (Nursing and Midwifery Council, 2004c). The development of health action plans should be supported by primary health care services (Department of Health, 2001) and, with this in mind, some primary care trusts in the UK have introduced annual health checks for people with intellectual disabilities.

Care programme approach

This is a method for assessing, planning and co-ordinating care and support for people identified as using mental health services (including some people with intellectual disabilities) by establishing the intervention needed and who can best provide this. It is usually employed when a person is vulnerable or presenting a risk to others and typically there have been various professionals and agencies involved in an individual's life. Thiru et al. (2002) have described the care programme approach as:

> 'a framework for heath and social care assessment, including risk assessment, within a comprehensive, person centred, multi-disciplinary care planning process.' (Thiru et al., 2002, p. 11)

In the standard model, a full review would take place at least annually, and six-monthly in the case of an enhanced care programme approach. Individual provider organisations may arrange for more flexible reviews as necessary; a person may move between care programme approach levels (see Chapter 7) as their needs change. Although they may initially appear to be in conflict, person-centred care planning and other more directive forms of care planning, such as the care programme approach, need not be mutually exclusive. Intellectual disability nurses supporting service users in a forensic setting, in which clients' freedom is restricted, must still integrate the principles of person-centred care planning into their daily practice. The key principles of the care programme approach – assessment, care co-ordination, care planning, evaluation and review – are also prominent in care management.

Life planning

To a lesser or greater extent we all think about and plan for our lives in different ways. Some of us have very clear ideas about what we want in life, why we want it and how we will achieve it. We all of us plan for children, careers and old age. Adopting a person-centred approach, life planning is about whom we are, what our needs, wishes and dreams are and how we go about trying to achieve them. We constantly make life plans around holidays, living arrangements, careers, money, shopping and relationships, and we talk of these plans to families and friends. Regardless of who we are, no one person is in complete control of all events in their life and neither is any one person at the complete mercy of destiny or fate. There is an interface between the extent which an individual can exert a greater or lesser influence over the course of their life. It is the extent of this influence that is of crucial importance for people with intellectual disability. For the most part a number of people with intellectual disabilities are quite capable of determining what they want from their lives, but some people may need considerable help from their family, friends and carers; sometimes intellectual disability nurses can contribute to this.

Summary

Within the context of this book, care planning and delivery will refer to a specific document that delineates a plan of care that is prescribed by a nurse, and that this plan can be followed and delivered by another nurse, or, in the context of intellectual disability service provision, this increasingly includes unqualified social care staff. There are at least four steps to the systematic construction of a care plan and its subsequent delivery. Firstly, a comprehensive needs assessment (physical, psychological, social and spiritual) has to be completed. If a nurse is required to work with someone with intellectual disabilities and/or their families, it is necessary that their needs are assessed and incorporated into the individual care plan, taking their desires, wishes and aspirations into account. The nurse will need to work closely with the clients' family, care providers and other professionals as this broad approach may bring very important and essential information to light for assessment, as well as care plan development, its approach, delivery and management. This first stage is followed by the construction of a written care plan that is then implemented and followed by ongoing review and evaluation.

The use of the nursing process and nursing models

The nursing process can best be described as a framework for planning individualised care for patients/clients with intellectual disabilities. It should be understood that because it is a *process*, this process never finishes, as the clients'/patients' needs constantly change and it is the nurses' responsibility to respond to these changing needs wherever necessary. The nursing process is usually depicted as comprising four or five stages depending on the resources available and work setting, and includes: diagnosis, assessment, planning, implementing and evaluation. Not only is the nursing process and its use critical to the success of a number of imperatives of professional and social policy, Fitness for Practice (UKCC, 1999), Making a Difference (Department of Health, 1999), and the National Health Service Plan (Department of Health, 2000b), but its use also enables nurses to construct and deliver their care in a systematic manner.

The nursing process should be undertaken using a collaborative and participative approach with other professionals, gathering and implementing resources, in order to improve the care process (Department of Health, 2000b; Department of Health, 2001). Jones (1999) has claimed that the intellectual disability nurse's approach to care is probably the best example of holistic care, as intellectual disability nurses

> 'support their clients' health needs, social inclusion, welfare, educational requirements and act as advocates mainly for people with poor or no communication skills.' (Jones, 1999, p. 61)

Assessment

Arguably assessment is the most important part of care planning and delivery. It includes areas such as health and health needs, daily living skills, activity programmes, mobility, mental health, risks to the client, finance, respite, social events/outings, support requirements, spiritual needs and, possibly, accommodation issues (Department of Health, 2000b; Sox, 2004a). If the assessment is not undertaken properly, or the information provided is not accurate, people with intellectual disabilities may miss out on many life opportunities.

Assessing the needs of people with intellectual disabilities is not an easy task. It is important to consider what kind of information is needed in order to complete the assessment successfully. It is a necessity for the professional performing the assessment to establish a good relationship and rapport with the client, his or her family and the care providers involved in the client's care in order to gain more detailed knowledge of the current and previous needs of the client. Because assessment plays such a major part in care planning in practice, nurses frequently use instruments and tools to assist them in assessing a person's needs and this is sometimes, although not always, combined with an appropriate nursing model used as a guide; this often depends on the care setting, area, resources, local policy and the purpose of the assessment.

In relation to the assessment of health many nurses, community learning disability teams and residential settings have developed their own health assessment forms or questionnaires or have adopted the now widely used 'OK' health check (Matthews, 2004). The 'OK' health check is helpful in identifying physical conditions found more frequently in clients with intellectual disabilities, such as dental disease, epilepsy, mental health problems, hearing and/or sight impairments (Matthews, 2004; Royal College of Nursing, 2004). Other sections include, for example, mobility, sexuality and necessary screenings and continence issues. Additionally, the 'OK' health check list identifies the health needs, staff training needs and action or areas needed for development in order to improve the health of people with intellectual disabilities living in the community (Matthews and Hegarty, 1997; Matthews, 2004). A part of the assessment also includes physical examination, which could be completed by a nurse or a general practitioner, including the measurement of biometric data, such as pulse, blood pressure and respiration rate.

Assessing an individual in a familiar or client-chosen environment may result in a better contribution from them and also may assist in obtaining more valid information for the assessment. In addition to this, offering convenient appointments and recognising and demonstrating sensitivity toward the personal, social and cultural circumstances of the client and all members involved in their care may enhance the foundation of the assessment further (Barr, 2003). The intellectual disability nurse performing the assessment must not be judgmental or critical, and must always act in a professional manner as described in the Nursing and Midwifery Council's *Code of Professional Conduct* (Nursing and Midwifery Council, 2004c). Accurately assessing clients' needs often depends on the assessor's ability to listen and observe, and their knowledge and use of verbal and non-verbal communication as well as the careful use of open and closed questions.

Before the assessment commences it is important to inform the client and everyone involved in the process about 'the rationale, scope and nature of the assessment, including clarification of the extent of confidentiality' (Barr, 2003), so that all those involved can decide how much information they want to provide.

It is important to clarify that the assessment can be both objective and subjective in nature. The intellectual disability nurse should look at the needs of the person with intellectual disabilities from different perspectives, bringing into the assessment views of others that will enrich the assessment. For example, there could be different emphases drawn on what the client needs from a professional view and the view of the client themselves, which could be addressed through a friend, relative, supporter or advocate. Once needs have been assessed and identified, the written planning of care should commence.

Planning

Care planning is an essential part of an individual's life (Sox, 2003b); Grant et al. (1998) have suggested that care plans:

'should respond to physical, psychological and social aspects identified in the assessment and provide opportunities for family members to build on existing strengths and develop coping resources.' (Grant et al., 1998)

A care plan must not be based on assumptions and therefore it must be realistic (Barr, 2004) and set goals that should be achievable and reviewed regularly, as the needs of the individual with intellectual disability may change. The process of care planning is also an opportunity to review existing services and resources in order to find the best possible service, which will suit the client's identified needs and provide the best possible care. The approach to the care planning throughout all of the stages of the nursing process must be person centred and this is especially so in the construction of a care plan (Department of Health, 2001).

The structure and format of care plans are variable; examples of different types of care plans are shown throughout this book. Some for example overtly adopt a nursing model that guides the content and ways in which the care plan is constructed (see Chapter 13); others are orientated toward using the nursing process approach to record the assessment, identified care needs, subsequent goals of intervention and plan of care followed by evaluation strategies (see Chapter 8), whereas others identify a more accessible client-centred approach (see Chapter 12). These are all variations on a theme and all are legitimate and all belong to the wider family of care plans as they all hold the person with intellectual disabilities as central to the care planning process. Whatever format is used, once the care plan is constructed it is important that everybody involved is provided with a copy of the care plan in an accessible format so they understand its context and can refer to it when necessary (Barr, 2003).

Implementation

Successful implementation of a care plan to meet the assessed needs of an individual is crucial and perhaps the most challenging part of the nursing process. Wherever appropriate it is vital for people with intellectual disabilities to be fully supported and involved throughout implementation of care in order for them to continue to make decisions and choices about their health and lifestyle as well as achieving any goals agreed in the care plan.

Target dates are set for the achievements of short- and long-term goals, and these should be reviewed on a regular basis during implementation of a care plan and reviewed regularly at review meetings. A care plan co-ordinator should be identified who will be responsible for the implementation of the care planning process; this co-ordinator could be a nurse, a social worker, a manager of the establishment where the client lives, a client's key worker or their health facilitator. Ideally the care plan co-ordinator should be known to all and easily approachable and contactable by everyone involved in the implementation of the care plan. Good communication plays a pivotal role in the success or otherwise of implementing care plans. Poor communication between the client, professionals involved, family and other carers may result in unnecessary stress and the withdrawal of important key individuals from care planning at a later stage. This can lead to a plan of care breaking down at the stage of implementation because of inconsistencies and, as Barr (2003) has suggested, unreliable management, poor communication channels and a lack of accountability may lead to loosening of the structure of the partnership between all involved.

Evaluation

Evaluation is concerned with the effectiveness of the assessment, the care plan itself and the implementation of that care. Before one arrives at a formal evaluation point for care it is desirable that care is reviewed and that interventions are monitored on an ongoing basis. All dates for such reviews should be agreed during the planning process and should be clearly documented on the care plan (Barr, 2003). In addition to these ongoing reviews more formal evaluation of care might take place as follows: 6 weeks after establishing a new care plan, then at 3 months, then at 6-monthly intervals. Everyone involved in the construction of the care plan and the implementation of that care should have the opportunity to prepare for and attend both the reviews and more formal evaluation events (Barr, 2003).

Evaluation of care provides an opportunity to re-examine and reflect on the process of nursing. This might typically include examining the accuracy and completeness of the initial assessment, reflecting whether the set goals are realistic and therefore achievable and the appropriateness of any agreed actions. Furthermore, it provides an opportunity for all of those involved in care planning and delivery to consider each other's contributions and to learn what types of support and interventions were more effective and helpful for the person with intellectual disabilities. Additionally team members have to be prepared to acknowledge that not all care planned or delivered meets the expectations of all those involved, and this makes it important that:

'the accountability for actions and omissions in services should be transparent to all involved.' (Barr, 2003)

Reader activity 1.1

Identify someone with intellectual disabilities you have recently worked with. Identify when their care plan was last formally evaluated. Who was involved in the process? What was the outcome of any action points generated by the evaluation? If there has not been a formal evaluation in the last 6 weeks, why this is, and what can be done to ensure regular and formal evaluation of care plans?

The use of nursing models

Models, within the context of nursing, have been variously defined; for example McFarlane (1986) has described them as 'a representation of reality', while other commentators use similar descriptions, such as 'ways of organising a complex phenomenon or some kind of conceptual or diagrammatic representation of what nursing means' (McKenna, 1997). In this book it is advocated that nursing models should be used as a flexible framework to stimulate and organise thoughts to assist in leading to the development of a logical care plan that is sufficiently robust and practical that it is likely to be used in practice settings. In response to both social and political influences the arena of intellectual disability care models and that of care planning have changed considerably: so, therefore, has the practice of intellectual disability nurses (Alaszewski et al., 2001). For example, during the last century, intellectual disability services were dominated by a medical model of care which emphasised the biological needs of people and the need to 'cure' physical problems in order to allow a person to function in society (Aggleton and Chalmers, 2000). The majority of people with intellectual disabilities have now moved out of long-stay hospitals, but there remains a concern that the powerful effects of the medical model continue to influence care provided in smaller community-based residences. Klotz (2004) has argued that the use of the medical model has pathologised and objectified people with intellectual disabilities leading to them being seen as 'less human'. Therefore, if nurses are to adopt some kind of model to guide their care in practice it must remembered that the use of such a model must hold the person with intellectual disabilities as central to any care-planning process, and that the nurse must be mindful they use such a model to promote what is best for that person.

There are numerous nursing models that can be adapted and used in a variety of health and social care settings. Some nursing models, such as Orem's self-care or Roper's activities of daily living, are well known and seemingly most used. It should be remembered that they may not be seen as relevant or ideal for all people with intellectual disabilities, but they can generally be adapted relatively easily and then become ideal frameworks for the assessment of health as well as more general needs. For example, it has been argued that some people with profound disabilities require considerable support with self-care (Kozier et al., 1998) and therefore the use of using Orem's self-care model may not be appropriate for them. However this is countered by an argument that Orem's self-care model focuses on learned behaviours of self-care ability (Orem, 1991) to maintain life, health and well-being (Mayo, 1997) and can be approached from different dimensions/perspectives. Therefore it offers guidance to a person considering their disability to regain or develop all or some level of self-care and it may also identify areas of self-care where the client will require support. As has been said there are numerous models of nursing and their use or otherwise is still very much contested (McKenna, 1997). Notwithstanding this, the reader is advised to seek additional and a much detailed treatment of this subject before forming any strong opinions on this matter (Meleis, 1997; McKenna, 1997). In this chapter we briefly explore three models of nursing but other examples of their use, along with the nursing process, are identified in more detail in Part 2 of this book.

Roper, Logan and Tierney (1980)

Roper et al. (2002) have described the course of life as something that starts at conception and lasts until death. During this course they identify activities of living that individuals engage in and these include maintaining a safe environment, communicating, breathing, eating and drinking, eliminating, personal cleansing and dressing, controlling body temperature, mobilising, working and playing, expressing sexuality, sleeping and dying (Roper et al., 2002). Each of these activities might be seen to be conceptualised as lying on a continuum from dependence to independence. At times during the course of life we may be more dependent on others to meet our needs and this, it is argued, is where the role of nursing is authenticated: in helping people move towards independence in all activities of daily living. Their model also identifies a range of factors that impact on the individual and affect their levels of dependence/independence and these include biological, psychological, socio-cultural, environmental and politico-economic variables. The activities of daily living themselves are not too dissimilar to a number of assessments commonly used in intellectual disability nursing and this model can therefore be adjusted accordingly (Gray, 2003). By way of contrast Brittle (2004) has claimed that this approach is not appropriate for intellectual disability nurses as it does not cover issues such as participation in the community, leisure, education, housing and employment. Notwithstanding this, in Chapter 13, an attempt is made to demonstrate how this model of nursing might be applied to the care of someone with profound intellectual disabilities and complex needs.

Peplau (1952)

This is a model of nursing where the individual is seen as a unique self system comprising the biological and physiological alongside interpersonal characteristics (Meleis, 1997). This model is often advocated for working with people with mental health problems because it is psychodynamic in nature and focuses on the nurse–client therapeutic relationship. This is developed through overlapping phases such as orientation, identification, exploitation and resolution (Forchuk et al., 1989). These phases are used in order to help a client to deal with certain behaviours or mental illness and direct them to further growth. As said, this model is mainly used for care planning of people with mental health problems; however, it can be adopted, once adjusted, in the care of people with dual diagnosis (see Chapter 8).

Aldridge (2004)

Aldridge (2004) has proposed a model for intellectual disability practice that he refers to as *Ecology of Health Model* and that was developed out of the *Ordinary Living Model* for intellectual disability nurses (Aldridge, 1987). This 'ecological' model takes into consideration all aspects of an individual's health and their and their families' relationship with their community (Jacques, 2004). In this model the person is seen as having physical and psychological components that form self and that exist in a social environment. This self interacts with the environment, and this interaction between self and environment forms an ecological system. Aldridge (2004) has proposed that this 'ecological' viewpoint informs the model's explanation of health, which maybe defined as:

'a dynamic and ever-changing state of individually defined optimal functioning and well-being, determined by the interplay between the individual's internal physiology and psychology and their external environment.' (Aldridge, 2004, p. 172)

Case illustration 1.1

Ayesha is 16 years old and attends a special school. She has just moved into the '16 plus' department where the focus will be on the development of social and independent living skills. She can stay on at school until she is 19, a rather prolonged sixth form perhaps, without an academic focus.

She lives with her parents and younger brother. She has a mild hemiplegia on her left side, which gives her an awkward gait. Ayesha often knocks things over and bumps into things and her over enthusiasm results in a lack of co-ordination and balance. Her speech is very difficult to understand even when the listener is reasonably familiar with her and very nearly impossible for strangers to understand. She uses a combination of Makaton and her own set of creative signs and gestures. Ayesha generally manages to show a remarkable level of persistence and patience with such 'stupid' others. She needs to, given that she loves to talk and fires incessant questions, being bright and endlessly curious about the world.

Ayesha can also become frustrated, impatient and angry; because of her lack of co-ordination, sometimes she does not seem to know how hard she pinches and grabs. This has caused much concern between the school and her family over the years, possibly more so now as she grows bigger and stronger. Her parents have attended many 'something must be done' meetings and still dread the notes home from school.

Like all teenagers, Ayesha wants relationships, both platonic and romantic. However, her lack of social skills sometimes makes this difficult and frustrating for her. Her humorous charm nevertheless often gains her favour and forgiveness. She, of course, rebels against parental authority in her own creative and unique ways. Her parents struggle, whether they are dealing with a normal teenager or a disabled teenager. Ayesha can go from charming and amusing to stubborn and back again very quickly. Her wilfulness can make life very difficult, but her parents also know that given her disabilities, such a trait is probably necessary in order for her to get on in her life.

Ayeshas' brother Zaffar has become somewhat emotionally distant from his sister. At times Zaffar has felt pushed out from the family. He does not bring his friends home and although very intelligent, he is regarded as something of an underachiever at school. He sometimes expresses resentment at what he regards as the preferential treatment of his sister, particularly in relation to discipline.

Ayesha is approaching an age when the notion of independence is becoming more relevant. Whilst life within the family remains a struggle at times, thoughts about Ayesha's future evoke mostly anxiety. How will she cope outside the protection of her family? Whilst she is developing the skills necessary for an independent life, her understanding of the responsibilities that come with this remains limited.

Reader activity 1.2

Spend some time reading Case illustration 1.1. A transitional meeting has been called at Ayesha's school and you have been asked to go along as the local community nurse. The agreement is to draw up some kind of care plan for her for the next few years. Think what your role might be at such a meeting. Would you need to develop a nursing care plan, or would you document your role into the overall construction of a person-centred care plan/life plan? Who should attend such a meeting, who will speak for Ayesha, if she needs anyone? What if any specific interventions could or should you offer Ayesha and her family?

The role of the intellectual disability nurse in care planning

Intellectual disability nurses have many dimensions and responsibilities within their role (UKCC, 1998); however, supporting people with intellectual disabilities to reach their goals in the form of living their lives as fully and independently as possible is by far the most vital. This role must always be practised in adherence to the Nursing and Midwifery Council Professional Code of Conduct (Nursing and Midwifery Council, 2004c) and this includes a range of practice-related issues that have direct bearing on care planning and delivery; these are shown in Box 1.1.

The Nursing and Midwifery Council Professional Code of Conduct was republished in November 2004 and replaced the United Kingdom Central Council for Nursing, Midwifery and Health Visiting Code of Conduct, together with the Scope of Professional Practice and the Guidelines for Professional Practice. As the regulatory body, the Nursing and Midwifery Council is

---

Box 1.1   Practice-related issues for care planning and delivery (UKCC, 1998)

- Accountability
- Consent
- Inter-disciplinary working
- Evidence-based practice
- Advocacy
- Autonomy
- Relationships
- Confidentiality
- Risk management

required to protect the public by ensuring that nurses, midwives and specialist community public health professionals provide, maintain and set high standards of education, training, conduct and performance to their clients and patients (Nursing and Midwifery Council, 2004a, b). Registered nurses and specialist community health practitioners are personally accountable for their own practice and they must be aware that their Professional Code of Conduct (Nursing and Midwifery Council, 2004c) requires them to:

- Treat clients as individuals and with respect
- Obtain consent before any treatment or care is given
- Protect confidential information
- Co-operate with others within the team
- Maintain own professional knowledge and competence
- Be trustworthy
- Identify and minimise potential risks to clients and patients

As registered professionals they have a duty of care and they have to act within the best interests of their clients at all times and this necessarily includes the planning and delivery of care. Therefore it is vital to document nursing care and this too should adhere to the requirements of the Nursing and Midwifery Council, and so should not contain abbreviations or jargon, should be accessible to clients, ensure confidentiality, be written clearly, be factual and accurate and should not be able to be erased (Nursing and Midwifery Council, 2002). Failure to maintain a good standard of record keeping of nursing care, or the use of the nursing process can lead to a breakdown in the quality of provided care (Nursing and Midwifery Council, 2002). Furthermore, this could also have legal implications following the misconduct of record keeping and a nurse could be removed from the professional register; the reader may wish to refer to Chapter 5 that deals with the legal and ethical aspects of care planning and delivery. Also of use to the reader is a text by Gates et al. (2004) that deals with general and specific issues related to accountability in nursing practice.

Reader activity 1.3

Spend some time locating as many different types of care plan format as you can. You may find it helpful to undertake this activity with a colleague or even as a group either on pre-registration or post qualifying programme of study. Identify what is common to each and what separates them. Are some more socially/medically/nursing orientated than others? How central to the care plan is the person with intellectual disabilities and what was involved in its construction? Which care plan is superior and what criteria would you use to make such a decision?

Conclusion

In this chapter the reader has been introduced to the nature of care planning, person-centred care planning, care management, health action planning and the care programme approach. The reader has also been introduced to some relevant and contemporary social policy as well as the Nursing and Midwifery Council's guidelines, competencies and expectations of professional practice as they apply to nursing and their planning and delivery. This chapter has also advocated the need for robust, professionally prepared care plans based on a systematic nursing assessment. In addition to this, reference has been made to nursing models and their appropriateness to care planning and delivery. In subsequent chapters of Part 1 of this text attendant issues that nurses must also consider in care planning and delivery are considered and these include integrated care pathways, life planning, person-centred care planning, legal and ethical issues of care planning and delivery, and, finally, risk assessment and risk management in intellectual disability nursing.

References

Aggleton, P. and Chalmers, H. (2000) *Nursing Models and Nursing Practice*, 2nd edn. Basingstoke: Palgrave.

Alaszewski, A., Motherby, E., Gates, B., Ayer, S. and Manthorpe, J. (2001) *Diversity and Change: The Changing Roles and Education of Learning Disability Nurses*. London: English National Board.

Aldridge, J. (1987) Initiating the use of a nursing model: the importance of systematic care planning – a ward clinician's perspective. In: *Mental Handicap: Facilitating Holistic Care* (Barber, P., ed.). London: Hodder and Stoughton.

Aldridge, J. (2004) Intellectual disability nursing: a model for practice. In: *Learning Disability Nursing* (Turnbull, J., ed.). Oxford: Blackwell Publishing.

Barr, O. (2003) Working effectively with families of people with intellectual disabilities. In: *Learning Disabilities: Toward Inclusion*, 4th edn, (Gates, B. ed.). Edinburgh: Churchill Livingstone.

Bonfenbrenner, V. (1979) *The Ecology of Human Development*. Cambridge, Mass: Harward University Press.

Brandon, D. and Towe, N. (1989) *Free to Choose: An Introduction to Service Brokerage*. Surrey: Hexagon Publishing.

Brittle, R. (2004) Managing the needs of people who have a learning disability. *Nursing Times* **100** (10), 28–9.

Circles Network (2004) *The Models of Disability* [online]. Available from: www.circlesnetwork.org/models_of_disability.htm. (Accessed 14 January 2005)

Department of Health (1999) *Making a Difference: Strengthening the Nursing, Midwifery and Health Visiting Contribution to Health and Healthcare*. London: Department of Health.

Department of Health (2000a) *Nurses, Midwives and Health Visitors (training) Amendment Rules: Approval Order 2000*. London: Department of Health.

Department of Health (2000b) *The NHS Plan*. London: Stationery Office.

Department of Health (2001) *Valuing People: a New Strategy for Learning Disability for the 21st Century. Towards Person Centred Approaches: Planning with People*. London: Department of Health.

Duffy, S. and Sanderson, H. (2004) Person centred planning and care management. *Learning Disability Practice* **7** (6), 12–16.

Elliott, J., Hatton, C. and Emerson, E. (2003) The health of people with intellectual disabilities in the uk: evidence and implications for the NHS. *Journal of Integrated Care* **11** (3), 9–17.

Forchuk, C., Beaton, S., Crawford, L., Ide, L., Voorberg, N. and Bethune, J. (1989) Incorporating Peplau's theory and case management. *Journal of Psychosocial Nursing and Mental Health Services* **27** (2), 35–8.

Gates, B. ed. (2003) *Learning Disabilities: Toward Inclusion*, 4th edn. Edinburgh: Churchill Livingstone.

Gates, B., Wolverson, M. and Wray, J. (2004) Accountability and clinical governance in learning disability nursing. In: *Accountability in Nursing and Midwifery* (Watson, R. and Tilley, S., eds.). Oxford: Blackwell Publishing.

Gilbert, P. (2003) *Social Care Services and the Social Perspectives* [online]. Medicine Publishing Company. Available from: www.intellectualdisability.info/values/social_care_pg.html. (Accessed 29 December 2004)

Grant, G., Ramcharan, P., McGrath, M., Nolan, M. and Keady, J. (1998) Rewards and gratifications among family caregivers: towards a refined model of caring and coping. *Journal of Intellectual Disability Research* **42** (1), 58–71.

Gray, C. (2003) *Supporting Independence for People with Intellectual Disabilities* [online]. Nurses Network. Available from: www.nursesnetwork.co.uk/envo/models.php?op=modload&name=News&file=article&sid=3. (Accessed 23 December 2005)

Howells, G. (1986) Are the health needs of mentally handicapped adults being met? *Journal of the Royal College of General Practitioners* **36** (2), 449–53.

Jacques, R. (2004) *Intellectual about Intellectual Disabilities and Health: Family Issues* [online]. Medicine Publishing Company. Available from: www.intellectualdisability.info/families/family_issues_rj.html. (Accessed 23 February 2005)

Jones, S. (1999) Learning disability nursing – holistic care at its best. *Nursing Standard* **13** (52), 61.

Klotz, J. (2004) Sociocultural study of intellectual disability: moving beyond labelling and social constructionist perspectives. *British Journal of Learning Disabilities* **32**, 93–4.

Kozier, B., Erb, G., Blais, K., Wilkerson, J.M. and Van Leuven, K. (1998) *Fundamentals of Nursing: Concepts, Process, and Practice*, 5th edn. Menlo Park, CA: Addison Wesley Longman.

Mansell, I. (2002) Intellectual aides. *Nursing Standard* **6** (17), 112.

Matthews, D.R. and Hegarty, J. (1997) The 'OK' Health Checks and health assessment checklist for people with learning disabilities. *British Journal of Learning Disabilities* **25** (4), 138–43.

Matthews, D.R. (2004) *The 'OK' Health Check: Health Facilitation and Health Action Planning*, 3rd edn. Preston: Fairfield Publications.

Mayo, A. (1997) *Orem's Self-Care Model: a Professional Nursing Practice Model*. Available from: http://members.aol.com/annmrn/nursing_portfolio_I_index.html. (Accessed 22 December 2004)

Mazrui, J. (2003) *Empowerment* [online]. Available from: www.empowermentzone.com. (Accessed 13 January 2005)

McFarlane, J.K. (1986) Looking to the future. In: *Models for Nursing* (Kershaw, B. and Salvage, J., eds.). Chichester: John Wiley and Sons.

McKenna, H. (1997) *Nursing Theories and Models*. London: Routledge.

Meleis, A.I. (1997) *Theoretical Nursing: Development and Progress*, 2nd edn. Philadelphia: Lippincott.

Mencap (2004) *Treat Me Right: Better Healthcare for People with an Intellectual Disability*. London: Mencap.

Newton, C. (1991) *The Roper–Logan–Tierney Model in Action*. Hampshire: MacMillan Press.

Nursing and Midwifery Council (2002) Guidelines for records and record keeping. London: Nursing and Midwifery Council.

Nursing and Midwifery Council (2004a) *About the NMC* [online]. Nursing and Midwifery Council: London. Available from: www.nmc-uk.org/nmc/main/about/$aboutUsMain. (Accessed 19 February 2005)

Nursing and Midwifery Council (2004b) *Complaints about Unfitness to Practice: A Guide for Members of the Public*. London: Nursing and Midwifery Council.

Nursing and Midwifery Council (2004c) *The NMC Code of Professional Conduct: Standards for Conduct, Performance and Ethics*. London: Nursing and Midwifery Council.

Orem, D.E. (1991) *Nursing: Concepts of Practice*. St Louis: Mosby.

Peplau, H.E. (1952) *Interpersonal Relationships in Nursing: A Conceptual Framework of Reference for Psychodynamic Nursing*. New York: G.P. Putnam & Son.

Roper, N., Logan, W. and Tierney, A. (2002) *The Elements of Nursing*, 4th edn. Edinburgh: Churchill Livingstone.

Royal College of Nursing (2004) Supporting people with intellectual difficulties [online]. London: Royal College of Nursing. Available from: rcn.org.uk/news/congress2004/display.php?ID=1060&N=25. (Accessed 23 January 2005)

Sanderson, H., Kennedy, K., Ritchie, P., and Goodwin, G. (1997) *People, Plans and Possibilities: Exploring Person-Centred Planning*. Edinburgh: Scottish Human Services Publications.

Sox, H.F. (2004a) *Care Plans. Comprehensive Care Planning for Long Term Care Facilities: A Guide to Resident Assessment Protocols (RAPs) and Interdisciplinary Care Plans*. Volume 1. Ohio: Robin Technologies Inc.

Sox, H.F. (2004b) *What is a Care Plan?* [online]. Westerville. Available from: www.careplans.com. (Accessed 23 December 2004)

Thiru, S., Hayton, P. and Stevens, E. (2002) Assertive outreach. *Learning Disability Practice* **5** (9), 10–13.

Thompson, J. and Cobb, J. (2004) Person centred health action planning. *Learning Disability Practice* **7** (5), 12–20.

United Kingdom Central Council for Nursing, Midwifery and Health Visiting (1998) *Guidelines for Mental Health and Learning Disabilities Nursing*. London: United Kingdom Central Council for Nursing, Midwifery and Health Visiting.

United Kingdom Central Council for Nursing, Midwifery and Health Visiting (1999) *Fitness for Practice*. London: United Kingdom Central Council for Nursing, Midwifery and Health Visiting.

van Schrojenstein Lantman de Valk, H.M., Metsemakers, J.F., Haveman, M.J. and Crebolder, H.F. (2000) Health problems in people with intellectual disability in general practice: a comparative study. *Family Practitioner* **17** (5), 405–7.

Walker, A. (1993) Community care policy: from consensus to conflict. In: *Community Care: A Reader* (Bornat J., Pereira C., Pilgrim D. and Williams F., eds.). Basingstoke: Macmillan/Open University.

Watson, R. and Tilley, S. (eds) (2004) *Accountability in Nursing and Midwifery*. Oxford: Blackwell Publishing.

Further reading and resources

Beardshaw, V. and Towel, D. (1990) *Assessment and Case Management: Implications for the Implementation of Caring for People*. Briefing paper No.10. London: King's Fund Institute.

Cambridge, P. (1999) Building care management competence in services for people with learning disabilities. *British Journal of Social Work* 29 June, 393–415.

Cambridge, P. and Carnaby, S. (eds) (2005) *Person Centred Planning and Care Management with People with Learning Disabilities*. London: Jessica Kingsley Publication.

Concannon, L. (2005) *Planning for Life: Involving Adults with Learning Disabilities in Service Planning*. London: Routledge.

Cesta, T. and Tahan, H. (2003) *Case Manager's Survival Guide: Winning Strategies for Clinical Practice,* 2nd edn. St. Louis: Mosby.

Challis, D., Chesterman, R., Luckett, R., Stewart, K. and Chessum, R. (2002) *Case Management in Social and Primary Health Care*. Ashgate: Aldershot.

Department of Health (1996) *CPA: Taking Stock and Moving on*. London: Department of Health.

Department of Health (1999) *Co-ordinating Care: The Care Programme Approach and Care Management*. London: Department of Health.

Department of Health/Social Services Inspectorate (1991) *Care Management and Assessment: Manager's Guide*. London: Stationery Office.

Duffy, S. and the Valuing People Support Team (2004) *Workbook on Person Centred Care Management: Person Centred Approaches: Next Steps*. London: Paradigm.

Ellis, J.R. (2004) *Managing and Coordinating Nursing Care*, 4th edn. Philadelphia: Lippincott Williams & Wilkins.

Gilbert, A.P. (2000) *Social Welfare: Care Planning and the Politics of Trust*. DPhil thesis. Buckingham: Open University.

Gilbert, T. (2003) Exploring the dynamics of power: a Foucaldian analysis of care planning in learning disabilities services. *Nursing Inquiry* **10** (1), 37–46.

Hogg, J. (1986) *Profound Retardation and Multiple Impairment*. Vol. 3: Medical and Physical Care and Management. London: Chapman and Hall.

Lewis, J., Bernstock, V., Bovell, V. and Wookey, F. (1997) Implementing care management: issues in relation to the new community care. *British Journal of Social Work* 27 Feb, 5–24.

Monks, K.M. (2003) *Home Health Nursing Assessment and Care Planning*, 4th edn. St. Louis: Mosby.

McNally, S. (2003) Helping to empower people. In: *Learning Disabilities: Toward Inclusion*, 4th edn, (Gates B., ed.). Edinburgh: Churchill Livingstone.

Paffrey, C. (2000) *Key Concepts in Health Care Policy and Planning: An Introductory Text*. Basingstoke: Macmillan.

Papadopoulos, A. (1992) *Case Management in Practice: An Introductory Guide to Developing Case Management Systems for Vulnerable People*. Bicester: Winslow.

Swearingen, P.L. (2003) *All-in-one Care Planning Resource Medical-surgical, Paediatric, Maternity and Psychiatric Nursing Care Plans*. St. Louis: Mosby.

Towell, D. and Beardshaw, V. (1991) *Enabling Community Integration: The Role of Public Authorities in Promoting 'An Ordinary Life' for People with Learning Disabilities in 1990s.* London: Kings Fund Institute.

Wilcock, P., Carnpion-Smith, C. and Elston, S. (2003) *Practice Professional Development Planning Guide for Primary Care.* Abingdon: Radcliffe Medical.

Useful websites

Healthcare Commission: hai.org.uk
Provides useful information on the performance of health care organisations.

Commission for Social Care Inspection: www.csci.org.uk
Provides useful information on the performance of social care organisations.

Department of Health: www.dh.gov.uk
Provides useful information on health and social care policy as well as guidance and publications.

www.intellectualdisability.info
This is an excellent resource with much useful information of intellectual disabilities and health. The site is maintained by Sheila Hollins, Jane Brenal and Jan Hubert.

Foundation for People with Learning Disabilities: www.learningdisabilities.org.uk
This site has a wealth of information on aspects as far ranging as publications, policy, news and events, as well as an excellent links page.

National Institute for Health and Clinical Excellence: www.nice.org.uk
This provides national guidance on the promotion of good health and the prevention and treatment of ill health.

Nursing and Midwifery Council: www.nmc-uk.org
Provides useful information and guidance for nurses.

American Nurses Association: www.nursingworld.org
Some useful material on care planning can be found here.

National Electronic Library for Health: www.nelh.nhs.uk
Excellent search and retrieval facilities on all aspects of health.

Chapter 2

Integrated care pathways in intellectual disability nursing

Hazel Powell and Elaine Kwiatek

Introduction

This chapter explores the concept of integrated care pathways. This will enable and facilitate readers to reflect on their practice and assist them in using integrated care pathways for people with intellectual disabilities. Promoting accessible healthcare through the use of patient passports and easier to read versions of patient information will also be explored to enable nurses to employ these models to ensure people with intellectual disabilities obtain high quality healthcare.

Integrated care pathways will be defined and their application is described. The evidence base relating to integrated care pathways will be investigated along with their constraints and benefits. The use of integrated care pathways for people with intellectual disabilities will be explored and suggestions are made for developing or improving their use in the area of intellectual disability nursing.

The emergence of the use of communication passports, both within intellectual disability services and as a means for accessing healthcare provision, will be described. There is an opportunity to examine the limited evidence for the use of these communication aids and to identify the benefits and challenges that are emerging as these are used increasingly within services. The literature concerning the communication needs of people with intellectual disabilities regarding healthcare information is reviewed. This leads to an overview of the use of accessible information and an exploration as to how this can be incorporated into everyday practice.

Background to integrated care pathways

Integrated care pathways initially evolved within the healthcare systems in the USA in the 1980s. These new pathways aspired to focus on the patient rather than the systems, identify measurable outcomes, demonstrate efficiency and meet the changing needs of healthcare (Allen, 1997; NELH, 2003). Integrated care pathways were introduced into the United Kingdom in the early

1990s when the NHS funded a patient-focused initiative to support organisational change (Kitchiner and Bundred, 1999). This led to the examination and expansion of concepts such as integrated care pathways, which are now used universally (NELH, 2003).

Originally the development of integrated care pathways concentrated on surgical procedures and medical conditions with a predictable sequence of events. In recent times, integrated care pathways are being used within more complex scenarios (Middleton et al., 2003), such as the care of people with drug or alcohol problems.

What is an integrated care pathway?

A number of terms are used interchangeably when referring to integrated care pathways, with many of the terms meaning slightly different things. This can lead to misunderstanding and confusion. Box 2.1 depicts some of the terms used when referring to integrated care pathways. It is important to be clear what is meant when the term integrated care pathway is used to avoid confusion. For the purpose of this chapter integrated care pathway will therefore be the term described.

'Integrated care pathways are structured multidisciplinary care plans which detail essential steps in the care of patients with a specific clinical problem.' (Campbell et al., 1998, p. 133)

The integrated care pathway can form all or part of a client's record and will consist of locally agreed standards based on the best available evidence, enabling the evaluation of outcomes and continuous quality improvement (Currie and Harvey, 1998; Kitchiner and Bundred, 1999; Syed and Bogoch, 2000). It is suggested that integrated care pathways address particular clinical problems within a multi-disciplinary approach (Norris and Briggs, 1999).

Box 2.1   Different terms for integrated care pathways

- Clinical pathways
- Anticipated recovery pathways
- Multi-disciplinary pathways of care
- Care protocols
- Clinical guidelines
- Critical care pathways
- Integrated care management
- Pathways of care
- Care packages
- Collaborative care pathways
- Care profiles
- Care Maps®
- Co-ordinated care pathways

Integrated care pathways describe the crucial steps to be followed by all relevant professionals at various stages of the healthcare journey (Syed and Bogoch, 2000).

Integrated care pathways aim to allow more predictable evidence-based care for clients, improving quality and enabling costs and efficacy to be evaluated by defining the optimal sequencing and timing of healthcare interventions (Lock, 1999; De Luc, 2001a). The goal of integrated care pathways is to provide comprehensive, systematic care in a proficient manner, thus reducing the costs of healthcare (Wilson, 1997; Syed and Bogoch, 2000).

Integrated care pathways aim to have the following (NELH, 2003):

- The right people
- Doing the right things
- In the right order
- At the right time
- In the right place
- With the right outcome
- All with attention to the patient experience
- And to compare planned care with care actually given

An authentic integrated care pathway will contain prearranged tracking of the planned care, what care is actually given and how this matches or deviates from the planned care. Unless the integrated care pathway has a mechanism for recording variations and deviations from the planned care it is not a true integrated care pathway (NELH, 2003; Wales, 2003). Norris and Briggs (1999) have described the key features of integrated care pathways as follows:

- Developed by the multidisciplinary team, to promote seamless care
- Based on guidelines and evidence, which establishes 'best practice'
- Designed in a manner that reflects both local needs and constraints
- Defining the standard that clients can expect from whoever is treating them
- Including variance tracking to detect and analyse for departures from the expected

---

Reader activity 2.1

Access the National Electronic Library for Health website http://libraries.nelh.nhs.uk/pathways/
Explore the site and read the knowledge zone section, 'About Integrated Care Pathways'.

Variance tracking and analysis

In relation to integrated care pathways variance has been described as the difference between what is expected to take place within a set timescale and what actually takes place (Zander, 2002). If the nursing care delivered varies from what is illustrated in the integrated care pathway this is documented as a variation (De Luc, 2001b). Variance reporting allows progress to be monitored and unexpected events to be identified and analysed. In turn this leads to appropriate responses given to client needs, the management of clinical risk, and the identification of areas for development and research (De Luc, 2001b; Middleton et al., 2003; ICPUS, 2004). Similarities in unexpected events or regular deviation from the expected norm, identified by variance tracking, would suggest an area for research; furthermore, variance tracking creates a mechanism for clinical audit.

Currie and Harvey (1998) have identified that there are usually three causes of variance:

- Client – for example a physiological problem
- Caregiver – for example omission or delay in completing the intervention
- System – for example institutional practice patterns, policies or procedures

Causes of variations may be avoidable or unavoidable. Unavoidable variances are those which others have no control over, for instance a person trying a new drug treatment for epilepsy experiences severe side effects. An example of avoidable variance could be a person with intellectual disabilities not fully understanding the instructions in relation to administering an inhaler for asthma, resulting in no improvement at review. Where there is an avoidable variance a solution should be sought (Kitchiner, 1997). Solutions for the person with the inhaler could be a tailored training programme involving a speech and language therapist and intellectual disability nurse, training carers to administer the inhaler or increasing support worker input at medication administration times.

Scrutiny and analysis of variations from the pathway provide information to the multi-disciplinary team on the overall effects and quality of care, enabling any patterns to be identified that may require further examination and allowing changes to be made to the pathway in response to the analysis.

Constraints

Some concerns surrounding fear of litigation have been expressed; the main concern appears to be having the integrated care pathway as a permanent record, and that this may make staff vulnerable (Currie and Harvey, 1998; ICPUS, 2004). However Tingle (1997) has argued that nursing care provided in a systematic manner, based on clinical guidelines is, in fact, protective. Current nursing guidance demands appropriate records of care are kept (Nursing and Midwifery Council, 2004); integrated care pathways do not change this requirement, or make it less or more likely that litigation will occur.

Time in relation to developing the integrated care pathway, reviewing guidelines, developing documentation, multi-disciplinary meetings, education and evaluation is recognised as a potential barrier to developing integrated care pathways to their full potential (McKee and Clarke, 1995; Herring, 1999; Syed and Bogoch, 2000).

Further concerns include a belief that integrated care pathways may over-emphasise the clinical condition at the expense of individual patient care (Kitchiner and Bundred, 1999). Integrated care pathways may discourage appropriate clinical judgements (Campbell et al., 1998) and are difficult to use with complex conditions (Sulch and Kalra, 2000), such as dual diagnosis. However, it is worth noting that other authors suggest integrated care pathways are particularly helpful for planning care in complex and costly situations. Lock (1999) has provided an example of using an integrated care pathway, evolved from existing practice, protocols and national guidelines, for the treatment of anorexia nervosa in adolescents. Formally structuring clinical care in a complex situation, the integrated care pathway identified treatment protocols and admission and discharge criteria. Lock (1999) found that the integrated care pathway demonstrated effectiveness, identified problem areas and supported arguments for changes in referral and treatment models.

Evidence base

One of the most commonly cited criticisms of integrated care pathways is the lack of empirical evidence to support the use of integrated care pathways. Campbell et al. (1998) have described how, despite integrated care pathways having first-rate principles, there have been few studies that have considered the effectiveness of integrated care pathways. There is a paucity of literature relating to integrated care pathways and people with intellectual disabilities or intellectual disability nursing. Therefore reviewing the wider literature is important to acquire an understanding of the topic, its key issues and relevant research.

For example Sulch and Kalra (2000) have reviewed the literature in relation to the role of integrated care pathways in stroke management; they have found the evidence to be weak with uncertainty around the effectiveness of integrated care pathways. Sulch et al. (2000) have found that integrated care pathway management for stroke rehabilitation offered no benefit over conventional multidisciplinary care in a randomised controlled trial. Kwan and Sandercock (2004) included the study of Sulch et al. (2000) when they considered randomised controlled trials and non-randomised studies, comparing care pathway care with traditional care planning in relation to stroke care. They found insufficient evidence to support the use of integrated care pathways within this field.

De Luc (2000) has described a mixed outcome from a quasi-experimental case study of two integrated care pathways for midwifery-led maternity care and breast disease. She concluded that there seemed to be changes for the better in the quality of care in some areas but not in others; positive outcomes included that integrated care pathways focused staff on improving clinical care. The Clinical Resource and Audit Group (CRAG) (1999) project evaluated 103 integrated care pathways at two hospitals and concluded that there was consistent and statistically significant evidence to support the effectiveness of integrated care pathways in the areas studied.

A number of proponents have cited improved communication and multidisciplinary working as benefits of integrated care pathways (Campbell et al., 1998; Kitchiner and Bundred, 1999). Atwal and Caldwell (2002) undertook quantitative and qualitative methods as part of their action research into whether integrated care pathways improved inter-professional collaboration. They concluded that, although integrated care pathways improved health outcomes, there was little evidence to suggest improved communication or inter-professional relationships. It is also suggested that staff compliance with integrated care pathways can be low (Kinsman, 2004). These examples of different authors reporting completely opposite findings further complicate understanding and subsequent adoption of integrated care pathways into practice.

Currie and Harvey (1998) have suggested further research is required to answer the following questions concerning the use of integrated care pathways in healthcare:

- Do care pathways result in quality improvements in patient care?
- Are resources used more effectively and efficiently?
- Are desirable outcomes achieved?

McKee and Clarke (1995) have suggested guidelines seldom supply all the answers and a scarcity of research-based evidence in many areas can be a difficulty. Box 2.2 identifies some examples of where health-related guidelines and research can be found.

Benefits

Guidelines are recognised as a method to support evidence-based practice (Kitchiner and Bundred, 1999; Thomson et al., 1995). Integrated care pathways can be used as a mechanism to incorporate local and national guidelines, thereby supporting evidence-based practice; furthermore they can be linked to the

---

Box 2.2   Health-related guidelines and evidence

- Scottish Intercollegiate Guidelines Network (SIGN) (www.sign.ac.uk)
- National Institute for Clinical Excellence (NICE) (www.nice.org.uk)
- National Service frameworks (www.nelh.nhs.uk/nsf/)
- Clinical Standards Board for Scotland (www.show.scot.nhs.uk/crag/topics/csbs/)
- NHS Quality Improvement Scotland (www.nhshealthquality.org)
- National Guideline Clearing House (www.guideline.gov/)
- Eguidelines (www.eguidelines.co.uk)
- Agree collaboration (www.agreecollaboration.org)
- Centre for evidence based medicine (www.cebm.utoronto.ca/)
- Centre for reviews and dissemination (www.york.ac.uk)
- The Cochrane Library (www.nelh.nhs.uk/cochrane)
- Research articles

organisational goals of clinical governance, clinical audit and clinical effectiveness (De Luc, 2001a; Middleton et al., 2003). Integrated care pathways encourage the conversion of national guidelines into local protocols by offering a structure for developing and implementing local protocols of care based on evidence-based guidelines (Campbell et al., 1998). Clinical governance has been defined as:

'A framework through which NHS organisations are accountable for continuously improving the quality of their services and safeguarding high standards of care by creating an environment in which excellence in clinical care will flourish.' (Donaldson and Gray, 1998, p. 38)

Herring (1999) has suggested that the process by which integrated care pathways are developed creates an optimum environment for research-based practices to underpin care, which in turn should ultimately lead to improved client outcomes (Johnson, 1997). With the recent publication of Scotland's Health Needs *Assessment for people with intellectual disabilities* (NHS Health Scotland, 2004) and a growing body of research within the field of intellectual disabilities, it may be that integrated care pathways could provide a vehicle to embed evidence-based practice into intellectual disability nursing.

Campbell et al. (1998) have suggested that integrated care pathways have the potential to promote teamwork in patient care. Middleton et al. (2003) and Walsh (1998) have agreed and have suggested integrated care pathways have the potential to enhance multi-disciplinary working, communication and patient involvement. By their very nature, integrated care pathways bring together all professional groups involved to arrive at a consensus about standards of care and expected outcomes (Walsh, 1998). Proponents have further described client involvement in the development of, the plan and the sharing of the plan with clients and carers as empowering, providing client-focused care (Walsh, 1998; Kitchiner and Bundred, 1999).

The Scottish Executive (2000) has recommended that people with intellectual disabilities are involved in anything that directly affects them. Person-centred planning has a history of use within intellectual disability services (Sanderson, 2003) as has multi-disciplinary working. It would appear that the underpinning philosophy and aims of integrated care pathways would readily fit into care planning practice for people with intellectual disabilities.

Integrated care pathways help to reduce unnecessary variations in patient care and outcomes. In practical terms the integrated care pathway can act as a single record of care, with each member of the multi-disciplinary team required to record his or her input on the integrated care pathway document, providing an appropriate method for monitoring overall care (Campbell et al., 1998; Brett and Schofield, 2002; Middleton et al., 2003). These single records have potential to develop into patient-held records. In addition streamlined documentation can reduce duplication and promote seamless patient-focused care (Norris and Briggs, 1999; Middleton and Roberts, 2000).

Currie and Harvey (1998) have suggested that nurses are best placed to act as facilitators of the integrated care pathway and that this role can enhance professional nursing practice. The role of integrated care pathway facilitator could easily fit within the existing role of the health facilitator, liaison nurse or community intellectual disability nurse.

Implementing an integrated care pathway

There is a number of stages to developing and implementing an integrated care pathway. Firstly, to undertake the development, a facilitator with credibility is required, alongside the development of a multi-disciplinary group and resources to support the process (De Luc, 2001b). The designated facilitator provides ongoing education and support and acts as a link between different professional groups. Currie and Harvey's (1998) description of the integrated care pathway facilitator is shown in Box 2.3.

The stages of developing and implementing an integrated care pathway include the selection of a topic and definition of the problem with specific inclusion and exclusion criteria. Following this, the multi-disciplinary team should review the evidence base and guidelines, undertake an audit of current practice and seek users' views on current services. The development of the integrated care pathway requires consideration of both local needs and constraints. Gathering samples of similar integrated care pathways from other areas avoids duplication and unnecessary work.

Thorough planning in the early stages should result in the development of the integrated care pathway describing the desired outcomes, decision points, procedures to follow and milestones to achieve. Variance tracking, analysis and review should also be detailed within the integrated care pathway, including the scheduling of audits. The documentation to support the integrated care pathway should be developed as multi-disciplinary documentation.

Following the development of the integrated care pathway a period of staff education is required. It is also advisable to pilot and review the integrated care pathway before final implementation, to address any issues which arise. Following implementation, ongoing support is required to ensure new staff are conversant with the integrated care pathway and to maintain and adjust the integrated care pathway following audits.

It is suggested that when developing and introducing integrated care pathways, it is important to incorporate them into organisational strategy, to

---

Box 2.3   Integrated care pathway facilitators

- Support clinical staff through the processes of developing and implementing care pathways
- Have a knowledge of the project
- Understand change management theories
- Have team building skills
- Facilitate group work

(Currie and Harvey, 1998)

be aware of the need for powerful champions, support of medical colleagues and education to develop team building skills, support understanding and promote ownership of the integrated care pathway (Currie and Harvey, 1998; Middleton et al., 2003). It should also be recognised that integrated care pathways are dynamic and change is to be expected in them as new evidence and guidelines emerge. Clearly effort is required to implement integrated care pathways successfully in practice.

Integrated care pathways and people with intellectual disabilities

In recognition of the sometimes complex journeys people with intellectual disabilities have to make through mainstream healthcare, many authors have identified the need for more tailored services, improved training, collaborative working and more comprehensive patient documentation for people with intellectual disabilities accessing health services (Bolland and Jones, 2002; Glasby, 2002; Hunt, 2004; Sweeney, 2004). Integrated care pathways may have a role in ensuring peoples' journeys are more straightforward and their healthcare needs are appropriately met.

Reader activity 2.2

Identify someone with intellectual disabilities who recently accessed primary or secondary healthcare services. Consider if an integrated care pathway would have improved this experience and think about what this integrated care pathway might look like. Discuss with your mentor or a colleague the usefulness of the integrated care pathway.

There are few examples in practice of integrated care pathways being used as part of care planning for people with intellectual disabilities. However some can be found, including an integrated care pathway for adults with intellectual disabilities whose challenging behaviour results in a crisis situation (Department of Health, 2004) and one for oral health care (Faculty of Dental Surgery, 2001).

It would appear that there are some misconceptions surrounding integrated care pathways, and perhaps these hinder their use generally and particularly in intellectual disability services. Case illustration 2.1 describes an integrated care pathway within an acute liaison nursing service. Intellectual disability nurses working within acute hospital settings within Scotland provide the acute liaison service. Although this example maps the patient journey from admission to discharge and indicates the optimal sequencing and timing of multi-disciplinary health interventions, it does not clearly demonstrate variance tracking and analysis. This lack of variance tracking means that this pathway is less likely to impact on the individual care or highlight areas of deficiency. Nevertheless, it would require little modification to incorporate variance tracking and the benefits this may bring. By ensuring the documentation highlighted changes from the expected journey and building in regular opportunities to analyse the documents and review any variance, the integrated care pathway should be more effective.

Case illustration 2.1   Acute Hospital Liaison Service

The purpose of the Acute Hospital Liaison Service is to ensure the specific needs of people with an intellectual disability are met within and by the secondary care services, ensuring throughout the 'patient journey' that services are working for them in an effective and seamless manner whilst respecting and valuing the person's wishes.

An individualist approach is taken with a full and ongoing assessment process being key in identifying:

- Treatment aims and implications on the person
- What are the person's understanding and expectations of treatment
- Required environmental and logistical adaptations

A personalised pathway is devised that incorporates assessment findings, allows for variables and works concurrently with established integrated care pathways in the secondary care services. In conjunction with a speech and language therapist, all patient information is assessed and adapted to enable accessibility; this is particularly crucial when managing consent issues. As a service, pathways in the form of flow charts are made within each clinical area, clarifying the approach and care to be given working with an individual who has an intellectual disability, and giving clear guidance on actions care providers can take within their clinical area to ensure an inclusive and flexible service is achieved.

Within the accident and emergency department an 'alert flag' allows for crucial information to be stored on the information technology system, which all healthcare staff have access to immediately an individual attends. This information is fully consented to by the individual and enables continuity of care across primary and secondary care and ensures staff have constructive advice at hand on how best to meet the person's needs and manage their care. This information is governed by a joint protocol between the intellectual disabilities service and the accident and emergency department and ranges from simple immediate contact details to extensive care plans and pathways.

Patient passports are an adjunct to the assessment process and are used for individuals who are frequently in contact with secondary services. Again a personalised and individual approach is taken in documenting information that staff will require to know about an individual's care.

Whereas there are few examples in practice of integrated care pathways being used for people with intellectual disabilities, there is even less written about integrated care pathways and people with intellectual disabilities. However, Ahmad et al. (2002a, b) have described developing integrated care pathways for epilepsy, hearing impairment and challenging behaviour for people with intellectual disabilities, demonstrating how integrated care pathways can be developed for people with intellectual disabilities with complex health needs. They initiated their developments by holding seminars to introduce the integrated care pathways and outline the areas to be developed. Working groups commenced with wide representation from a range of stakeholders and a facilitator; these groups then developed a mission statement, reviewed current research and guidelines before developing their integrated care pathways and relevant documentation for piloting. Integrated care pathways have potential to identify the gaps in relation to evidence base and direct future research.

Reader activity 2.3

Access, read and review copies of:

Ahmad, F., Bissaker, S., De Luc, K., Pitts, J., Brady, S., Dunn, L. and Roy, A. (2002a) Partnership for developing quality care pathway initiative for people with learning disabilities. Part 1: Development. *Journal of Integrated Care Pathways* **6** (2), 9–12.

Ahmad, F., Bissaker, S., De Luc, K., Pitts, J., Brady, S., Dunn, L. and Roy, A. (2002b) Partnership for developing quality care pathway initiative for people with learning disabilities. Part 2c: Epilepsy. *Journal of Integrated Care Pathways* **6** (2), 90–93.

Consider these articles in relation to how these could be replicated in your own practice area or current placement.

A contemporary issue in intellectual disability care is the emerging understanding that people with intellectual disabilities may have different patterns of illness and healthcare needs; for instance, in cancer care it is suggested that people with intellectual disabilities have different patterns of malignancies, when compared with the rest of the population (NHS Health Scotland, 2004). These differing patterns of health needs coupled with higher levels of unmet health needs, and known barriers to accessing healthcare increase health inequalities in people with intellectual disabilities (NHS Health Scotland, 2004). People with intellectual disabilities may find that the resources and healthcare policies are not focused on the areas that affect them the most. Integrated care pathways, which take into account the evidence base and adapt this to local need, provide one potential solution to bridge this gap.

Alongside the emerging health needs evidence in the field of intellectual disabilities is a range of mainstream guidelines that could easily be adapted for people with intellectual disabilities. One example would be developing a multi-disciplinary group to consider and adapt the Scottish Intercollegiate Guidelines Network (SIGN) guideline for epilepsy care and treatment. This multi-disciplinary group could cross primary, secondary and specialist care spectrums, with the guideline adapted to consider the local and specific needs of people with intellectual disabilities and epilepsy. Similar approaches could be adopted to consider obesity, diabetes, schizophrenia, dementia and a range of other conditions that affect people with intellectual disabilities.

Reader activity 2.4

Identify a specific condition or illness that you have encountered in some-one with an intellectual disability. Look for best practice guidelines and research evidence that could be used in an integrated care pathway in man-aging their care for this condition or illness.

Communication passports

The English White Paper, *Valuing People* (Department of Health, 2001a), has asserted that people with intellectual disabilities should be enabled to access a health service designed around their individual needs. It also suggests that additional support should be given wherever necessary. Yet many people with intellectual disabilities are still not receiving basic routine healthcare (Whoriskey and Brown, 2002; NHS Health Scotland, 2004). The reasons for this range from health professionals' lack of knowledge about and willingness to treat this population, to perceived problems in communicating effectively with the group. Primary care staff often do not have the necessary training and skills to deal sensitively with people with intellectual disabilities or have the equipment and motivation to organise their services to ensure that people with intellectual disabilities are fully included (Fitzsimmons and Barr, 1997; Barr et al., 1999; Hemsley et al., 2001).

Valuing People (Department of Health, 2001a) has suggested that health facilitators have a primary responsibility for facilitating access to primary care. It also identified that, by 2002, a Patient Advocacy and Liaison Service (PALS) would be established in every NHS trust. In Scotland *'The Same as You?'* (Scottish Executive, 2000) has suggested that each acute service employ a liaison nurse. Whichever scheme is used, it should mean that individuals will have an identifiable person to whom they can turn to if they have a health problem or need information.

Cumella and Martin (2000a, b and 2004) have identified a range of problems that people with intellectual disabilities experience when they are admitted to acute care and these include:

- Poor communication
  - Inadequate information prior to admission
  - Inadequate information about hospital procedures

- — Poor transmission of information within the hospital
- — Poor information at discharge
- — Limited information about choices within the hospital
- Fear and distress
  - — Traumatic experiences
  - — Unfamiliar environment
  - — Lack of comprehensible information
  - — Lack of support
- Lack of appropriate care
  - — Difficulty in making 'concessions' to the individual needs of the inpatients
  - — Lack of space
  - — Lack of flexibility
  - — Lack of adapted facilities
  - — Lack of responsiveness
  - — Inferior treatment

The main solutions identified by Cumella and Martin (2000a, b and 2004) were:

- Improved communication
- Patient held data – communication passports
- Preparation for admission
- Information to accompany the person into hospital
- Improved information about choices while in hospital
- Improved transfer of information within hospital

This suggests that the use of a communication passport along with the implementation of a patient advocacy and liaison service scheme or the creation of liaison posts along with the development of more accessible information would improve the healthcare journey for people with intellectual disabilities.

Background to communication passports

A major problem when considering the use of communication passports for people with intellectual disabilities is that different people use this term to describe different kinds of passports. Furthermore, different terms are used to describe inherently similar documents. Looking at the relatively sparse literature it becomes apparent that, despite the confusion over terminology and meaning, there are three major types of passports.

Type 1 personal communication passports

The first type to be considered are the personal communication passports which were developed by Sally Millar, a specialist speech and language therapist at the Communication Aids for Language and Learning (CALL)

Centre, University of Edinburgh, in 1991–1992 (CALL Centre, 2003). Millar and her colleagues have done much to advocate the use of these passports for people who have communication difficulties in services for people with intellectual disabilities in Scotland. This type of passport contains information about all aspects of the person's life (Caldwell et al., 1995). It is a useful tool in enabling the person to have a say and to make real choices. HM Inspectors of Education now recommend this type of personal communication passport as good practice in some school inspections; the Social Work Services Inspectorate highlight the need for communication passports in the *Draft National Standards of Care* document (Social Work Services Inspectorate, 2001).

Type 2 personal communication passports

This type of personal communication passport is used to support access between two services that is, prior to treatment at an outpatient appointment or an admission. It is a snapshot of the person's individual needs at the time of access and should change as the person's needs change (Kent, 2004). This type does not focus on all aspects of the person's life but solely on the health needs of the person. Harrison and Berry (2005) provide an example of this type of record, which they call a 'health profile'. These profiles contain the client's main health information and provide an active record for staff to make notes in (Harrison and Berry, 2005). These records are useful for focusing clients and staff on the person's health history and health needs. They are developed in partnership and fully include the client in identifying needs and planning to improve their health. A health action plan is contained within the profile and this is fully discussed with the client in terms they will understand. The client is facilitated in identifying their own health needs and formulating a simple plan to meet those needs. The core of the process is providing the clients with choices about their health and lifestyle and facilitating healthy choices where possible. This type of record is very similar to the 'patient passport' which was developed by The Royal Shrewsbury Hospitals, Hull Hospital and Shropshire Community Mental Health Trust (Cumella and Martin, 2000b), the 'patient passport' used by South Warwickshire NHS Primary Care Trust, the personal health records described by Turk and Burchell (2003), and the personal passports described in *Speak Up* (Ontario Trillium Foundation, 2005).

It is suggested that this type of personal portable health record should accompany people with intellectual disabilities who become patients in general hospitals (Sweeney, 2004) and that this should become a minimum standard within the NHS (Lindsay, 1998). Indeed the Department of Health Valuing People Support Team has produced written advice which gives accessible information about health passports or personal health records that could be used by practitioners wishing to develop the use of communication passports (see further reading and resources for web address). There is also guidance for lead planners which sets out a framework to make personal health records become more commonplace.

Combination of types 1 and 2

PAMIS is a Scottish voluntary organisation working with people with profound and multiple learning disabilities, their family carers and professionals who support them. On its website this organisation provides an overview of a communication passport which is a combination of the two types of communication passports described above. This could then be used within intellectual disability services to enhance communication and increase personal decision making, whilst also including a section on health needs which could be used to enhance access to healthcare. PAMIS has stressed that the health needs section should contain information on safety issues related to things like feeding, thus enabling nurses to give informed care.

Reader activity 2.5

Access the website below and look in particular at the section on passports: www.scope.org.uk/earlyyears/parents/resources.shtml
   Now answer the following:

(1)   What do you think of this resource?
(2)   If you were going into hospital is this the kind of information you would want the caregivers to have?
(3)   Are there other things that you think it would be important for caregivers to know about you?

Case illustration 2.2   A good practice example of the use of a personal health record

Gloucestershire Partnership NHS Trust has developed a 'hospital assessment' for people with intellectual disabilities. It is a simple three-page document that uses a traffic light system: red, amber, and green. The cover of this assessment identifies that if the person accesses healthcare they should take the assessment with them and that they should make sure that all the nurses that look after the person should read it.

   The red alert page identifies the things that are most important and includes information on current medication and current medical conditions. It also contains information on how specific medical interventions should be approached with that person. The amber page contains information about things that are really important to the person and includes information on how to communicate with the person, how the person takes medication and how you would know that the person is in pain. The green page has information on things the person would like to happen and what the person likes and dislikes.

Features of a passport

Millar and Caldwell (1997) have asserted that communication passports provide a special and efficient way of sorting and presenting information that is accessible to a wide variety of readers. Passports should, in their view, present the highly personal information in a way that is both positive and empowering.

The CALL centre can be easily accessed (see further reading and resources for web address) and gives advice on how to go about creating a type 1 passport. The passport starter (CALL Centre, 2003) can be freely used. They suggest a photo of the person should be inserted on the first page along with the person's name and instructions for people on how to read the document. South Warwickshire NHS Primary Care Trust produces a type 2 passport in two formats, one which could easily be carried in a handbag and a second pocket-sized version. They both contain information on:

- Personal contact details
- Professional contact details (e.g. social worker, community nurse, doctor)
- Medical history
- Communication details
- Language
- Faith
- Likes and dislikes
- Current medication
- Allergies
- Issues around consent

The degree to which communication passports use symbols will depend on a person's level of ability. Millar (2003a) has suggested that they may include photographs and other graphic material, since this will make the passport more accessible to the passport holder. All key information should be detailed and illustrated, when description alone is inadequate. She has also suggested that the passport should be in clear simple language and that it should be both bright and attractive.

Benefits of passports

Millar and Caldwell (1997) and Millar (2003a) have asserted that passports are a positive manner of supporting people with intellectual disabilities and communication problems. They gather together important and complex information about the person and make this information accessible to others. The benefits of using a passport include (Millar and Caldwell, 1997):

- Supporting the person
- Ensuring continuity of care
- Orientating new staff quickly

- Enabling people to observe more competently
- Empowering the person
- Valuing everyone's contribution to care
- Enhancing relationships
- Providing a focus of discussion with families and staff

Kent (2004) has suggested that they also:

- Make a connection with the people who know the patient best
- Respond to individual needs of the person
- Speed up access
- Make the best use of the skills of the nurses
- Improve treatment and care

The result of research undertaken by Hannon (2004) has clearly identified that the use of pre-admission assessment improves the care of people with intellectual disabilities when they are admitted to hospital for a problem unrelated to their disability. It is apparent, however, that this information must be shared sensitively with professionals responsible for the care of people with intellectual disabilities during their stay in hospital.

Constraints of passports

Passports do not have legal status, however Millar (2003b) has identified that they are recommended in guidance from the Scottish Executive. The legality of this document could cause some ethical problems for healthcare professionals. Passports contain highly personalised information about the person and their health needs. In some instances they may be compiled by the person themselves or in other cases by parents or carers. It has already been identified that the passport may contain information on current medication and that this could be used by healthcare professionals during an inpatient stay. What if, however, the information within the passport is flawed? Healthcare professionals may then be basing their care on flawed information contained in a passport that has no legal status.

Reader activity 2.6

List all the ethical challenges you can think of in using a communication passport.

Service delivery

People with intellectual disabilities have an important part to play in the improvement of service delivery. They have, for example, been involved in the development of a video of the patient's journey through their local acute hospital, which has then been used for teaching sessions within services for people with intellectual disabilities. Further information about this project can be found at takingpart@btinternet.com.

The Disability Discrimination Act (HMSO, 1995) mandates the removal of discriminatory barriers to public services including those in buildings, communication systems and transportation. Brown and Gill (2002) have reported that there are some promising directions in research and practice but these require careful nurturing. Millar (2003a) has identified that a supportive and successful environment can be created in schools if there are the following:

- A coherent communication policy in the organisation
- Strategic use of official documentation
- Training for staff
- Effective interdisciplinary working

All of these could be used within the NHS. For example a coherent communication policy could mean that pictorial images accompany all ordinary signs within the NHS, and all appointments and letters could be presented in simple language with symbols as well as words. Support to access services in this way is identified in the benchmarks of good practice outlined in Essence of Care (Department of Health, 2001b). Indeed Edinburgh City Council, Scotland, has just completed redesigning symbols for Roodlands Outpatients Clinic in East Lothian and these are available from the Bonnington Symbol System (Edinburgh City Council, 2005).

Case illustration 2.3

When looking at enhancing a person's experience with healthcare, Shropshire County Primary Care Trust (2002) have recommended the following:

- User-friendly information sheets
- Risks vs benefits information sheets on surgical procedures
- The use of augmentative and accessible communication systems
- Photographs or videos of the patient's journey
- Audio cassette recordings with familiar voices (also suggested by Lothian Universities Hospitals Trust and Lothian Primary Care NHS Trust 2002)
- Menu cards made more user-accessible through the use of symbols or in different formats – Braille, audio cassette, large print
- Information sheets for patients about their healthcare needs
- Reassessment of signposting, directions and maps (Braille maps, user-friendly maps, colour coded areas)
- Consideration of lines on floors and walls, colour coded (located at eye level for wheelchair users)
- Pre-admission books to be sent to the patient

The *Health Needs Assessment* (NHS Health Scotland, 2004) has stated that existing methods for eliciting the views of people with intellectual disabilities often fail to address how people with additional communication disabilities can be included in discussions concerning their care. Information systems that have been developed by users will often incorporate areas that would otherwise be forgotten or inappropriately prepared solely by healthcare professionals (Shropshire County Primary Care Trust, 2002). Graphic recording has been used successfully to enable some people with intellectual disabilities and communication problems to tell their story. Audio recording and transcription can also be used but it is suggested that pictures are more recognisable and give a person a true record of what they say or think. Carr (2004) has developed a questionnaire designed to glean the views of people with intellectual disabilities using picture communication symbols. The information gathered was used to develop a policy for the care of people with intellectual disabilities in acute hospitals.

Accessible information

As long ago as 1994, Robillard had identified that people with severe communication impairment reported a lack of power and expressed feelings of overwhelming anxiety when reflecting on their experiences of attempting to communicate with nurses when they were in hospital. The Mental Health Foundation, in their report, *Building Expectations* (Mental Health Foundation, 1996), concurred with this view, suggesting that a stay in hospital is often a very unnerving and frightening experience for a person with a intellectual disability. This report identified that better information in more accessible formats could make this experience better. Mencap (1998, 2004) have reported that poor communication, lack of information and appropriate supports are some of the problems faced by people with intellectual disabilities when accessing acute hospital care. It seems that acute care staff lack confidence in working with people with intellectual disabilities.

An estimated 26% of people with an intellectual disability are admitted to general hospitals every year compared with 14% of the general population (NHS Health Scotland, 2004); the Scottish Executive (2000) have estimated that 50% of people with intellectual disabilities have a significant communication problem, and that 80% have some communication problem. Thus there is not only an increased likelihood that people with intellectual disabilities will be admitted to acute care, but, whilst there, they may have difficulty asking for help when they are ill, in pain or need to describe symptoms, because of their associated communication problems. People with intellectual disabilities within an acute hospital setting are vulnerable yet they have the right to the same level of care as that provided to the general population (NHS Health Scotland, 2004). Their care must be flexible and responsive and any diagnosis or treatment must take into account the specific needs generated by their intellectual disabilities. Yet Hemsley et al. (2001) have identified that in most cases there was no policy in the workplace pertaining to communicating with patients with a severe communication difficulty. Indeed, Hemsley et al. (2001) have further suggested that this has led to longer recovery times for people with intellectual disabilities. It seems that meeting the communication and information needs more effectively could lead to reduced recovery times as well as enhancing the person's healthcare journey. It should be noted that some areas are actively trying to support staff in this area. In Glasgow, for example, specially designed training packs enable staff to support people with intellectual disabilities more effectively (Findlayson et al., 2004).

People with intellectual disabilities can be a challenging group to work with; some have reasonable literacy skills whereas some have very limited ability to benefit from the written word, and some people, such as those that are deaf or blind, are severely disadvantaged (Walmsley, 2004). A key message is that different people benefit from different strategies. Shakespeare (1996) has suggested that the messages must be made as simple as possible and no simpler.

People with intellectual disabilities are arguably disadvantaged in any health screening procedures because of the reliance on written materials to communicate health promotion information (Meehan et al., 1995). Watson et al. (2003) have suggested that any information needs to be presented in an accessible format, and not just in a tokenistic way, such as an increase in the font of the printed materials. NHS guidelines have identified the provision of accessible illustrated information as an important function in the healthcare of people with intellectual disabilities (Department of Health, 1998, 2001b; Lindsay, 1998).

A study undertaken by Broughton and Thomson (2000) to elicit the views of women with intellectual disabilities on cervical smears identified that 70% of the women in the study did not understand the purpose of the cervical smear test. They also suggested that careful preparation for this type of health screening is vitally important. As well as allocating extra time, staff need to use straightforward language and materials that are meaningful to women. They recognise that women with intellectual disabilities and their carers need much more information about the importance of the procedure and its relevance for them. Thus the development and use of teaching packs like those described by Poynor (2003) for breast self-examination and screening services for women with intellectual disabilities have the potential to cross this communication gap.

All the guidelines for improving written material for people with limited reading skills suggest that pictures and symbols should be used in order to improve understanding and accessibility. However there are few picture books that are available for adults and adolescents who cannot read or who have difficulty reading. Books Beyond Words (see further reading and resources) is a series of picture books, which have been developed to make communication and discussion easier for people with intellectual disabilities. The stories are told through colour pictures that include mime and body language to communicate simple explicit messages. They include:

- A Guide for GPs and the Primary Care Team
- Going to the Doctor
- Going into Hospital
- Going to Outpatients

The Royal Institute for the Blind, as well as producing booklets and tapes on 'Getting your eyes tested' and 'Getting new glasses', have written excellent guidelines for the preparation of a person with a visual impairment for surgery called 'Having a cataract operation' (see further reading and resources). These could easily be modified to suit the needs of people with intellectual disabilities.

Reader activity 2.7

Access www.cancernorth.nhs.uk/infoprint.asp

- What do you think about the information about cancer written for people with intellectual disabilities that is on the website?
- Are the messages clear?
- Would they help you to explain about cancer to a person with an intellectual disability?

The *Guide and Directory to Health and Medicines Information* (see further reading and resources) helps people with intellectual disabilities understand the type of medication they are prescribed and helps them formulate appropriate questions about that medication. Strydom et al. (2001) have asserted that the information presented in most patient information leaflets that are supplied with all dispensed medicines is complex and has a poor level of readability, making them unsuitable for people with intellectual disabilities. In their study Strydom et al. (2001) identified that the participants wanted a leaflet that they could read and understand with their medication. They went on to design leaflets in partnership with the people with intellectual disabilities utilising 'The writing symbols' software (Widget Software, 1997) to illustrate key words in the text. This software was entirely appropriate and was shown to meet the information needs of the people in the study. PAMIS have also produced a checklist for people to take with them when they go to the doctors, which helps them ask relevant questions about their medication.

Describing the type and the intensity of pain can be difficult for anyone. Foley and McCutcheon (2004) have stressed the importance of using alternative methods in the assessment of pain in people with intellectual disability. Donovan (2002) has reported that a form of symbolic expression has been used successfully with people with intellectual disabilities to enable them to tell staff when they are in pain. Shropshire Primary Care Trust has produced a pictorial leaflet to help identify areas of pain (Shropshire County Primary Care Trust, 2002). It can be deduced that these aids help a person to describe their pain and therefore enable healthcare professionals to respond appropriately. St Oswald's Hospice in Gosforth, Newcastle upon Tyne, has created a 'distress assessment tool' which assists staff in examining the patient who may have poor communication skills and be unable to communicate the pain and discomfort that they may be experiencing.

Millar (2003a) has described how pictures and symbols can be used dynamically in consultations to help people with communication difficulties indicate their views and preferences. Sorting and rating activities for use with children are described by Aitken and Millar (2002). They suggested the use of a smiley face for like, a sad face for doesn't like and a mid position for okay or not bothered. They explained how some of the children marked the face of their choice whilst others pointed or eye-pointed. This type of communication aid could be used to assess pain and in a variety of other situations in order to help the person with intellectual disabilities have their say or make a choice.

Cameron and Murphy (2002) and Watson et al. (2003) have all described the use of Talking Mats™. This is an interactive resource used to concentrate attention and interaction on thirteen life-planning topics. The group in the study undertaken by Watson et al. (2003) found that they had been useful in the process of life planning. Bell and Cameron (2003) have demonstrated that these mats along with an adapted 'Not a Child Anymore' (Fraser, 1987) package can be used to work with those people who have severe intellectual disabilities with poor communication and have described how the mats were used to assess a person's sexual knowledge. It was suggested that this type of assessment would be useful in a variety of situations, including protecting people from abuse or inappropriate sexual advances. They also, in their view, enhance carers' understanding of any allegations of sexual abuse. Pound and Hewitt (2003) have referred to this kind of resource as 'communication ramps' since in their view they provide access to social conversation. It is suggested that with careful thought and planning, the ideology of Talking Mats™ could be adapted to enable better communication between healthcare professionals in acute and primary care and people with intellectual disabilities.

Literature suggests that, although health information can be readily accessed through the use of focus groups, this method is rarely used with people with intellectual disabilities (Fraser and Fraser, 2001). Martin et al. (1997) have suggested that a range of communication aids or ramps were needed to enable people with intellectual disabilities understand health. Goodman (1998) has identified that focus groups could be used with those with communication problems if drawings, role play, video and posters are used in a creative way. In two separate research studies undertaken by Thornton (1999) and Barr et al. (1999) it was identified that the community intellectual disability nurse has a central role in health promotion. This role could be made more effective by facilitating focus groups, which enhance the understanding of health, health promotion and health screening.

Creating your own accessible information

It has been clearly identified there are different mortality and morbidity patterns in people with intellectual disabilities than those in the general population (Turner and Moss, 1996; Barr et al., 1999; NHS Health Scotland, 2004). This means that it is especially important that information related to health is accessible for people with intellectual disabilities. It may also mean that the information required for a person with intellectual disabilities, the healthcare journey will need to be created on an individual basis.

Creation of individualised information can have its pitfalls. Some authors have shown that symbol messages can be confusing if these are not used correctly (Garrett, 1999). Others have shown that even simple pictograms can be problematic if not developed with sensitivity to an appropriate educational level or cultural experience (Dowse and Ehlers, 1998). Indeed, LeGrys (2004) has clearly identified the challenges of providing pictorial information for people with intellectual disabilities. Macdonald (1998), however, has suggested that symbols can be used effectively on many communication aids. Symbols may, according to Cornwallis and Peacock (1998), be imported into other documents giving clients with literacy difficulties access to information.

Access to over 6000 symbols can be achieved by using Boardmaker and its Addendum libraries. However, these are only symbolic representations and people with learning disabilities may have difficulty in making the connections. Gibb (2003) has asserted that real pictures help with understanding and has suggested that they can be used to make more personal meaningful resources. Gibb (2003) has advocated the use of the Internet, free clip art and clip art CDs, digital cameras, photo CDs and pictures from a scanner. People with intellectual disabilities may more easily understand Photosymbols, which are designed for people who cannot read. They are made with real pictures of people with intellectual disabilities (see further reading and resources).

Over the last 25 years a number of symbol systems have been produced. These are either a substitute for speech or provide additional support for those with linguistic problems. They also meet the needs of many people with intellectual disabilities (Cornwallis and Peacock, 1998). Three common symbol systems and the associated software are identified within Box 2.4.

Millar and Larcher (1998) have described a number of utilities for producing symbols materials including Access Bliss, Bliss for Windows, BlissWrite/ Internet, Boardmaker, COMPIC, Gridmaker and Makaton explorer. The website for the Bonnington Symbol System includes symbols for outpatient clinics, which can be downloaded free of charge. This can be explored at http:// www.modemoperandi.co.uk/symbols/news.htm.

> **Box 2.4   Symbols systems**
> - Rebus
> - Gridmaker and Writing with symbols
> - Picture Communication System
> - Boardmaker
> - Blissymbols
> - Blissymbols for Windows

It is suggested that the many sites that offer free downloads of symbols, photographs and the like could be easily accessed and the images imported into many of the information and health promotion leaflets, information packs and, indeed, integrated care pathways.

Benefits of accessible information

Millar and Caldwell (1997) have suggested that using accessible information will lead to the following:

- Seamless approaches to care
- Better communication
- Reductions in anxiety and stress
- Better preparation
- Reductions in risks
- Increased choice
- Increased participation by patients in their own care
- Better information for patients

Conclusion

There is a wealth of evidence to support the need to improve the experience of people with intellectual disabilities accessing healthcare (Bolland and Jones, 2002; Hunt, 2004). Integrated care pathways are an established process for care planning within acute health settings. There appears to be potential for their use in health services for people with intellectual disabilities. To ensure integrated care pathways are used to their full capacity it is important that nurses working with people with intellectual disabilities have a sound understanding of integrated care pathways and their implementation. There is also a growing body of evidence that the use of communication passports and the provision of accessible information can improve the quality of the person's healthcare journey. It has been shown that this is already common practice in some areas. It is imperative that the areas that have not already examined the kind of environment they provide should learn lessons from these flagship healthcare facilities.

References

Ahmad, F., Bissaker, S., De Luc, K., Pitts, J., Brady, S., Dunn, L. and Roy, A. (2002a) Partnership for developing quality care pathway initiative for people with learning disabilities. Part 1: Development. *Journal of Integrated Care Pathways* **6** (2), 9–12.

Ahmad, F., Bissaker, S., De Luc, K., Pitts, J., Brady, S., Dunn, L. and Roy, A. (2002b) Partnership for developing quality care pathway initiative for people with learning disabilities. Part 2c: Epilepsy. *Journal of Integrated Care Pathways* **6** (2), 90–93.

Aitken, S. and Millar, S. (2002) *Listening to Children with Communication Support Needs.* Edinburgh: Sense Scotland.

Allen, C.V. (1997) *Nursing Process in Collaborative Practice,* 2nd edn. Stamford: Appleton and Lange.

Atwal, A. and Caldwell, K. (2002) Do multidisciplinary integrated care pathways improve interprofessional collaboration. *Scandinavian Journal of Caring Science* **16**, 360–7.

Barr, O., Gilgun, J., Kane, T. and Moore, G. (1999) Health screening for people with learning disabilities by a community learning disability nursing service in Northern Ireland. *Journal of Advanced Nursing* **29** (6), 1482–93.

Bell, D. and Cameron, L. (2003) The assessment of the sexual knowledge of a person with a severe learning disability and a severe communication disorder. *British Journal of Learning Disabilities* **3** (13), 123–33.

Bolland, R. and Jones, A. (2002) Improving care for people with learning disabilities. *Nursing Times* **98** (35), 38–9.

Brett, W. and Schofield, J. (2002) Integrated care pathways for patients with complex needs. *Nursing Standard* **31** (16), 36–40.

Broughton, S. and Thomson, K. (2000) Women with learning disabilities: risk behaviours and experiences of the cervical smear test. *Journal of Advanced Nursing* **32** (4), 905–14.

Brown, A. and Gill, C. (2002) Women with developmental disabilities; health and ageing. *Current Women's Health Reports* **2**, 219–25.

Caldwell, M., Calder, J., Aitken, S. and Millar, S. (1995) Use of personal passports with deaf blind people. *Talking Sense* Autumn. Available from: www.sense.org.uk/tsarticles/passports.html (Accessed 4 December 2004)

CALL Centre (2003) Passport Starter. Available from: www.callcentrescotland.org.uk (Accessed 10 January 2005)

Cameron, L. and Murphy, J. (2002) Enabling young people with a learning disability to make choices at the time of transition. *British Journal of Learning Disabilities* **30** (3), 105.

Campbell, H., Hotchkiss, R., Bradshaw, N. and Porteous, M. (1998) Integrated care pathways. *British Medical Journal* **316**, 133–7.

Carr, S. (2004) *Helping People in Hospital: Developing a Policy for the Care of People with Learning Disabilities in Acute Hospitals.* Inverurie: Inverurie Hospital.

Clinical Resource and Audit Group (CRAG) (1999) *Clinical Audit and Quality Using Integrated Pathways of Care.* Project CA96/01. Glasgow West: Glasgow Hospitals.

Cornwallis, P. and Peacock, A. (1998) *Use of Symbol Software in CALL Centre (1998), Augmentative Communication in Practice.* Edinburgh: CALL Centre.

Cumella, S. and Martin, D. (2000a) Community care for learning disabled. *The All Ireland Journal of Nursing and Midwifery* **2** (4), 18–19.

Cumella, S. and Martin, D. (2000b) *Secondary Healthcare for People with a Learning Disability.* A report completed for the Department of Health. London: Department of Health.

Cumella, S. and Martin, D. (2004) Secondary healthcare and learning disability: the results of consensus development conferences. *Journal of Learning Disabilities* **8** (1), 30–40.

Currie, L. and Harvey, G. (1998) Care pathways development and implementation. *Nursing Standard* **12** (30), 35–8.

De Luc, K. (2000) Care pathways: an evaluation of their effectiveness. *Journal of Advanced Nursing* **32** (2), 485–96.

De Luc, K. (2001a) *Developing Care Pathways: The Handbook.* Abingdon: Radcliffe Medical Press.

De Luc, K. (2001b) *Developing Care Pathways: The Tool Kit.* Abingdon: Radcliffe Medical Press.

Department of Health (1998) *Signposts for Success in Commissioning and Providing Health Services for People with Learning Disabilities.* London: The Stationery Office.

Department of Health (2001a) *Valuing People: A New Strategy for Learning Disability for the 21st Century.* Norwich: The Stationery Office.

Department of Health (2001b) *Essence of Care: patient focussed benchmarking for healthcare practitioners.* London: The Stationery Office.

Department of Health (2004) *Herefordshire Council: care pathway for adults with learning disabilities whose challenging behaviour results in a crisis situation.* Available from: www.dh.gov.uk/PolicyAndGuidance/HealthAndSocialCareTopics/SocialCare (Accessed 23 October 2004)

Donaldson, L.J. and Gray, J.A.M. (1998) Clinical governance: a quality duty for health organisations. *Quality in Health Care* **7** (suppl), 37–44.

Donovan, J. (2002) Issues and innovations in nursing practice: learning disability nurses' experiences of being with clients who may be in pain. *Journal of Advanced Nursing* **38** (5), 458–68.

Dowse, R. and Ehlers, M.S. (1998) Pictograms in pharmacy. *International Journal of Pharmacy Practice* **6**, 109–18.

Edinburgh City Council (2005) *Bonnington Symbol System.* Available from: www.modemoperandi.co.uk/symbols/free.htm (Accessed 28 February 2005)

Faculty of Dental Surgery (2001) *Clinical Guidelines and Integrated Care Pathways for the Oral Health Care of People with Learning Disabilities.* London: Faculty of Dental Surgery. Available from www.rcseng.ac.uk/dental/fds/clinical_guidelines/ (Accessed 4 November 2004)

Family Advice and Information Resource (2002) *Keep Yourself Healthy – A Guide to Having a Healthy Heart.* Edinburgh: Health Education Board.

Foley, D. and McCutcheon, H. (2004) Detecting pain in people with an intellectual disability. *Accident and Emergency Nursing* **12** (4), 196–200.

Findlayson, J., Cooper, S. and Morrison, J. (2004) Learning disabilities: enhancing care for adults. *Practice Nurse* **28** (10), 21–7.

Fitzsimmons, J. and Barr, O. (1997) A review of reported attitudes of health and social care professional towards people with learning disabilities; implications for education and further research. *Journal of Learning Disabilities for Nursing Health and Social Care* **2**, 57–64.

Fraser, J. (1987) *Not a Child Anymore.* London: Brooke Advisory Service.

Fraser, M. and Fraser, A. (2001) Are people with learning disabilities able to contribute to focus groups on health promotion? *Journal of Advanced Nursing* **33** (2), 225–38.

Garrett, S. (1999) Careless use of 'Writing with Symbols' software. (Letter) *British Journal of Learning Disability* **27** (29).

Gibb, S. (2003) Gathering images. In: *Augmentative Communication and Inclusion* (Wilson, A., ed.). Edinburgh: CALL publications.

Glasby, A.M. (2002) Meeting the needs of people with learning disabilities in acute care. *British Journal of Nursing* **11** (21), 1389–92.

Goodman, K. (1998) Service user involvement. In: *Developing and Maintaining High Quality Services for People with Learning Disabilities* (Burton, M. and Kellaway, M. eds.). Aldershot: Ashgate.

Hannon, L. (2004) Better pre-admission assessment improves learning disability care. *Nursing Times* **100** (25), 44–7.

Harrison, S. and Berry, L. (2005) Improving primary care services for people with a learning disability. *Nursing Times* **101** (1), 38–40.

Hemsley, B., Sigafoos, J., Balandin, S., Forbes, R., Taylor, C., Green, V. and Parmenter, T. (2001) Nursing the patient with severe communication impairment. *Journal of Advanced Nursing* **35** (6), 827–37.

Her Majesty's Stationery Office (1995) *Disability Discrimination Act*. London: HMSO.

Herring, L. (1999) Providing care using care pathways. *Nursing Standard* **13** (47), 36–7.

Hunt, C. (2004) Access to secondary care for people with learning disabilities. *Nursing Times* **100** (3), 34–6.

ICP Users Scotland (2004) *Introducing Integrated Care Pathways*. Available from: www.icpus.ukprofessionals.com/leaflet1.html (Accessed 23 October 2004)

Johnson, S. (ed.) (1997) *Pathways of Care*. Oxford: Blackwell Publishing.

Kent, A. (2004) *Using a Passport to Access Acute Services for People with a Learning Disability*. Available from: www.nnldn\A2A-AccesstoAcute\App4–DisablingPractice.doc (Accessed 11 November 2004)

Kinsman, L. (2004) Clinical pathway compliance and quality improvement. *Nursing Standard* **18** (18), 33–5.

Kitchiner, D. (1997) Analysis of variation from the pathway In: *Pathways of Care* (Johnson, S. ed.) Oxford: Blackwell Publishing.

Kitchiner, D.J. and Bundred, P.E. (1999) Clinical pathways, a practical tool for specifying, evaluating and improving the quality of clinical practice. *Medical Journal of Australia* [online] **170**, 54–5. Available from: www.mja.com.au/public/issues/jan18/kitchner/kitchner.html (Accessed 12 October 2004)

Kwan, J. and Sandercock, P. (2004) *Hospital Care Pathways for Stroke* (Cochrane Review), In: The Cochrane Library. Chichester: Wiley & Sons.

LeGrys, P. (2004) A way out of the information ghetto. *Learning Disability Practice* **7** (8), 36–7.

Lindsay, M. (1998) *Signposts for Success in Commissioning and Providing Health Services for People with Learning Disabilities*. London: NHS Executive.

Lock, J. (1999) How clinical pathways can be useful: an example of a clinical pathway for the treatment of anorexia nervosa in adolescents. *Clinical Child Psychology and Psychiatry* **4** (3), 331–40.

Lothian University Hospitals and Lothian Primary Care Trust (2002) *A Collaborative Approach for Patients with a Learning Disability in the Acute Hospital*. Edinburgh: Lothian University Hospitals and Lothian Primary Care Trust.

MacDonald, A. (1998) *Symbol Systems in CALL Centre, Augmentative Communication in Practice*. Edinburgh: CALL Centre.

Martin, D.M., Roy, A., Wells, M.B. and Lewis, J. (1997) Health gain through screening – users' and carers' perspectives of health care; developing primary health care services for people with an intellectual disability. *Journal of Intellectual & Development Disability* **22**, 241–9.

McKee, M. and Clarke, A. (1995) Guidelines, enthusiasms, uncertainty and the limits to purchasing. *British Medical Journal* **3** (10), 101–4.

Meehan, S., Moore, G. and Barr, O. (1995) Specialist services for people with learning disabilities. *Nursing Times* **91** (13), 33–5.

Mencap (1998) *NHS For All*. London: Mencap.

Mencap (2004) *Treat Me Right: Better Healthcare for People with a Learning Disability.* London: Mencap.

Mental Health Foundation (1996) *Building Expectations: Opportunities and Services for People with a Learning Disability.* London: Mental Health Foundation.

Middleton, S. and Roberts, A. (eds.) (2000) *Integrated Care Pathways: a Practical Approach to Implementation.* Oxford: Butterworth Heinemann.

Middleton, S., Barnett, J. and Reeves, D. (2003) *What is an Integrated Care Pathway?* Available from: www.evidence-based-medicine.co.uk (Accessed 12 October 2004)

Millar, S. (2003a) Pictures and symbols: planning, consulting and documenting. In: *Augmentative Communication and Inclusion* (Wilson, A., ed.). Edinburgh: CALL Publications.

Millar, S. (2003b) *Personal Communication Passports: Guidelines for Good Practice.* Edinburgh: CALL Publications.

Millar, S. and Caldwell, M. (1997) Personal Communication Passports. In: SENSE Conference, Dundee, 13 September 1997. Edinburgh: CALL Publications.

Millar, S. and Larcher, J. (1998) *Symbol Software*. Edinburgh: CALL Publications.

National Electronic Library for Health (2003) *Care Pathways Know-how Zone.* Available from: www.nelh.nhs.uk/carepathways/icp_about.asp (Accessed 12 October 2004)

NHS Health Scotland (2004) *Health Needs Assessment People with Learning Disabilities in Scotland.* Glasgow: NHS Health Scotland.

Norris, A.C. and Briggs, J.S. (1999) Care pathways and the information health strategy. *Health Informatics Journal* **5**, 209–12.

Nursing and Midwifery Council (2004) *Guidelines for Records and Record Keeping.* London: Nursing and Midwifery Council.

Ontario Trillium Foundation (2005) *Speak Up*. Available from: www.aacsafeguardibg.ca/index.htm (Accessed 28 February 2005)

Pound, C. and Hewitt, A. (2003) Conversation Partners and Communication Access; a Roadmap to Inclusion. In: Communication Matters Symposium, Lancaster.

Poynor, L. (2003) Being breast aware. *Learning Disability Practice* **6** (4), 10–14.

Robillard, A.B. (1994) Communication problems in the intense care unit. *Qualitative Sociology* **17**, 383–95.

Sanderson, H. (2003) Person centred planning. In: *Learning Disabilities: Toward Inclusion,* 4th edn, (Gates, B., ed.). Edinburgh: Churchill Livingstone.

Scottish Executive (2000) *The Same as You? A Review of Services For People with Learning Disabilities.* Edinburgh: Stationery Office.

Shakespeare, T. (1996) Rules of engagement: doing disability research. *Disability and Society* **11** (1), 115–20.

Shropshire County Primary Care Trust (2002) *Access to Acute (Secondary) Care; Supporting People with a Learning Disability on Admission to Hospital.* Shropshire: Shropshire

County Primary Care Trust. Available from: www.shropshirepct.nhs.uk (Accessed 28 February 2005)

Social Work Services Inspectorate (2001) *Draft National Standards of Care.* London: Stationery Office.

South Warwickshire NHS Primary Care Trust (2004) *Patient Passport.* Warwick: South Warwickshire NHS Primary Care Trust.

Strydom, A., Forster, M., Wilkie, M., Edwards, C. and Hall, I.S. (2001) Patient information leaflets for people with learning disabilities who take psychiatric medication. *British Journal of Learning Disabilities* **29** (2), 29–33.

Sulch, D. and Kalra, L. (2000) Integrated care pathways in stroke management. *Age and Ageing* **29**, 349–52.

Sulch, D., Perez, I., Melbourn, A. and Kalra, L. (2000) Randomised controlled trial of integrated (managed) care pathway for stroke rehabilitation. *Stroke* **31**, 1929–34.

Sweeney, J. (2004) Beyond rhetoric: access to mainstream health services in Ireland. *Learning Disability Practice* **7** (1), 28–33.

Syed, K.A. and Bogoch, E.R. (2000) *Integrated Care Pathways in Hip Fracture Management: Demonstrated Benefits are Few.* Available from: www.jrheum.com/abstracts/editorials/200806.html (Accessed 12 October 2004)

Thomson, R., Lavender, M. and Madhok, R. (1995) Fortnightly review: how to ensure guidelines are effective. *British Medical Journal* **3** (11), 237–42.

Thornton, C. (1999) Effective health care for people with learning disabilities; a formal carers' perspective. *Journal of Psychiatric and Mental Health Nursing* **6** (5), 383–94.

Tingle, J. (1997) Clinical guidelines and the law. In: *Integrated Care Management: The Path to Success?* (Wilson, J., ed.). Oxford: Butterworth Heinemann.

Turk, V. and Burchell, S. (2003) Developing and evaluating personal health records for adult with learning disabilities. *Tizard Learning Disability Review* **8**(4), 33–41.

Turner, S. and Moss, S. (1996) The health of adults with learning disabilities and the Health of the Nation strategy. *Journal of Intellectual Disability Research* **40**, 438–50.

Wales, S. (2003) Integrated care pathways – what are they and how can they be used? *Clinical Governance Bulletin* **4** (2), 2–4.

Walmsley, J. (2004) Involving users with learning difficulties in health improvement: lessons from inclusive learning disability research. *Nursing Inquiry* **11** (1), 54–68.

Walsh, M. (1998) *Models and Critical Pathways in Clinical Nursing,* 2nd edn. London: Baillière Tindall.

Watson, J., Cameron, L. and Murphy, J. (2003) Don't just make the font bigger. *Learning Disability Practice* **6** (7), 20–3.

Whoriskey, M. and Brown, M. (2002) *The National Review of the Contribution of Nurses to the Care and Support of People with Learning Disabilities.* The Complex Needs Subgroup report to the Scottish Executive. Edinburgh: Scottish Executive.

Widget Software (1997) *Writing with symbols (Symwrite) (Version 2.0).* Leamington Spa: Widget Software Ltd.

Wilson, J. (ed.) (1997) *Integrated Care Management: The Path To Success?* Oxford: Butterworth Heinemann.

Zander, K. (2002) Integrated care pathways: eleven international trends. *Journal of Integrated Care Pathways* **6**, 101–7.

Further reading and resources

Additional policy documents

Department of Health (1999) *Clinical Governance: Quality in the New NHS*. Available from: www.doh.gov.uk/clinicalgovernance/hsc065.pdf (Accessed 30 November 2004)

Department of Health (1998) *The New NHS Modern and Dependable: A National Framework for Assessing Performance*. Available from: www.doh.gov.uk/pub/docs/doh/nhsnfrm.pdf (Accessed 30 November 2004)

Books

De Luc (2001a,b) are two practical guides which reflect the latest experience and incorporate best practice in developing and using care pathways, with contributions from members of the National Pathways Association.

Middleton and Roberts (2000) provides a practical guide to developing, implementing and evaluating integrated care pathways and is written by people with understanding and experience of integrated care pathways.

Full details of both references can be found in the reference list above.

Journals and articles

Journal of Integrated Care Pathways is a forum for exploring a wide range of issues relating to integrated care pathways, including implementation, evaluation and strategic issues such as informatics, risk management and quality. See particularly the articles by Ahmad et al. (2002a, b), full details of which can be found in the reference list above.

Videos and learning packs

Faculty of Dental Surgery (2001) *Clinical Guidelines and Integrated Care Pathways for the Oral Health Care of People with Learning Disabilities*. London: Faculty of Dental Surgery. Available from: www.rcseng.ac.uk/dental/fds/clinical_guidelines

Thompson, J. and Saunders, M. (1999) *Audit in Teams: The Contribution of Integrated Care Pathways in Services for People who have a Learning Disability*. Nottingham: APLD Publications
This resource package is designed to support collaborative working and partnerships and describes an approach to developing audit practices using integrated care pathways. The package also addresses the need to involve users in developing services as well as key issues in effective change management within services. It includes example documentation, further reading, activities and overheads.

Useful websites

www.doh.uk/learningdisabilities/easy-to-read.pdf
This site provides advice on accessible information which could be used to develop communication passports.

www.rcn.org.uk/publications/pdf/ClinicalGovernance2003.pdf
A resource on clinical governance. The guide summarises the key themes of clinical governance and provides, where available, real life case studies that show clinical governance in action.

www.cgsupport.nhs.uk
NHS clinical governance support team website that aims to help clinicians implement clinical governance.

Integrated Care Pathways Users Scotland: www.icpus.ukprofessionals.com
This organisation is an established network of NHS staff from all over Scotland who use integrated care pathways in many different clinical areas. The site provides information on related events, a series of leaflets and useful links.

National Pathways Association: www.the-npa.org.uk
This organisation provides members with a network of professionals interested in developing, sharing and promoting the use of integrated care pathways. The website includes some frequently asked questions about integrated care pathways and some useful links.

www.nelh.nhs.uk/carepathways/icp_about.asp
National Electronic Library for Health page on integrated care pathways.

www.smartgroups.com/groups/carepathways
This group is designed for mental health professionals who are using, developing or implementing care pathways in their workplace. The group can exchange information and ideas to assist in combating some of the challenges of setting up care pathways and present work such as papers, essays and example pathways on the site.

www.intellectualdisability.info
Tips for doctors on good consultation practice with people with learning disabilities, including speaking in language that the person can understand and using communication aids in the form of pictures and symbols.

www.askaboutmedicines.org
The 'Guide and Directory to Health and Medicines Information' helps people with intellectual disabilities understand the type of medication they are prescribed and helps them formulate appropriate questions about that medication.

Royal National Institute for the Blind: www.rnib.org.uk
Contains a section on preparing for a cataract operation. The page www.rnib.org/access/provides advice on planning and designing accessible information.

www.communityliving.org.uk
Documents and leaflets can be sent to the site which will make them accessible.

www.plain-facts.org
38 leaflets in plain English including some on healthcare.

www.realvoice.org
Specialists in accessible information. They work with people with learning disabilities to produce accessible print, audio, multimedia and web design.

www.rcpsych.ac.uk/publications/bbw
Books Beyond Words, a series designed to make communication easier, and to enable discussions about difficult topics.

www.changepeople.co.uk
A UK-based organisation run by disabled people.

Mental Health Media: www.mhmedia.com
Training on how to make videos for people with learning disabilities.

Communication Aids for Language and Learning: www.callcentrescotland.org.uk
Provides information on how information and communication technology can aid people with disabilities or special education or communication needs. It includes a section giving advice on creating a type 1 passport.

www.dundee.ac.uk/pamis/projects/passports.htm
PAMIS website gives examples of communication passports.

www.photosymbols.com/dynamic/photosymbols80.jsp
Photosymbols are designed for people who cannot read. They are made with real pictures of people with intellectual disabilities.

www.plainenglish.co.uk/A-Z.html
Provides a free booklet of alternative words that people with intellectual disabilities may find easier to use and understand.

Chapter 3

Life planning

Carmel Jennings, Declan Courell and
Dympna Walsh Gallagher

Introduction

The care of individuals with intellectual disabilities has seen fundamental changes over the last 30 years, moving from a model of care that was primarily institutional and medically focused, to one that supports community presence and inclusion. Much of this change has been influenced by the work of Wolfensberger (1972), and later by O'Brien's five service accomplishments (O'Brien and Lyle, 1987). According to Burton and Sanderson (1998) a number of guides, plans and instructions for practice were born from the principles of normalisation, including work by Brechin and Swain (1987), Firth and Rapley (1990) and O'Brien (1987). Although these plans and guides have numerous names,

> 'such as individualized person plan, individualized service plan or individual programme plan, they may have many common features.' (Radcliffe and Hegarty, 2001, p. 87)

Rowe and Rudkin (1999) confer with this and have suggested that:

> 'all approaches to organized support for the social, health and ongoing educational needs of people with intellectual disabilities, could be regarded as lifestyle planning.' (p. 148)

Life planning styles

We all think about and plan for our lives in different ways. Some people have very clear ideas about what they want in life, why they want it and how they can achieve it. Other people may dream and try to make their dream a reality. Life planning is about whom we are, what our needs, wishes and dreams are, and how we can go about achieving our needs, wishes and dreams.

> 'Most of us spend a good deal of our time thinking and talking about what we plan to do now and in the future.' (Kingdon, 2004, p. 14)

We constantly make life plans around holidays, living arrangements, careers, money and shopping, and we talk about these plans to families and friends. Regardless of whom we are, or the process used, no one person is in complete control of all events in life. Neither is any one person at the complete mercy of destiny or fate. There is an interface between the two extremes in which a person can exert, to some extent, greater or lesser influence over the course of their lives (Kingdon, 2004).

It is this balance that we are trying to achieve in supporting people with intellectual disability in life planning. For the most part:

> 'Life planning with people who have a learning disability is concerned with the organisation and monitoring of ongoing social educational and health support for individuals.' (Rudkin and Rowe, 2001, p. 22).

Indeed the majority of people working in the area of intellectual disability now support some form of life planning (Iles, 2003).

Reader activity 3.1   Life planning exercises

- Describe yourself
- Describe where you are now in life
- Outline any future plans or dreams you may have for the next 5 years
- Identify the training/education/experience you will need to make your plans/dreams a reality
- List the resources and supports that will be needed to make these plans/dreams happen
- Identify any obstacles standing between you and your plan/dream
- Take each obstacle and write up one or more ways it could be overcome
- Outline key principles that are important for you when making a life plan

---

History of the development of life planning

In the 1970s service planners felt the need to move away from traditional models of planning for individuals with intellectual disabilities. Traditional models of planning tended to be service rather than service-user focused. The desire to develop a more person-centred planning led to the development of individual programme plans.

Individual programme planning

Individual programme plans were first developed in the United States, and later developed in the United Kingdom. O'Brien and Lovett (1992), Felce et al. (1998), Crosby (1976) and Schachter et al. (1997) used the term 'individualised programme plan' with reference to service and skill-building programmes that a client required.

Kaplan and Kauffman (1990) have described an individual programme plan as a:

> 'road map for the individual's future. Individual programme plans clearly state who will do what and when, it establishes responsibility and account- ability. It is the basis of reviewing progress and is a record for achievement.' (p. 145)

The individual programme planning (IPP) approach involves three distinct phases: assessment, goal setting and review. A named individual from the multi-disciplinary team is given the responsibility of co-ordinating the process. It is intended that the client and significant others in the client's life are involved in planning for the future, with the expressed aim of improving quality of life. The intention is that individual plans are client-centred and focus on the client's wishes, needs and wants.

However, some authors have criticised the IPP process, suggesting that it tends to focus on professional assessment and legal requirements, is service led and has a tendency to focus on negative aspects of individuals' lives (Wilcox and Bellamy, 1987; Crocker, 1990; Spooner and Millard, 1999; Rudkin and Rowe, 2001). Further criticisms and dissatisfaction with this system concerned the level of commitment from professionals, particularly in using the docu- mentation and in goal setting (Greasly, 1995). In addition Greasly (1995) has suggested that the growth of the self-advocacy movement, and the growing ability of people to self advocate, rendered IPP inadequate for meeting service user's needs.

This led to the evolution of life planning styles that were more explicitly person centred. Such approaches placed the person with intellectual disability firmly at the centre of the planning process, irrespective of communication and other intellectual impairments (Rudkin and Rowe, 2001).

As a result of some of the criticism deriving from IPP, other models of planning were developed that attempted to be more user, rather than service or professional, focused. Alexander and Hegarty (2001) have suggested that there is general agreement that the client should be involved in planning for their future. Taking this into account, new models of life planning assert to emphasise a more person-centred approach that encourages and supports the client to make decisions about what is important to them.

Shared action planning

An alternative method to the IPP process developed in the United Kingdom is that of shared action planning (Brechin and Swain, 1987). Shared action planning placed emphasis on choice and expressing wishes and desires through effective communication and the development of relationships. To facilitate this, meetings are small in size and focus on confirming plans and informing individuals rather than being based around making decisions (Rowe and Rudkin, 1999). Shared action planning is a life planning style that built on the positive aspects of the IPP process. Compared to the IPP process, shared action planning placed more emphasis on choice and facilitating people to express their wants and needs (Rowe and Rudkin, 1999; Rudkin and Rowe, 2001).

However, Radcliff and Hegarty (2001) have cautioned that decisions to change from more traditional modes of planning may have been based on:

> 'impressions of current systems, or on ideological grounds, rather than on objective evidence that individual planning approaches are not working well.' (p. 89)

Radcliffe and Hegarty (2001) have suggested that there is probably no one best way of providing individual planning, rather that the focus should be on improving systems that are already being used in practice. Similar criticisms were levelled at shared action planning as IPP, with the result that a family of approaches to life planning was developed made up of several different styles of life planning called person-centred planning (PCP).

Person-centred planning

PCP is another approach in the family of life planning systems. Its central premise is the belief that individuals with intellectual disabilities are able to make choices about their lifestyle and once this has been achieved the role of services/professionals is to ascertain how these aspirations or choices can be achieved. The principles underpinning PCP are drawn from the philosophies of O'Brien's (1987) five service accomplishments which advocate inclusion and valued experiences for individuals with intellectual disabilities.

There are several different styles of PCP. These include: personal futures planning (Mount, 1990), essential lifestyle planning (Smull and Burke-Harrison, 1992), Planning Alternative Tomorrows with Hope (PATH) (Pearpoint et al., 1991), making action plans (Forest and Pearpoint, 1992) and personal outcomes (The Council on Quality and Leadership, 2000). All of these approaches to PCP are based on the principles identified by Sanderson (2003) and Thompson and Cobb (2004) and are highlighted in Box 3.1.

Reader activity 3.2   Application of the principles of person-centred planning

- How do the principles of PCP compare to the key principles that were important for you when making a life plan?
- How many of the above principles are you applying to your practice in supporting people with intellectual disabilities?
- Based on these principles, how could you improve the way you are currently supporting people with intellectual disabilities?

> **Box 3.1   Principles of person-centred planning**
>
> - The person we are planning with is at the centre of the process. They are consulted throughout and they choose who they wish to involve. They also decide when and where the meetings take place. The process is rooted in the principle of shared power
> - Family members and friends are partners in the planning
> - The plan reflects what is important to the person and their capacities and the actual support they require
> - The plan results in actions that are about life. The actions reflect what is possible not just what is available. The focus is on inclusion and change
> - The plan results in ongoing listening, ongoing learning and the development of further actions
> - A PCP approach takes as its basis the view that a person with intellectual disabilities can benefit from and contribute to the community by being valued and listened to by their chosen network of support. The fundamental belief is that consumers define services (Rowe and Rudkin, 1999)

The various styles of PCP share common features that reflect their origins in the normalisation movement. These

> 'shared themes include: choice, the avoidance of depersonalising, negative labelling; listening to the person and those who know them best and in PCP terminology, "honouring those voices", building relationships; individualizing supports based on high expectations of the person's development and capabilities, and demanding that service systems change to meet the person's needs rather than trying to fit the person into existing services.' (Iles, 2003, p. 66)

Whichever style or combination of styles is used to support a person with an intellectual disability, these qualities must be reflected in the process.

Personal futures planning

Personal futures planning was developed by Mount in 1987 (Mount, 1990). It provides a means of describing a person's life now and identifies what they would like in the future (Sanderson, 2003). This was the reason that personal futures planning was the preferred PCP approach to transition planning from child to adult services (Rowe and Rudkin, 1999).

Personal futures planning involves its participants in developing a comprehensive description of the individual through interviews between a facilitator and the individual and those close to the person (Rowe and Rudkin, 1999). It aims to build support among family, friends and the local community by joining people in the personal futures planning process (Kilbane and Sanderson, 2004). From these interviews a series of personal profiles are created covering relationships, living and working environments, health, choices, dreams, nightmares and respect, with optional tools for communication (Rowe and Rudkin, 1999). Following such interviews the planning meeting takes place. This revolves around discovering, with the individual, a vision of a desirable future compiled out of the personal profile. An action plan is created, which identifies obstacles and opportunities, strategies for implementation and the priorities with which to commence. The final step is a review of how the existing system will deal with the desired future of the individual (Rowe and Rudkin, 1999).

Essential lifestyle planning

Smull and Burke-Harrison (1992) have developed essential lifestyle planning in the context of people moving from long-term institutions to the community. Essential lifestyle planning is a method of assessing essential and important factors within the everyday life of an adult with intellectual disabilities and identifying how their life can be improved (Sanderson, 2003). If a person is unable to use words to communicate, a communication section is developed early in the planning process (Rowe and Rudkin, 1999; Sanderson, 2003). Information is gathered under seven headings including: what someone must have in their life, what they must not have and negotiables; preferences; what the person enjoys; and what people who know and care about the person say. Once this information is gathered through dialogue with the client and key people in their life, it is recorded within a lifestyle plan.

The plan is written under a number of headings, including positive accounts of the person with intellectual disabilities and what others need to know or do to support the individual successfully. Further headings are 'unresolved issues' and 'negative reputation' (Rowe and Rudkin, 1999). The focus here is on how to help the person stay healthy and safe. The written plan is then reviewed and the essential lifestyle planning meeting held. As the plans are living and changing, they are regularly reviewed and evaluated (Rowe and Rudkin, 1999). Essential lifestyle planning is useful as a start to get to know the person and to begin to build a team or circle of support around the person (Sanderson, 2003). It is a very helpful system to ensure a consistent approach to an individual amongst different members of staff (Sanderson, 2003).

Planning Alternative Tomorrows with Hope

Planning Alternative Tomorrows with Hope (PATH) was developed by Pearpoint et al. (1991), as a planning style tool for both individuals and organisations (Kilbane and Sanderson, 2004). PATH is a goal-directed method of PCP, aimed at achieving immediate change for the person (Rudkin and Rowe, 2001). PATH is not a way of gathering information about a person but a way of planning direct and immediate action (Kilbane and Sanderson, 2004). PATH helps people who are already committed to supporting the individual to sharpen their sense of a desirable future and to plan how to make progress. PATH requires that the person can articulate his or her dream, or that someone who knows the person very well can articulate the dream on behalf of the person. A practical and pragmatic tool, it requires a skilled facilitator to ensure that the dreams are those of the person and not the team.

Making action plans

Developed in 1987, making action plans (MAPs) arose from the need to support families in getting a place for their child with intellectual disability in a mainstream school setting (Forest and Pearpoint, 1992). MAPs revolve around the belief that all children, regardless of disability, belong in a school community and should be given the opportunity to form relationships within a school community (Rowe and Rudkin, 1999). MAPs are a useful tool for getting to know the person.

> 'The MAPs process allows people to express both their hopes for the future, in the dreaming section, and their fears about the future in the nightmares section. The action plan is about working towards the dream and away from the nightmare.' (Sanderson 2003, p. 379)

The MAPs process brings together the person, their peers, school staff and family in a planning meeting where seven key questions are addressed, including dreams, nightmares, description of an ideal day at school and feedback from the making action plans team (Rowe and Rudkin, 1999). With its emphasis on integration, the involvement of peers without a disability is a necessary feature of the making action plans process.

Personal outcome measure

The personal outcome measure was developed by the United States Council on Quality and Leadership in 1996 as a method of measuring how well a service meets the needs of a person with intellectual disability (The Council on Quality and Leadership, 2000). Through interviews with 2500 people with disabilities, key areas of concern were identified. These included autonomy, attainment, affiliation, identity, safeguards, rights, health and wellness.

There are 25 outcomes as determined by The Council on Quality and Leadership; for example under the category of autonomy, outcomes include choosing daily activities, opportunities for privacy, using the environment and deciding when to share personal information. In the three-part process of applying the personal outcome measure there is a learning stage where the individual employees, teams and the organisation use the outcomes to learn about the person with an intellectual disability. Once there is a clear sense of the person's definition of their desired outcomes, the next stage is to organise the resources and co-ordinate the services and supports that will facilitate these outcomes. In the third stage the organisation aligns services and supports and then returns to the person to determine if they have achieved the outcome expressed. Many services and organisations are now using personal outcomes as a quality system to ensure that services are person-centred and responsive to the needs of service users.

Reader activity 3.3

- Describe what you understand by life planning
- Outline the different styles of life planning and describe how they may contribute to supporting people with intellectual disabilities
- Describe your role in supporting life plans for people with intellectual disabilities

---

The established tools for life planning offer a broad range of useful approaches enabling professionals, care workers, families and communities to facilitate people with intellectual disabilities exercise power and control over their own lives.

Life planning in practice

Although a variety of styles has been developed, all are based on the same principles:

'They all start with who the person is and end with specific actions to be taken.' (Kilbane and Sanderson, 2004, p. 19)

The indicator of a good life plan is the outcome for the person, and Parley (2001) has shown that the implementation of a PCP model resulted in more choice for clients and has also shown that it resulted in staff being more respectful to clients. Holburn et al. (2004) conducted a longitudinal comparative evaluation of PCP processes and outcomes for 20 individuals with intellectual disabilities and behaviours that challenge, and a matched control group, who received individual programme planning. Outcomes reported favourable changes in living arrangements, choice making, relationships, daily activities, satisfaction, and in the commitment to a vision by the team of the PCP process. Rowe and Rudkin (1999) conducted a systematic review of the qualitative evidence for the use of lifestyle planning in people with intellectual disabilities and these findings reported that PCP was successful in ensuring that plans are more person-centred than those produced by non-PCP approaches. However, they also suggested that there is no convincing evidence that any one form of life planning provides better outcomes for clients than any other. Therefore we can conclude that life planning styles can lead to a better life for a person with intellectual disabilities, but facilitators need to be informed, educated and supported in using the different styles, picking, choosing and combining styles to give the best options for the person with intellectual disability. Findings also suggest that in practice, most people have some form of life planning, but that it is often informal and unorganised (Parley, 2001).

Furthermore, Coyle and Maloney (1999) have identified that shifting from one model of service delivery to another model based on life planning could place conflicting demands on staff, and may impact on the extent of positive outcomes experienced by service users. This is an important factor for consideration in developing and implementing any life planning style. Parley (2001) has stated that:

> 'Despite gains achieved through the implementation of the person-centred model, little progress was made in involving people in planning their care on a power-sharing basis.' (p. 299)

This begs the question of the power base when using any style of life planning: how can a real shift of power be incorporated into the process?

Rowe and Rudkin (1999) have suggested that there is a need to establish quantitative and qualitative outcome data if different forms of life planning are going to be used in an informed and appropriate way:

> 'In order to move practice on in a constructive way, it could be argued that we need more evidence and less ideology.' (Rowe and Rudkin, 1999, p. 154)

These findings are supported by Iles (2003) who, in addition, suggests that much of the effectiveness of PCP is in the form of anecdotes and stories which are:

> 'powerful and describe positive change in people's lives (but however) lack of clear academic rigour in terms of subjecting such claims to critical analysis leaves their status as evidence in doubt.' (Iles, 2003, p. 71)

Discovering the real person

Individual life planning is a process of continual listening and learning. The main focus is on what is important to a person now and in the future, and acting on this information with their family, professionals and friends. This process offers a variety of approaches that can be used to highlight areas of a person's life, as they share stories, describe their dreams and plans for their future. Helping people to achieve the life plan that they desire now, and the hopes they have for the future requires time to find out who they are as people and what is important in their lives. This is time that is well spent, as it provides an opportunity to break through stereotypes, professional roles and impersonal approaches, and to find a new way to see people for who they are, that is people with abilities not disabilities.

Individual life planning gathers a lot of different information about a person, for example their history, likes/dislikes, hobbies, friends, family and work situations. It also illustrates the person's experiences and achievements as well as their dreams and hopes for the future. When people are supported to tell their own story, it can give them more control over what they want to say and share about their lives, rather than someone else describing their life for them. By listening to the person and learning from them and other close members we can form rich, colourful details that can be added to the pen picture of who the individual really is. However, if individuals cannot communicate verbally, discovering the ways in which they express themselves is vital. This involves spending time and 'being with' individuals, talking to them, asking them questions and observing their reactions. In some cases it may be necessary to talk to significant people in the individuals' lives.

Whatever method is employed to gather information about a person the first step should always be to find out good things about that person. This may be by asking the person themselves what they like best about themselves and then asking others what they like and admire most about them in order to get a picture of the real person. The overall aim is to find out what is important to the person now and for the future, and what help and supports that person needs. This will highlight actions that need to be taken from different people's perspectives by their family, friends and/or professionals.

Having considered all the above factors and their importance in individual life planning let us now look at Peter who needs your assistance in developing his individual life plan.

Case illustration 3.1   Peter's story

Peter is a 32-year-old man who has Down's syndrome and a moderate intellectual disability. Peter suffers from recurrent respiratory tract infections and has type II diabetes. Recently Peter has shown signs of deterioration in self-help skills and short-term memory. He lives in the North Western region of Ireland, in campus-style accommodation with four other male colleagues. Cheryl (Peter's key worker) and Peter worked together for 12 weeks to help Peter think about what was and is important in his life and aspects of it that he would like to change. Cheryl spent a total of 12 hours with Peter averaging out at 1 hour per week. They talked about things he liked and disliked about his job and his family, and together they made up a portfolio.

When Cheryl first met Peter, she was informed by staff that since his mother passed away Peter didn't like to talk about his family as it upset him. However, Cheryl discovered that Peter loved to talk about his family, especially his mother, showing off photographs of her that he kept hidden away in a case under his bed. He showed Cheryl many of the presents and cards that his mother and father gave to him. For Peter these were his most precious possessions. Other staff were not even aware of their existence.

Peter decided he wanted to put one photo of him and his mother in the portfolio and one other photo with all the family in the portfolio too. Peter also wanted a photo of himself taken while he was working on his computer at his workshop. Currently Peter is only able to work on the computer for an hour on Tuesdays and Fridays as the computer is shared between 12 people. By giving Peter the opportunity to think about what was important to him, he informed Cheryl that he hated sharing his bedroom as he had no privacy. He liked to meditate quietly and look over his favourite possessions frequently.

When Peter and Cheryl had finished outlining what is important to him, they had clear ideas about what Peter wanted to change and wanted to talk about with other people. This portfolio was used to prepare a lifestyle planning meeting to suit Peter. Peter decided he would like to have the meeting at his house while his fellow housemates were at work. Peter chose who he wanted to invite to the meeting. They included members of his family, his social worker, two key workers, the manager of the workshop that he attends and two friends from home.

Cheryl raised the point at the meeting that Peter's health status may have an impact on his life plan. With Peter's agreement a referral was made to a clinical psychologist to assess Peter's recent memory and skill loss. With Peter's permission, it was also agreed at the meeting that his key worker would support him to attend his general practitioner for a full physical examination and to discuss with the doctor his problems with recurrent respiratory tract infections.

The social worker agreed to discuss Peter's living arrangements with the service provider, in particular his request for more privacy and to have his own room. The social worker also agreed to approach the day service that Peter was attending to discuss the possibility of increasing his time on the computer. Peter's key worker agreed to co-ordinate all aspects of his life plan. She, along with his family, also agreed to help him choose a photograph of his mother and his family for his portfolio.

Peter enjoyed showing off different sections of his portfolio at the meeting and talking about issues that were important to him. The staff commented on how much they learned about Peter, even though some of them had worked with him for many years. They discovered aspects of him that they were not aware of previously.

At previous planning meetings for Peter, staff were in control and only very occasionally did Peter get the opportunity to voice his opinion about how own life. Too often it was all pre-prepared and Peter's life plan was completed without his involvement. The review date for Peter's next lifestyle planning meeting was set for 4 months' time.

Reader activity 3.4

The family and the health professionals in Peter's life had different degrees of involvement and consequently made different contributions. Can you summarise the different degrees of involvement and the contributions of others using the following two headings:

- Professional involvement
- Person-centred approach or style

Case illustration 3.2   Cathy's story

Cathy lives at home with her parents, sister and four brothers. She is a very attractive woman in her mid-thirties. She lives in an urban area in Northern Ireland and her family is a very close Roman Catholic family.

Cathy has cerebral palsy due to prolonged labour at birth. Contrary to what the doctors then believed, Cathy is of high intelligence and communicates very well using a communication board, some hand gestures and the use of symbols. Cathy is confined to a specially designed wheel chair; however Cathy has said that she would like to have an electric wheel chair so that she can be more independent.

Cathy is very well cared for and presents with no medical complaints or complications. She was educated at home by her parents for the first 12 years of her life. Then for 2 years a special needs teacher came into her home 5 days a week for 2 hours. Cathy is always treated as one of the family and is allowed make choices and decisions for herself. However, Cathy relies on her mother to meet her physical needs.

Her communication board includes photographs of her family with their names underneath, numbers from 0–100, the alphabet, names of close friends and the names of places where she loves to go, for example, Lourdes, Knock, Doon Well, Galway, England, Scotland and France. She has visited these places with her mother, father and sister. Cathy has expressed a desire to have a talking computer to assist with her communication.

Cathy is a 35-year-old woman with great aspirations and really enjoys having a laugh. She attends a local adult training service and enjoys meeting her friends and socialising. However, when Cathy was talking about her weekly activities at this service she told the life planning meeting that she didn't enjoy the dinners there and that most days she had very little to eat, but drank plenty of fluids. She also said that she would like to do more arts and crafts, as a lot of the day she was bored. Cathy's physical disability often precluded her from participating in sports and the Special Olympics. Cathy requested that staff help support her to become more involved in these activities.

Reader activity 3.5

In Cathy's individual life plan she illustrated what is important to her now. These things included:

- Being involved in all family decisions and occasions as usual
- Socialising at least two times a week
- Her desire to have an electric wheel chair and a talking computer
- Attending the adult training centre
- Being involved in arts and crafts and Special Olympics
- Working on the computer and writing letters to people on it
- Visiting her friends Marie, Nora, Sean, Philomena, Sr. Simon . . . at least once a month
- Going to mass every Sunday and all holy days and anniversaries
- Going away for weekends and holidays

Describe the supports that need to be put into place in order for Cathy's life plan become a reality. In your answer you may need to consider the following:

- The need for occupational therapist involvement with regard to her request for an electric wheelchair
- The need for a speech therapist to assess Cathy's suitability for a talking computer
- The need for a dietician to be involved to assist and advise Cathy's key worker on aspects of her diet
- The need for the key worker to develop a range of social activities for Cathy, including involvement in Special Olympics, arts and crafts, going to mass, visiting her friends, and to support Cathy's use of the computer so that she can write to her friends

---

Conclusion

It is very important that intellectual disability nurses help people understand what individual lifestyle planning is about. It is a way of assisting people to work out what they want in alliance with family, friends and professionals to get the support they require in order to achieve their life plan. Life planning requires a fundamental shift of thinking from a 'power over' relationship to a 'power with' relationship.

As has been outlined in this chapter, over the last 30 years many different approaches to life planning have emerged. However, they all share the view that the person concerned has a voice, has the right to be heard and to be placed at the centre of the process. Life planning enables individuals to express their desires, needs dreams and aspirations. The role of the intellectual disability nurse is to ensure that health and social care professionals listen carefully to the voice of individuals who are risk of being silenced, and to put into place supports and interventions that will assist service users attain their dream and to live their life to the full.

References

Alexander, M. and Hegarty, J.R. (2001) Measuring client participation in individual programme planning meetings. *British Journal of Learning Disabilities* **29**, 17–21.

Brechin, A. and Swain, J. (1987) *Changing Relationships: Shared Action Planning with People with a Mental Handicap.* London: Harper and Row.

Burton, M. and Sanderson, H. (1998) Paradigms in learning disability: compare, contrast, combine. *Journal of Applied Research in Intellectual Disability* **11** (1), 44–59.

Carnaby, S. (1997) What do you think? A qualitative approach to evaluating individual planning services. *Journal of Intellectual Disability Research* **41** (3), 225–31.

Coyle, K. and Maloney, K. (1999) The introduction of person-centred planning in an Irish agency for people with intellectual disabilities: an introductory study. *Journal of Vocational Rehabilitation* **12**, 175–80.

Crocker, T. (1990) Assessing client participation in mental handicap services: a pilot study. *British Journal of Mental Subnormality* **36** (2), 98–107.

Crosby, K.G. (1976) Essentials of active programming. *Mental Retardation* **14**, 3–9.

Falvey, M., Forsest, M., Pearpoint, J. and Rosenberg, R. (1994) Building connections. In: *Creativity and Collaborative Learning. A Practical Guide to Empowering Students and Teachers* (Thousand, J., Villa, R. and Nevin, E., eds.). Baltimore: Paul H Brookes Publishing.

Felce, D., Grant, G., Todd, S., Ramcharan, P., Beyer, S., McGrath, M., Perry, J., Shearn, J., Kilsby, M. and Lowe, K. (1998) *Towards a Full Life. Researching Policy Innovation for People with Learning Disabilities.* Oxford: Butterworth-Heinemann.

Firth, H. and Rapley, M. (1990) *From Acquaintance to Friendship.* Kidderminster: BIMH Publications.

Forest, M. and Lusthaus, E. (1987) The kaleidoscope: challenge to the cascade. In: *More Education/integration* (Forest, M., ed.). Ontario: G Allen Roeher Institute.

Forest, M. and Pearpoint, J. (1992) Commonsense tools: MAPs and circles. In: *The Inclusion Papers: Strategies to Make Inclusion Work* (Pearpoint, J., Forest, M. and Snow, J., eds.). Toronto: Inclusion Press.

Greasley, P. (1995) Individual planning with adults who have learning difficulties. *Disability Society* **10**, 353–67.

Holburn, S., Jacobson, J.W., Schwartz, A.A., Flory, M.J. and Vietze, P.M. (2004) The Willowbrook Futures Project: a longitudinal analysis of person-centered planning. *American Association on Mental Retardation* **109** (1), 63–76.

Iles, I.K. (2003) Becoming a learning organization: a precondition for person centred services to people with learning difficulties. *Journal of Learning Disabilities* **7** (1), 65–7.

Kaplan, C.M. and Kauffman, C.S. (1990) Developing the individual program plan. In: *Program Issues in Developmental Disabilities* (Gardner, J.F. and Chapman, M.S., eds.). Baltimore: Paul H. Brooks.

Kilbane, J. and Sanderson, H. (2004) 'What and how': understanding professional involvement in person centred planning styles and approaches. *Learning Disability Practice* **7** (4), 16–20.

Kilbane, J. and Thompson, J. (2004) Never ceasing our exploration: understanding person centred planning. *Learning Disability Practice* **7** (3), 8–31.

Kingdon, A. (2004) Person centred planning & the care programme approach. *Learning Disability Practice* **7** (7), 14–15.

Mount, B. (1987) *Personal Futures Planning: Finding Directions for Change* (Doctoral dissertation, University of Georgia, 1987). Ann Arbor, MI: UMI Dissertation Information Service.

Mount, B. (1990) *Making Futures Happen: A Manual for Facilitators of Personal Futures Planning*. Minnesota: Governor's Council on Developmental Disabilities.

O'Brien, J. (1987) A guide to personal futures planning. In: *A Comprehensive Guide to the Activities Catalogue: An Alternative Curriculum for Youth and Adults with Severe Disabilities* (Bellamy, G. and Willcox, B., eds.). Baltimore: Paul H Brookes.

O'Brien, J. and Lovett, H. (1992) *Finding a Way Towards Everyday Lives: The Contribution of Person Centred Planning*. Harrisburg, PA: Pennsylvania Office of Mental Retardation.

O'Brien, J. and Lyle, C. (1987) *Framework for Accomplishments*. Available from: Responsive System Associates, 93-D Treeview Lane, Decatur, GA 30038.

Parley, F.F. (2001) Person-centred outcomes. Are outcomes improved where a person-centred care model is used? *Journal of Learning Disabilities* **5** (4), 299–308.

Pearpoint, J., O'Brien, J. and Forest, M. (1991) *PATH: A Workbook for Planning Positive Possible Futures*. Toronto: Inclusion Press.

Radcliffe, R. and Hegarty, R.J. (2001) An audit approach to evaluating individual planning. *The British Journal of Developmental Disabilities* **47** (2), 87–97.

Rowe, D. and Rudkin, A. (1999) A systematic review of the qualitative evidence for the use of lifestyle planning in people with learning disabilities. *Journal of Learning Disabilities for Nursing, Health and Social Care* **3** (3), 148–58.

Rudkin, A. and Rowe, D. (2001) Planning For life. *Learning Disability Practice* **3** (5), 22–6.

Sanderson, H. (2003) Person-centred planning. In: *Learning Disabilities: Toward Inclusion*, 4th edn, (Gates, B., ed.). Edinburgh: Churchill Livingstone.

Schachter, M., Kennedy, J., Ritchie, P. and Godwin, G. (1997) *People, Plans and Possibilities: Exploring Person Centred Planning*. Edinburgh: SHS Ltd.

Smull, M. and Burke-Harrison, S. (1992) *Supporting People with Severe Reputations in the Community*. Virginia: National Association of State Directors of Developmental Disabilities Services.

Spooner, B. and Millard, C. (1999) A person-focused system for people with learning disabilities. *Nursing Times* **95** (38), 50–1.

The Council on Quality and Leadership (2000) *Personal Outcome Measures*. Maryland: Towson.

Thompson, J. and Cobb, J. (2004) Person centered health action planning. *Learning Disability Practice* **7** (5), 12–15.

Thornicroft, G. (1991) The concept of case management for long term illness. *International Review of Psychiatry* **31**, 125–32.

Wilcox, B. and Bellamy, G.T. (1987) *A Comprehensive Guide to the Activities Catalogue: An Alternative Curriculum for Youths and Adults with Severe Disabilities*. Baltimore: Paul H Brookes.

Wolfensberger, W. (1972) *The Principles of Normalisation in Human Services*. Toronto: The Canadian Institute on Mental Retardation.

Yates, J. (1980) *Program Design Sessions*. Carver: Jack Yates.

Chapter 4

Person-centred planning in intellectual disability nursing

Steve McNally

Introduction

All care planning must place the person with intellectual disabilities at the heart of decision making and, ideally, this should include everyone, whatever their level of disability. This chapter will further explore particular issues concerning person-centred planning (PCP) building on the previous chapter. Initially, the nature of PCP and its prominence in policy is reviewed. The benefits and limitations of PCP approaches are explored. The chapter will also attempt to articulate some of the inherent tensions which exist between the professional and personal perspectives of care planning. What actually happens for a person will depend to some extent on availability of, and access to, resources to provide appropriate support to lead a fulfilling life. The implications for professionals will be explored, including the need for facilitation of PCP to be acknowledged as sound professional practice. Facilitation of PCP is a role that can be integrated with the therapeutic relationship between intellectual disability nurses and people with intellectual disabilities. Additionally this chapter will draw on research data from a study on the practice of self advocacy. Group members' views on rights, choice, independence and inclusion will be presented to provide a user perspective concerning the delivery of these principles, central to PCP, to their lives. A case illustration is also included to demonstrate essential lifestyle planning in practice.

What is person-centred planning?

Person-centred planning (PCP) is best described as a cluster of concepts guiding good practice rather than a single entity. Proponents have claimed that PCP is:

> 'based on a completely different way of seeing and working with people with learning disabilities.' (Sanderson, 2003, p. 369)

This assertion certainly warrants scrutiny; it perhaps reflects the fervor of its apologists. Given this claim to being completely different to any previous approach, authors have sought to identify the distinguishing features of PCP. Among the nuances cited in the literature are the three characteristics described below.

PCP aims to consider the:

> 'aspirations and capacities expressed by the service user or those speaking on their behalf, rather than needs and deficiencies.' (Mansell and Beadle-Brown, 2004, p. 1)

The plan should be in the control of the focus person or their nominated facilitator. This is a key aspect, because power issues, such as the relative powerlessness of service users, have been significant in the development of intellectual disability services. The application of PCP could help to address the imbalance of power between service users and professionals.

Secondly, it attempts to include and mobilise the individual's family and wider social network, as well as statutory services. Although one can see the advantages of this approach, one might question whether the use of such natural supports fills a gap left by statutory provision. A third distinctive aspect of PCP identified by Mansell and Beadle-Brown (2004) is that it places an emphasis upon the support needed to achieve goals. In a PCP context, the plan needs to be responsive to the person's changing needs and aspirations. This contrasts with the tendency within more traditional services to limit goals to those which the agency can manage.

PCP has been described as a:

> 'process of continual listening and learning, focused on what is important to someone with learning disabilities now, and for the future, and acting upon this in alliance with the person's family and friends.' (Sanderson, 2003, p. 370)

It is characterised as a family of approaches which are fundamentally different to previous forms of care planning, such as individual programme planning, because it emphasises power sharing and community inclusion. However, it has been noted that PCP 'shares many characteristics with previous attempts at individual planning' (Mansell and Beadle-Brown, 2004, p. 17).

The most established approaches to PCP include essential lifestyle planning, personal futures planning, making action plans, and Planning Alternative Tomorrows with Hope (PATH), as described in Chapter 3, 'Life planning' (pp. 53–67). All share a value base founded on inclusion. They involve the following processes (Sanderson et al., 2002):

- Finding out what is important to the person (in their everyday life and in the future)
- Identifying what support they require
- Developing an action plan to facilitate the above
- Continuing to reflect and act on the actions and the plan

The policy context of person-centred planning

Legislative developments affecting people with an intellectual disability in the United Kingdom during the past decade have assumed an increasing focus on the person. Statutes, including the Disability Discrimination Act 1995, Human Rights Act 1998 and Race Relations [Amendment] Act 2000, reflect an emphasis on the rights and autonomy of the individual. Policy related specifically to people with an intellectual disability, namely the Government White Paper, *Valuing People* (Department of Health, 2001), and the guidance document, *Planning with People* (Department of Health, 2002), strongly advocate a person-centred approach.

PCP has become an increasingly influential idea underpinning how services should be formulated (O'Brien, 2004; Mansell and Beadle-Brown, 2004). It has been characterised as a medium for creating positive change, realising the Government's vision expressed in *Valuing People* (O'Brien, 2004). The relevant policy documents affecting people with an intellectual disability in the other home nations of the United Kingdom – Wales (*Fulfilling the Promises*, 2002), Scotland (*The Same as You?* 2000) and Northern Ireland (*Equal Lives*, 2004) – are discussed in Chapter 10, which discusses care planning in community nursing settings.

PCP gained great impetus from its appearance in the Government White Paper, *Valuing People* (Department of Health, 2001), as a mechanism for implementing the objectives of rights, independence, choice and inclusion. Its prominence in policy meant that it has received substantial attention from managers and policy makers locally via learning disability partnership boards.

PCP embodies important principles but its emergence can be perceived as an evolution which is traceable through earlier ideas, such as the 'ordinary life' model (King's Fund, 1980) and the shared action planning of Brechin and Swain (1987). The former was far-sighted and person-centred in the context of its era. The shared action plan formulation acknowledged the importance of a holistic approach, and involved an emphasis on objectives, with responsibility for follow-up action (Brechin and Swain, 1987). Other important influences in the development of PCP include normalisation and social role valorisation (Wolfensberger, 1972, 1983), self advocacy (Williams and Shoultz, 1982; Goodley, 2000), the 'five accomplishments' (O'Brien, 1987) and supported living (Kinsella, 1993).

Person-centred planning in practice: a critical review

It is beyond question that support services should be designed to meet, and be generated from, individual needs. In this respect the importance of PCP cannot be underestimated. The former pattern of professionally dominated care planning is now changing. *Valuing People* (Department of Health, 2001) has provided a national framework with local involvement geared towards the centrality of the person with an intellectual disability to the planning process.

Although the government has embraced PCP for people with intellectual disabilities (Department of Health, 2002), there is a lack of empirical evidence for the effectiveness of PCP. Success stories have been recounted largely from case studies (Rudkin and Rowe, 1999; Parley, 2001). Nevertheless, PCP has taken hold as the 'big idea' underpinning policy and services for people with an intellectual disability. Would any contemporary professional in the field of intellectual disability declare themselves to be other than person-centred in their practice? Person-centredness as a concept is open to wide interpretation – my version may be different to yours. This is not to suggest that standardisation is desirable or achievable, any more than having a template for a 'standard' therapeutic relationship, but to emphasise that the term covers a range of meanings. A professionally led model of planning could be administered in a person-centred way; conversely a support staff team could produce an apparently comprehensive plan without the person's involvement.

It has been argued that quality, not quantity, should be prioritised in implementing PCP. There appears to be a sound case, given a belief in its likely effectiveness and benefits for the person and the service system, for advocating access to PCP for some individuals. Any new initiative has to be introduced gradually. However, one might question the quality of life for the majority of service users with an intellectual disability in a system which facilitates access to PCP only for a minority of individuals (Mansell and Beadle-Brown, 2004). A further issue to have been identified is that few people have an individual plan of any description (Mansell and Beadle-Brown, 2004).

A criticism of PCP is that it may comprise an activity trap with the danger of a focus on the paper plan rather than the person. Service managers have taken up person-centred approaches enthusiastically in recent years, encouraging their staff to implement the system. An unintended consequence which can ensue is the situation in which a support team has agonised over, for example, an individual's essential lifestyle plan, with the resultant document growing to monolithic proportions. This phenomenon is to be avoided. Staff members generally learn to deal with this process more succinctly as their skills have developed.

The forms of documentation associated with PCP are of themselves a secondary factor. The most important element is the process and the way in which appropriate user participation is ensured. This presents a challenge for professionals and agencies. For many people who use services, relaxed informal approaches will tend to be successful, in contrast with more formal meetings. O'Brien has posed the question:

'Can PCP can be used to make improvements, even in the absence of positive policies and sufficient resources?' (O'Brien, 2004)

The answer is potentially 'yes', as has always been the case in human services. Innovative, caring practitioners have, historically, practised effectively to uphold the rights and wishes of service users, even within organisational structures which failed to encourage such practice. Good work has taken place in spite of systems which have been professionally led and task orientated. Aspects of good practice have been recognised in much earlier conceptual work, for example Peplau's work in devising a nursing model with an emphasis on interpersonal relations (Peplau, 1952).

Assumptions underlying the implementation of effective PCP include the availability of sufficient, flexible funding through the care management system. Care management operates on a model of individual planning but its bureaucratic procedures can be interpreted as a form of control of access to resources, i.e. rationing. Such resource issues can lead to frustration and tensions for service users, their families and, indeed, professionals. Care management concentrates on assessment and re-assessment and as a process it is weighted heavily towards the assessment phase. It has been argued that service provision has been adversely affected by the loss of provider social work time with the advent of care management roles, in effect a 'retreat from professionalism' (Lymbery, 1999).

Another possible criticism of PCP is that it involves a reliance on the family and social networks rather than paid carers, perhaps mirroring the debate on community care itself. Social care is often in reality care provided not by statutory or voluntary sector service providers but by ordinary people with the bulk of support delivered by close relatives (Barclay Report, 1982; Parker, 1992). Two types of caring activity have been distinguished, with informal helpers such as neighbours, who may provide practical help for a few hours to others each week, being differentiated from 'people who are substantially involved, providing personal and physical care, as well as many other types of assistance, in their own households and for long hours' (Parker, 1992, p. 14).

A danger of PCP is the possibility that it becomes a meaningless buzz term, whereby managers and supporters focus on the paperwork, instead of the person, for the purpose of inspection or audit. An impressive plan may be in place but it is crucial that action follows. Therefore, implementation has to be pursued vigorously. Professionals and support staff should to be aware of the pitfall of too much concentration on the plan and planning phase at the expense of intervention and action.

Service users should play a role in selecting the model of planning. It may be more appropriate and effective to ensure access to a brokerage or direct payments model. Arguably this would feature a greater level of power for the person but there have been difficulties in access.

PCP assumes a high level of communication skill on behalf of staff in facilitating the wishes of people who use non-verbal communication and in co-coordinating the process. Perhaps a major danger is that PCP itself is perceived as a panacea which obviates other approaches.

Case illustration 4.1

Peter is 37 and lives in supported housing which is provided by a private profit-making organisation. The community team professionals involved in Peter's support consider that he might be better supported in another setting, but they respect Peter's choice to live there. A community intellectual disability nurse became involved in supporting Peter in response to a request for health advice, specifically on epilepsy, and also advising the mainly inexperienced staff giving 'social care'. James, the nurse, talked with Peter to establish things which are essential to Peter, those which are important to him and those activities he enjoys. It was found that Peter was leading a rather solitary and introspective life. He spent much of his time in his bedroom, or walking the streets of the town. James worked with the staff team to identify what was required. It was necessary to adopt the elements of essential lifestyle planning (see below). A process was developed of matching staff skills and interests to Peter's needs.

Elements of the essential lifestyle plan

- Essential (Non-Negotiables)
- Important (Strong Preferences)
- Enjoys (Highly Desirable)

People who know Peter would say . . .
Peter's reputation says . . .
To be successful in supporting Peter, we must . . .
How Peter communicates with us . . .
To help Peter stay healthy we must . . .
To help Peter stay safe we must . . .
Unresolved issues . . .

Outcomes of using a person-centred approach for Peter

An outline activity and support plan was devised. A named person was made responsible for ensuring the implementation of plans. Activities were monitored, although it is important to consider that this is meaningful only if the activities are valued by the target person, in this case Peter. To support Peter's music interest he was accompanied by Dave, a final year intellectual disabilities nursing student, to music gigs locally.

The essential lifestyle planning approach had a positive influence on activities and Peter's level of inclusion in his local community. He developed the confidence to participate in activities such as attending music concerts and eating out rather than meandering around the local area, passing time. Peter became involved with a local self-advocacy group. He subsequently took on the role of selecting and providing music for social events and selected background music for the Annual Conference of the Partnership Board.

Intellectual disability nurses as facilitators of person-centred planning

Intellectual disability nurses, as an occupational group, are in a particularly strong position to implement and refine PCP. Among nurses' assets are the specialist nature of intellectual disability nurse training and the high proportion of time spent with people who have an intellectual disability; this compares with other professionals who may make a single visit for assessment purposes, but spend an insufficient time to develop a relationship. However, the greatest contribution of nursing is its emphasis on interpersonal skills and the therapeutic relationship (Peplau, 1952). Although nurses generally must balance service users' freedom with the professional, ethical 'duty of care', they have a philosophical history of supporting service users' autonomy (Gadow, 1980; Millette, 1989).

There is debate in the literature about the extent to which nurses, as paid employees of service organisations, can advocate for service users (Gates, 1994; UKCC, 1998; Blackmore, 2001). This is sometimes referred to as 'professional advocacy' (Brandon, 1995). It has been asserted that:

> 'Learning disability nurses are ideally suited to advocate for clients during person-centred planning. That is, exploring all aspects of their life with them, from collaboration to community care, and what assistance they may require.' (Llewellyn, 2004, p. 16)

Research findings from a study of self-advocacy groups

To explore the issues of PCP further, some extracts from interviews conducted with self advocates are presented and discussed in the context of contemporary developments in policy and practice. These group interviews were carried out in the context of an investigation into the development of self-advocacy groups and the experience of self advocacy for people with intellectual disability in an English region. The objectives of the study included analysis of the influence of membership of selected self-advocacy groups and eliciting service users' views of their experience as self advocates.

The policy context and the rights agenda affecting people with intellectual disability have seen significant legislative developments in the past decade, including the Disability Discrimination Act 1995 (HMSO, 1995), Human Rights Act 1998 (HMSO, 1998) and *Valuing People* (Department of Health, 2001). The findings of a regional study of self-advocacy groups for people with intellectual disabilities in England anticipated the thrust of recent policy initiatives (McNally, 2005). The self-advocacy groups who participated in this study emphasised the act of 'speaking up' and choice, inclusion, independence, and rights – the key principles of *Valuing People* (Department of Health, 2001).

People with intellectual disability are becoming more aware of their rights and entitlements and are insisting on being involved in decision making affecting their lives. Themes from the group interviews included concerns about racism in services for people with an intellectual disability, and in society generally.

Speaking up

Speaking up or speaking out is a central idea in self-advocacy practice. Three distinct contexts for speaking out emerged: within the group, in the life of the individual and speaking up for others. In the group context of this study speaking up involved learning or refining communication skills, gaining greater knowledge of rights and becoming more confident. The following is an excerpt from a conversation between a researcher and some group members.

> Researcher: *'Would anyone like to give an example of how being in the group has helped them in changing something, or feeling more confident, or just speaking up to get something done?'*
> Group member 1: *'We just speak up for ourselves.'*
> GM2: *'We got results. We always speak up for like the problems that we, we always speak up for ourselves, we also speak up for people in wheelchairs, ones who can't speak at all, so we speak up for them as well.'*
> GM1: *'We speak up for the whole centre here, don't we? And they do it there.'*

Another group member offered the following definition of self-advocacy:

> GM3: *'Well, self advocacy in action means that – like I've said before – helping, speaking up for yourself, speaking for other people, going to conference meetings or whatever and getting people's ideas from them and them getting ideas from us. Be more assertive in yourselves as people . . .'*

Another member returned to the theme of representing others.

> GM4: *'Some people are not confident to say something. You have to have somebody else speak up for them.'*

A member of a committee representing service users within a day service explained their role:

> GM5: *'We are the voices to speak up for them. Whatever they complain, and they don't want to say it in there, that's fair enough. We are the voices for the whole centre here.'*
> R: *'Would you say it has helped you being in the group?'*
> GM5: *'It's helped me a lot. In two things.'*
> R: *'In what way do you think it's helped you?'*
> GM5: *'Confident to know and talk.'*

Speaking up and making choices and decisions are closely associated. Contributions on the importance of exercising choice included:

'We enjoy coming to the group and we enjoy getting involved in decision making.'
[Choice is about] *'How a service should be run – not the bosses telling us how it should be run.'*

Independence

'College is all right because the tutor don't tell you what to do, not like when you're at school. At school the teachers tell you off every five minutes.'
'I like the course because it teaches you how to be independent. . . . it teaches you that one day you could be independent for yourself and you won't be living at home.'
'That's what we come here for isn't it, to be independent?'

It is important to take account of the idea of mutuality in carer–client relationships. It is seldom the case that a member of support staff simply delivers care to a client, without receiving positive feedback and reinforcement from the service user. Although it would not be healthy or desirable for a professional to be emotionally dependent on clients, it is relevant to acknowledge the concept of interdependence.

Taking users' views into consideration, listening to them and consulting them is important but no longer acceptable unless people are actively involved in the planning and commissioning of services (Redworth and Phillips, 1997). In recent years, service policies have been developed which support this notion of active involvement, and emphasise the importance of person-centredness in the development, delivery and evaluation of services (Department of Health, 2001). Despite this progress, it has been observed that a gap continues to exist between policy generation and implementation.

Rights

Nine of the groups in this study referred to rights during the interviews. This may reflect a growing awareness of civil rights, and of statutory developments including the Human Rights Act 1998, which came into effect in October 2000.

This Act primarily consolidated existing rights into the United Kingdom constitution, but it may have important implications for services for people with intellectual disability. Combined with this has been the influence of the White Paper, *Valuing People* (Department of Health, 2001), emphasising the rights agenda most clearly, supported by the principles of independence, choice and inclusion. A thought-provoking quote regarding the legal rights and responsibilities of people with intellectual disability emerged from a group member with a strong sense of justice.

'We should be treated equally . . . people with learning problems know what's right and wrong. We know what's right and wrong.'
[Self-advocacy] *'It's about speaking up for yourself and sticking up for yourself, and about how everyone's got rights.'*

The contributions cited above are consistent with the notion of 'rights as empowerment' that has been discussed by Means and Smith (1994), who identified two other strategies – 'exit' and 'voice' – which refer to the concepts of effecting change by actively opting out of an unsuitable service or the act of speaking up to create positive change within existing services.

Inclusion

People with intellectual disability are susceptible to aspects of social exclusion, such as low income or being caught in the 'benefits trap', with consequent difficulties in access to good quality housing; lack of awareness of rights or of the assertiveness skills needed to assert these; and problems with access to primary health care (Keywood et al., 1999).

> 'Social inclusion is the process by which efforts are made to ensure that everyone, regardless of their experiences and circumstances, can achieve their potential in life. To achieve inclusion income and employment are necessary but not sufficient. An inclusive society is also characterised by a striving for reduced inequality, a balance between individuals' rights and duties and increased social cohesion.' (Centre for Economic and Social Inclusion, 2002)

Leisure and work are key aspects of social inclusion. The groups interviewed in the present study did not actually use the term 'leisure' but this emerged as a theme with groups referring to a range of social activities including spending time with friends in pubs, social clubs and discotheques. The following comments were made by group members.

> *'There's always pubs'* [member of new group discussing a social outing].
> *'We try to meet up in pubs'* [member of independent group].
> *'Organise a lunch or go for a pub meal'*
> *'I go to two clubs in the work'* [member of college-based group referring to work experience].
> *'We have discos'*

The above statements on the social activities promoted and sponsored by self-advocacy groups are consistent with previous studies (Sutcliffe and Simons, 1993; Goodley, 2000). The development of PCP can be linked to the influential ideas mentioned above, including the 'five accomplishments' model (O'Brien, 1987), which is itself derived from earlier conceptual work on social role valorisation and normalisation (Wolfensberger, 1972 and 1983). The accomplishments model does not represent a new definition or theory but it does provide a framework for exploring the implications of normalisation for organisations which provide human services. O'Brien identified five major accomplishments which services should achieve for their users: community presence, community participation (which pivots on support for developing and maintaining networks of friends and relatives), choice, competence and respect (positive promotion of the image of people with intellectual disability), all of which are central to PCP. The theme of 'relationships' applies to all of the accomplishments. The comments below illustrate group members' ideas and aspirations regarding close personal relationships and how these should be conducted.

> 'I says to J, "Have one – not half-a-dozen."' [girlfriends].
> 'I travel on me own a lot because on Sundays I go and see me girlfriend.'

Work featured in all 15 of the interviews, possibly bearing out its strong link with self-esteem. There were two main contexts: self-advocacy work relating to the group and individuals' paid work. In some cases, there was also paid work for training and service evaluation.

> 'I went to a day centre. . . . I was told what to do and when to do it. You had to do what they told you and I got fed up with it. I went to see my social worker and asked them to find me something else other than the day centre.'
> 'We are looking for work and things like that. Shop work and for work experience.'
> 'Some of the work I didn't like.'

Eight of the groups discussed college. Two of the participating groups were college-based; in other cases, people talked of specific courses attended, competencies achieved and certificates attained. Group members were relatively uncomplaining about lack of money, a finding which echoes previous studies (Simons, 1992). This may be attributable to low expectations concerning income, or even to the knowledge of being caught in the 'poverty trap'.

Racism

Initiatives revealed in this study included the development of groups for black and Asian service users, with a mission of sharing their culture with others and dealing with racial harassment. These findings from the work of black service users' groups interviewed in this study are consistent with information emanating from Government, acknowledging that services have not met the needs of ethnic minority members.

> 'Government Departments know about the concerns of people from black and ethnic backgrounds with learning disabilities and the worries that these people are not being included.' (Department of Health, 2004, p. 12)

Members of black and ethnic minority service user groups were positive about the self-advocacy group of which they were members, although some individuals reported negative experiences (of racism in many cases).

> 'It makes me meet different people like Asians, like different religions. That's the best thing really.'
> 'Religion comes first.'

A group member recalled being abused verbally by another service user:

'I felt very angry and hurt. He shouldn't say things like that. Then. . . . I went to see somebody to sort them out.' [Went to see a staff member to explain what had happened.]

This resolution of the situation contrasts with the experience of a member of a group based at a day service.

'So when they say "Paki", what do you say to them?'
'I would rather leave it, there is no point in fighting.'

Another group member expressed his frustration at the attitude of some peers:

'Because I was an Egyptian they called me "Camel" and stuff . . . It's not right at all. I could be teaching people how to read Arabic.'

The above excerpts tend to support the observation that:

'Minority ethnic communities face substantial inequalities and discrimination in employment, education, health and social services.' (Mir et al., 2001, p. 2)

The Department of Health and the Valuing People support team are developing advice to be provided to partnership boards on improving this dimension of services locally. For ethnic minority members who have an intellectual disability the experience of simultaneous disadvantage related to race, impairment and, for women, gender, is common. An important issue in the future application of PCP in the UK is likely to be how it works for people from ethnic minorities.

Conclusion: towards an integrated model

There seems little doubt that the family of approaches known collectively as PCP has the potential to offer a positive contribution to the lives of people with intellectual disability. However, the value of PCP lies not in its format or procedures but the integration of its tenets into practice. It is unlikely to matter to the person whether they have, for example an essential lifestyle plan or 'PATH'.

Their concerns are more likely to be whether they think their housing and support networks are suitable, and if they have the opportunities to pursue education, employment or leisure activities of their choice. PCP requires proper resources despite a climate of financial constraints. It is the way in which the PCP process is managed and support is provided which is crucial. PCP principles should be embedded in professional nursing practice with relevant prominence in professional curricula and organisational in-service training programmes. PCP should be an integral part of practice, which flows naturally from the therapeutic relationship.

Person-centred principles should be applied in the personal development plans for support staff. Higher status managers and academics guide practitioners, but support staff may have challenging posts with very modest pecuniary reward. As is the case for people with intellectual disability, they need a 'circle of support'. Person-centred models of supervision may develop and be practised to the benefit of support staff and service users. PCP has an important role to play but it is part of an evolving overall picture in the development of styles of support for people with an intellectual disability. There will be continuing resource implications of PCP for provider agencies, including how they will address the issues of time and staff resource implications in working in partnership with people with profound or multiple disabilities.

PCP has a potential role to play in improving the access of people with an intellectual disability to direct payments. Whereas there are barriers to be overcome in the employment of personal assistants, such as selection, difficulties in asserting wishes and risk of exploitation, it could act as a lever for progress in this area in which uptake has been low. The Government needs to address problems with low uptake of direct payments by people with intellectual disability (Department of Health, 2004). The service brokerage model, in which the person has both the funds to purchase their own service and the support of a service broker to assist them in this endeavour, may be relevant in this connection (Brandon and Towe, 1989).

Organisations must place the emphasis on service delivery through good practice, and PCP approaches can facilitate this. The values associated with PCP are not only compatible with good professional practice; they are essential to effective practice. Documents associated with PCP should not be too lengthy because too much detail may obscure the important points and create a focus on the forms used. We must ensure that person-centred principles are integral to professional practice rather than being mere presentational 'spin'. Recording and administration have their place but client–staff interaction, not a mountain of paperwork, is at the core. Caution needs to be exercised in expectations of families and informal networks. Their input will be extremely valuable, depending on the needs and wishes of the person, but they should not be expected to take the pressure off service providers. In fact families have a key role to play in lobbying for the setting up of new service initiatives.

The term PCP has been in use for some years and, at this stage, agencies and professionals should be concentrating on implementation in practice rather than just planning. Indeed, professionals should be moving a step further towards integrating PCP in their professional practice. It remains to be demonstrated that practice matches the rhetoric of person-centredness. Indeed, it has been noted that there is an:

> 'implementation gap. . . . there are sufficient grounds in the literature cited to be concerned that person-centred planning (or any other kind of individual planning) is largely a paper exercise.' (Mansell and Beadle-Brown, 2004, p. 5)

PCP has the potential to help improve the person's quality of life, but it may be that the process will need to be adapted for some people with intellectual disabilities and their families. It is vital that service providers do not take ownership of PCP because is about the person's choice, not how services are delivered. It will be interesting to see how PCP is operated nationally, given its importance in the delivery of services to people with an intellectual disability. Service planners must be aware that the low pay and low status of direct care staff can result in care provision by devalued staff members who take refuge in reverting to a task-orientated approach (Brewster and Ramcharan, 2005).

PCP stresses circles of support, neighbourhood and community, not defining individuals according to their need to use services. Although the aspiration is good, and may indeed be successful for some individuals, it could be said to offer a naively rosy view of 21st century post-industrial society. For instance, many people in urban areas of south-east England barely know their neighbours. There are variations across the United Kingdom. In Northern Ireland, for example, the sense of community is almost palpable.

PCP is a potentially fertile area for participatory research. There is scope for employing inclusive research methods to evaluate the user experience of the planning process and the support provided (Richardson, 2000; Walmsley, 2001).

Professionals should not over-elaborate on whether to use personal futures planning, PATH, making action plans or another person-centred planning tool. An eclectic approach to use of the range of PCP approaches would be appropriate according to individual circumstances. What matters is the quality of the process and how it is conducted, allied to realism and honesty regarding the achievability of outcomes. The approaches themselves are merely vehicles to facilitate the expression of choice, listening and acting upon these choices by providing suitable supports. It is the continuing PCP process itself, with its attendant focus on the person and their evolving needs and aspirations, which can be a catalyst for positive change.

References

Barclay Report (1982) *Social Workers: Their Role and Tasks.* London: National Institute for Social Work/Bedford Square Press.

Blackmore, R. (2001) Advocacy in nursing: perceptions of learning disability nurses. *Journal of Learning Disabilities* **5** (3), 221–34.

Bradford District NHS Care Trust (undated) *The Care Programme Approach.* Bradford: Bradford District NHS Care Trust.

Brandon, D. (1995) *Advocacy – Power to People with Disabilities.* Birmingham: Venture Press.

Brandon, D. and Towe, N. (1989) *Free to Choose: An Introduction to Service Brokerage.* Surrey: Hexagon Publishing.

Brechin, A. and Swain, J. (1987) *Changing Relationships: Shared Action Planning with People with a Mental Handicap.* London: Harper, Row.

Brewster, J. and Ramcharan, P. (2005) Enabling and supporting person-centred approaches. In: *Learning Disability. A Life Cycle Approach to Valuing People* (Grant, G.,

Goward, P., Richardson, M. and Ramcharan, P., eds.). Maidenhead: Open University Press.

Centre for Economic and Social Inclusion (2002) *What is Social Exclusion?* Available at cesi.org. (Accessed 20 July 2004)

Department of Health (2001) *Valuing People: a New Strategy for Learning Disability for the 21st Century.* London: The Stationery Office.

Department of Health (2002) *Valuing People: A New Strategy for Learning Disability for the 21st century. Towards Person-Centred Planning Approaches: Planning With People: Guidance for Implementation Groups.* London: Department of Health.

Department of Health (2004) *Valuing People: Moving Forward Together.* The Government's Annual Report on Learning Disability 2004, HC507. London: The Stationery Office.

Department of Health, Social Services and Public Safety (2004) *Equal lives: Review of Policy and Services for People with Learning Disabilities in Northern Ireland.* Belfast: Stormont.

Gates, B. (1994) *Advocacy: A Nurses' Guide.* Middlesex: Scutari.

Gadow, S. (1980) Existential advocacy: philosophical foundation of nursing. In: (Spicker S. and Gadow S., eds.). *Nursing: Images and Ideals.* New York: Springer.

Goodley, D. (2000) *Self-Advocacy in the Lives of People with Learning Difficulties.* Buckingham: Open University Press.

Her Majesty's Stationery Office (1995) *Disability Discrimination Act.* London: Her Majesty's Stationery Office.

Her Majesty's Stationery Office (1998) *Human Rights Act.* London: The Stationery Office.

Her Majesty's Stationery Office (2000) *Race Relations [Amendment] Act.* London: The Stationery Office.

Keywood, K., Fovargue, S. and Flynn, M. (1999) *Best Practice? Health Care Decision-Making by, with and for Adults with Learning Disabilities.* Manchester: National Development Team.

King's Fund (1980) *An Ordinary Life.* London: King's Fund.

Kinsella, P. (1993) *Supported Living – A New Paradigm?* Manchester: National Development Team.

Llewellyn, P. (2004) Nursing and advocacy in person centred planning. *Learning Disability Practice* **7** (9), 14–17.

Lymbery, M. (1999) The retreat from professionalism: from social worker to care manager. In: *Professionalism, Boundaries and the Workplace* (N. Malin, ed.). London: Routledge.

Mansell, J. and Beadle-Brown, J. (2004) Person-centred planning or person-centred action? Policy and practice in intellectual disability services. *Journal of Applied Research in Intellectual Disabilities* **17**, 1–9.

McNally, S. (2005) *Advocacy and Empowerment: Self-Advocacy Groups for People with a Learning Disability.* Unpublished PhD Thesis. London: South Bank University.

Means, R. and Smith, R. (1994) *Community Care: Policy and Practice.* London: Macmillan.

Millette, B. (1989) *An Exploration of Advocacy Models and the Moral Orientation of Nurses.* Unpublished PhD Thesis. Massachusetts: University of Massachusetts.

Mir, G., Nocon, A., Ahmad, W. and Jones, L. (2001) *Learning Difficulties and Ethnicity.* London: Department of Health.

National Assembly for Wales (2002) *Fulfilling the Promises: Proposals for People with Learning Disabilities. Consultation Documents.* Cardiff: National Assembly for Wales.

O'Brien, J. (1987) A guide to personal futures planning. In: *A Comprehensive Guide to the Activities Catalog: An Alternative Curriculum for Youth and Adults with Severe Disabilities* (Bellamy, G. and Wilcox, B., eds.). Baltimore: Paul JH Brookes.

O'Brien, J. (2004) If person-centred planning did not exist, *Valuing People* would require its invention. *Journal of Applied Research in Intellectual Disabilities* **17**, 11–15.

Parker, G. (1992) Counting care: numbers and types of informal carers. In: *Carers: Research and Practice* (Twigg, J., ed.). London: Her Majesty's Stationery Office.

Parley, F. (2001) Person-centred outcomes. Are outcomes improved where a person-centred care model is used? *Journal of Learning Disabilities* **5** (4), 299–308.

Peplau, H.E. (1952) *Interpersonal Relations in Nursing.* New York: Putnam.

Redworth, M. and Phillips, G. (1997) Involving people with learning disabilities in community care planning. *British Journal of Learning Disabilities* **25**, 31–5.

Richardson, M. (2000) How we live: participatory research with six people with learning difficulties. *Journal of Advanced Nursing* **32** (6),1383–95.

Rudkin, A. and Rowe, D. (1999) A systematic review of the qualitative evidence for the use of lifestyle planning in people with learning disabilities. *Journal of Learning Disabilities for Nursing, Health and Social Care* **3** (3), 148–58.

Sanderson, H. (2003) Person centred planning. In: *Learning Disabilities: Toward Inclusion,* 4th edn, (Gates, B., ed.). Edinburgh: Churchill Livingstone.

Sanderson, H., Jones, E. and Brown, K. (2002) Active support and person-centred planning: strange bedfellows or ideal partners? *Tizard Learning Disability Review* **7** (1), 31–8.

Scottish Executive (2000) *The Same as You? A Review of Services for People with Learning Disabilities.* Edinburgh: The Stationery Office.

Simons, K. (1992) *Sticking up for Yourself – Self Advocacy and People with Learning Difficulties.* York: Joseph Rowntree Foundation.

Sutcliffe, J. and Simons, K. (1993) *Self Advocacy and Adults with Learning Difficulties – Contexts and Debates.* Leicester: National Institute of Adult Continuing Education.

Towell, D. and Sanderson, H. (2003) Person-centred planning in its strategic context: reframing the Mansell/Beadle-Brown *critique. Journal of Applied Research in Intellectual Disabilities* **17** (1), 17–21.

United Kingdom Central Council for Nursing, Midwifery and Health Visiting (1998) *Guidelines for Mental Health and Learning Disabilities Nursing.* London: UKCC.

Walmsley, J. (2001) Normalisation, emancipatory research and inclusive research in learning disability. *Disability and Society* **16** (2), 187–205.

Williams, P. and Shoultz, B. (1982) *We Can Speak for Ourselves.* London: Souvenir Press.

Wolfensberger, W. (1972) *The Principle of Normalization in Human Services.* Toronto: National Institute of Mental Retardation.

Wolfensberger, W. (1983) Social role valorization: a proposed new term for the principle of normalization. *Mental Retardation* **21**, 234–9.

Further reading and resources

Alexander, M. and Hegarty, J.R. (2001) Measuring client participation in individual programme planning meetings. *British Journal of Learning Disabilities* **29**, 17–21.

American Association on Mental Retardation. Fact Sheet: *Self-Advocacy.* Article from the Internet Homepage of AAMR. Washington: AAMR. Available at: www.aamr.org/Policies/faq_advocacy.shtml

Gates, B. (ed.) (2003) *Learning Disabilities: Toward Inclusion*, 4th edn. Edinburgh: Churchill Livingstone.

Malin, N. (ed.) (1999) *Professionalism, Boundaries and the Workplace.* London: Routledge.

People First London, Change, Speaking Up in Cambridge and Royal MENCAP (2000) *Nothing About Us Without Us – The Learning Disability Strategy: The User Group Report.* London: Department of Health.

The Care Programme Approach Association, Walton Hospital, Whitecotes Lane, Chesterfield, S40 3HW. Tel: 01246 552889; Fax: 01246 552896; email cpa.association@chcsnd-tr.trent.nhs.uk

Useful websites on issues related to person-centred planning

www.nursing-standard.co.uk/archives/ldp_pdfs/ldpvol7-6/ldpv7n6p1216.pdf
www.nursing-standard.co.uk/archives/phc_pdfs/phcvol15-06/phcv15n06p1820.pdf
www.valuingpeople.gov.uk/pcpresources.htm
http://www.bild.org.uk/factsheets/person_centred_planning.htm
http://www.doncaster.gov.uk/Living_in_Doncaster/social_services/learning_disabilities_adults/Person_Centred_Planning_Implementation_framework.asp

Chapter 5

The legal and ethical implications of care planning and delivery for intellectual disability nursing

Susan Harvey and Vicky Stobbart

Introduction

Nurses are required to safeguard the interests of their clients at all times (Nursing and Midwifery Council, 2004) and this requires the intellectual disability nurse to be clear about their scope of professional practice. They must practice in an anti-discriminatory and anti-oppressive way, remaining alert to the legal, moral and ethical implications of their practice. Intellectual disability nurses must operate in a non-parentalistic way, whilst recognising that they have a duty of care. It is widely recognised that the role of the intellectual disability nurse is diverse, reflecting policy changes leading to the closure of long-stay hospitals (Department of Health, 1971; Jay, 1979; Alaszewski et al., 2001). The recent White Paper, *Valuing People* (Department of Health, 2001a), has helped consolidate the diversity of this role, with the four key central principles of rights, choice, independence and inclusion having a direct impact on the practising intellectual disabilities nurse. In addition, changing practice has also been influenced by the Disability Discrimination Act (Department of Health, 1995) and the Human Rights Act 1998 section 2 (Department of Health, 1998).

This chapter will explore these issues and will also focus on treatment issues, consent and the Nursing and Midwifery Council's Code of Professional Conduct (Nursing and Midwifery Council, 2004). It is not anticipated that this chapter will provide solutions to all of the legal and ethical challenges faced by practising intellectual disability nurses but that it may be useful as the basis for discussion about practice dilemmas and a guide for reflection towards post-registration education and practice requirements.

Scope of practice

The foundation of intellectual disability nursing practice is the unique bond between the nurse and the person with an intellectual disability, created by working in partnership with the person over a period of time (Sines, 1995). In the United Kingdom, intellectual disability nursing is governed by the Nursing and Midwifery Council's Code of Professional Conduct (Nursing and Midwifery Council, 2004). Central to this chapter will be the use of this code, which acts as an ethical guide for nursing practice and aims to:

'. . . inform the professions of the standards of professional conduct required of them in the exercise of their professional accountability and their practice; and inform the public, other professionals and employers of the standard of professional conduct that they can expect of a registered practitioner.' (Nursing and Midwifery Council, 2004, standards 07.04, clause 1.1, p. 4)

The Nursing and Midwifery Council came into effect in June 2002, replacing the UK Central Council of Nursing, Midwifery and Health Visiting (UKCC) and the National Boards in England, Scotland, Wales and Northern Ireland. Prior to the Nursing and Midwifery Council, the UKCC published *Guidelines for Mental Health and Learning Disabilities Nursing* (UKCC, 1998). At the time of writing, this document is currently under review by the Nursing and Midwifery Council. This guide covers issues such as ethical, legal and professional guidance, consent, communication and team working. It is suggested the guidelines should be read in conjunction with the Nursing and Midwifery Council's Code of Professional Conduct (Nursing and Midwifery Council, 2004).

Serving and protecting the public is integral to legal and ethical issues. The Nursing and Midwifery Council was established for this purpose to improve the standard of nursing and midwifery care. The Nursing and Midwifery Council's key tasks are to:

- Maintain a register of qualified nurses and midwives (registrants)
- Set standards and guidelines for education, practice and conduct
- Provide advice on professional standards
- Consider allegations of misconduct or unfitness to practise due to ill health (Nursing and Midwifery Council, 2004)

The Nursing and Midwifery Council's Code of Professional Conduct (Nursing and Midwifery Council, 2004) makes clear that in caring for clients and patients as a registered nurse, midwife, or specialist community public health nurse, you must:

- Respect the patient or client as an individual
- Obtain consent before you give any treatment or care
- Co-operate with others in the team
- Protect confidential information
- Maintain your professional knowledge and competence
- Be trustworthy
- Act to identify and minimise the risk of patients and clients

A list of Nursing and Midwifery Council publications is provided in Box 5.1.

Box 5.1   Nursing and Midwifery Council publications

The NMC Code of Professional Conduct: Standards for Conduct, Performance and Ethics
Guidelines for Records and Record Keeping
Guidelines for the Administration of Medicines
The PREP Handbook
Employers and PREP
Complaints about Unfitness to Practise: A Guide for Members of the Public
Practitioner–Client Relationships and the Prevention of Abuse
Professional Advice from the NMC

(For further information visit www.nmc-uk.org)

Contemporary intellectual nursing disability practice

This section considers the role that the intellectual disability nurse plays in promoting anti-discriminatory practice. Taking the role of the community learning disability nurse as an example, anti-discriminatory practice and advocating for the rights of the person to use mainstream services has been a feature of this role prior to Disability Discrimination Act (Department of Health, 1995), Human Rights Act (Department of Health, 1998) and *Valuing People* (Department of Health, 2001a). A study by Alaszewski et al. (2001) has considered the development of intellectual disability nursing and concluded that changes in policy and societal attitudes have had a direct impact on the role of the intellectual disability nurse.

The identity of the intellectual disability nurse is defined by creativity, flexibility, adaptability and a pioneering spirit to practise in health and social care settings. Turnbull (2004) has questioned how many professions have members who would be prepared to do this, stating that this is:

'. . . . indicative of the loyalty that learning disability nurses feel towards people with learning disabilities'. (Turnbull, 2004, p. 6)

Due to the diversity of intellectual disability nurse practice, it is imperative that there is clarity regarding the scope of professional practice.

In line with the new strategic direction for learning disability services (Department of Health, 2001a), intellectual disability nurses operate within a framework of person-centred planning, which can bring about a certain level of tension and conflict between health and social care professionals, family carers and the person with an intellectual disability. Such complexities may lead to a fundamental difference about approaches to care and support for the individual. Differences often arise when an issue is of an ethical nature, as demonstrated in Case illustration 5.1. In this example, the decision-making process applies to a person with an intellectual disability having a blood test. Central to the role of the intellectual disability nurse is the ability to respect differing opinions in such scenarios, whilst ensuring adherence to professional codes and working within a legal and ethical framework.

Case illustration 5.1   Pearl

Pearl is a woman with mild intellectual disabilities who requires an annual blood test to identify any potential problems with her thyroid function. Over the last 6 months it has been noted that Pearl is becoming more lethargic, has put on 2 stone in weight and is frequently absent from work. A blood test may determine the root cause of the problem.

Different opinions that may emerge concerning Pearl

(A)   Pearl's opinion: that the blood test is not important, will cause pain and will require missing half a day's work

(B)   Opinion of Pearl's parents: that the blood test should be undertaken while Pearl is heavily sedated, to ensure that she is not aware of it and experiences no pain

(C)   Opinion of Pearl's residential home manager (a registered intellectual disability nurse working in a social care setting): Pearl needs to receive accessible information highlighting reasons for having the blood test and consequences of not having it, so that Pearl can make an informed decision about whether she consents to the invasive procedure

(D)   Opinion of GP: the presenting symptoms point to problems with thyroid function, which, if not treated in a timely way, will lead to a deterioration of health effecting Pearl's quality of life and independence

---

Considering the opinion of Pearl's residential home manager (C), the intellectual disability nurse may have personal values and beliefs about what may be in Pearl's best interest. However, this will have been made within the context of the Nursing and Midwifery Council's code of conduct framework, the Department of Health Consent Guidelines (Department of Health, 2001b), Human Rights Act (Department of Health, 1998) and local policy context. It is this legislation and guidance that serves to protect and act as a safeguard for people with intellectual disabilities, whilst guiding the practice of the qualified nurse.

Working with people with intellectual disabilities requires a knowledge of ethical decision making, as this forms the basis of several of the decisions that the intellectual disability nurse will make in practice. As already mentioned, nurses may find themselves working in diverse care settings. An intellectual disability nurse may be employed as a prison nurse, health promotion specialist, health facilitator, day resource manager, short breaks team leader, deputy registered home manager, advocacy co-ordinator, community nurse or forensic liaison nurse. Ethical principles can be used as guides to moral decision making and moral actions. This centres on the formation of moral judgements in professional practice (Beauchamp and Childress, 2001).

Intellectual disability nurses are required to clarify and articulate their own point of view as well as advocating for the person they are supporting. Nurses need to understand the potential conflict that may arise when advocating for people with intellectual disabilities. The role of advocate may be in direct conflict with a nurse's professional and personal opinion. An individual's viewpoint reflects societal, cultural and religious influences. Understanding one's own values and seeking to understand the value systems of others may help to reduce conflict during the care planning process (Potter and Perry, 2003).

This brief introduction to issues surrounding ethical decision making has highlighted some of the complexities involved when supporting people with intellectual disabilities. The next section will discuss in more detail a framework for ethical decision making when care planning.

Ethics and care planning

Ethical dilemmas may present in the care planning and care delivery process. This is usually when it is not clear what the right thing to do is or when healthcare professionals, family carers and a person with an intellectual disability are not in agreement about a course of action. In some cases this may be more complex to resolve due to the severity of the intellectual disabilities and difficulties with communication.

Ethical dilemmas involving care planning for people with intellectual disabilities may demand that the nurse negotiates many differing points of view. It is important that the intellectual disability nurse constantly reflects on their own set of values, beliefs and attitudes. This will better enable them to support the care planning process. If ethical problems arise the intellectual disability nurse must ensure that they strive to understand the other person's point of view. This will help in effectively supporting the person when different opinions emerge.

Ethics is concerned with what people see as good or bad and arises from values and personal points of view:

> 'The use of ethics in decision making strives to go beyond personal preferences and to establish standards on which individuals, professions and societies agree.' (Potter and Perry, 2003, p. 50)

There is a range of ways to approach ethical issues and below is a framework for ethical thinking that may be used when care planning. One approach to healthcare ethics which is widely recognised is a set of fundamental principles which need to be taken into account when ethical judgements are made. This is called the 'four principles framework', proposed by Beauchamp and Childress (2001) and outlined in Box 5.2. This framework reflects ethical decision making which may be used in a clinical nursing environment and also across a variety of health and social care settings.

Box 5.2   The four principle framework (Beauchamp and Childress, 2001)

Principle 1	Respect for autonomy	Respecting the decision-making capacities of autonomous persons; enabling individuals to make reasoned informed choices
Principle 2	Beneficence	This considers the balancing of benefits of treatment against the risks and costs; the healthcare professional should act in a way that benefits the patient
Principle 3	Non-maleficence	Avoiding the causation of harm; the healthcare professional should not harm the patient. All treatment involves some harm, even if minimal, but the harm should not be disproportionate to the benefits of treatment
Principle 4	Justice	Distributing benefits, risks and costs fairly; the notion that patients in similar positions should be treated in a similar manner

Resolving an ethical dilemma is similar to the nursing process as it involves deliberate, systematic thinking (Millar and Babcock, 1996). As previously mentioned, due to the diverse nature of intellectual disability nursing, a nurse may work outside the National Health Service (NHS) and in some cases in isolation. This may make it more difficult to ascertain relevant local guidelines and policies for ethical decision making. For nurses employed by a NHS organisation, the following may provide support in legal and ethical dilemmas:

- Local ethics committee
- Director of nursing/clinical governance
- Risk assessment managers
- Medical advisor
- Trust solicitors
- Multi-disciplinary teams
- Nursing peers
- Patient advisory liaison service

For qualified nurses employed by private and voluntary organisations, the support networks may be less clearly defined than for those employed by the NHS. In such situations it is imperative to use the Nursing and Midwifery Council Code of Professional Conduct, Human Rights Act (Department of Health, 1998), Disability Discrimination Act (Department of Health, 1995), current draft of Mental Capacity Bill (HM Government, 2005) and Department of Health Consent Guidelines (Department of Health, 2001b) as a foundation for all care planning and care delivery decisions.

Case illustration 5.2 is used to demonstrate the practical application of the four ethical principles of Beauchamp and Childress (2001).

Case illustration 5.2   Shaheen

Shaheen is a 42-year-old woman with intellectual disabilities. Over the last 12 months she has been admitted to an acute hospital on three different occasions with pneumonia. A video-fluoroscopy examination has identified that Shaheen is at risk of aspirating on both food and fluid. The speech and language therapist has recommended that Shaheen becomes *nil by mouth* with immediate effect and that a percutaneous endoscopic gastrostomy (PEG) tube is inserted to reduce the risk of choking and likelihood of developing aspiration pneumonia. The physiotherapist has recommended positioning and chest drainage (postural drainage). After a multi-disciplinary review with hospital health professionals, community learning disability team members, the general practitioner, family members and Shaheen, it has been agreed that a PEG tube will be inserted. Two days later, whilst a doctor is explaining the proposed procedure to Shaheen, it becomes apparent that Shaheen will not give consent. The refusal is on the basis that the general anaesthetic would require a needle being inserted into her arm. She indicated to the doctor that she is afraid of needles. The gastroenterologist's opinion is that if the PEG tube is not inserted Shaheen will be at risk of future chest infections which may lead to aspiration pneumonia, highlighted as a leading safety risk for people with intellectual disabilities by the National Patient Safety Agency (National Patient Safety Agency, 2004). Given the risk of dehydration, malnutrition, aspiration pneumonia and the potential for a continuation of her current health status to be life threatening, the multi-disciplinary team supporting Shaheen agree that it is in Shaheen's best interest to have the operation.

Reader activity 5.1

Consider the hypothetical case dilemma in Case illustration 5.2 and think about how you may apply the four ethical principles previously identified. Do ensure that you also consider religious, cultural and quality of life issues, reflected in the person-centred plan and health action plan.

The next section uses the four principles framework (Beauchamp and Childress, 2001) to explore some of the legal and ethical dilemmas facing the intellectual disability nurse supporting Shaheen.

Principle 1: respect for autonomy

Nurses and nurse practitioners in constructing care plans and preparing their delivery must consider taking into full account Shaheen's view on her treatment. Do remember that autonomy is not an all or nothing concept; it is possible that Shaheen may not be fully autonomous (and not legally competent to refuse the proposed treatment), but this does not mean that ethically the nurse should ignore her wishes which have been expressed clearly. The intellectual disability nurse's role in offering Shaheen support is to ensure that all information is accessible, comprehensive and comprehendible. As an intellectual disabilities nurse it may be useful to work in partnership with a speech and language therapist to seek advice on the best way to make information accessible for Shaheen.

Principle 2: beneficence

Intellectual disability nurses need to be clear about the benefits to Shaheen of having the PEG tube inserted both in the short and long term. Often this principle clashes with respect for the individual's autonomy. In Shaheen's case in the short term, she is frightened to have a needle inserted into her arm. In the longer term she will benefit from having a PEG tube inserted as this will mean less risk of serious health concerns which may be life threatening, such as aspiration and choking.

From a legal perspective, the multi-disciplinary team will need to be clear about whether Sheehan is competent to consent for treatment. It may be helpful to work in partnership with psychology and psychiatry colleagues to assess Shaheen's level of competency and explore her fears and concerns about needles. If she is competent, the multi-disciplinary team will not be able to override Shaheen's wishes under the principle of 'best interest'. It may be helpful at this point to familiarise yourself with the Nursing and Midwifery Council Code of Professional Conduct (Nursing and Midwifery Council, 2004), clause three, along with the Department of Health guidelines on seeking consent for people with learning disabilities (Department of Health, 2001b).

Principle 3: non-maleficence

Within this principle the intellectual disability nurse needs to consider which actions would cause the least harm to Shaheen. The options for Shaheen are to have a needle inserted into her arm for the general anaesthetic and PEG tube inserted or for no action to take place. If no action is taken there is the possibility that Shaheen's health will continue to deteriorate, with the likelihood of future episodes of pneumonia and an increased risk of early death.

The intellectual disability nurse will need to consider that in order for Shaheen to have the PEG tube inserted, a needle will have to be used whether the procedure is undertaken using a local or general anaesthetic. It may be that physical restraint or chemical sedation may need to be considered, which may leave Shaheen psychologically traumatised with a mistrust of health professionals.

The intellectual disability nurse will need to gather evidence-based information to determine whether the procedure is likely to be successful for Shaheen.

If non-compliant she may continue to take food and fluid orally or dislodge her PEG. To ensure safety following insertion of the PEG tube and to increase the adherence of the guidelines and advice from the dietician, speech and language therapist and physiotherapist, it is highly likely that training will need to be arranged for Shaheen and her carers. It is imperative for successful delivery of the care planning process to engage Shaheen and her carers fully in all stages to increase the chances of safety and compliance of the PEG tube feeds.

Principle 4: justice

The intellectual disability nurse needs to think about alternative treatments for Shaheen and whether the proposed treatment impacts on the quality of life, cultural, religious and any legal factors. Be aware that Shaheen may be viewed as a woman with intellectual disability and that this intellectual disability may lead to her being discriminated against (Mencap, 2004). This may lead to a delay of the proposed procedure. In addition this may have a negative impact on the timeliness of Shaheen's medical intervention. It is suggested that the reader refers to the Human Rights Act (Department of Health, 1998) and the Disability Discrimination Amendment Act (Department of Health, 1995) should they not be familiar with this legislation and find themselves faced with a similar dilemma.

Reader activity 5.2

Consider the legal and ethical dilemmas that Case illustration 5.2 may pose for the community learning disability nurse using the four principles framework.

Ethical decision making

In addition to the four principles framework for healthcare ethics it may also be useful to consider the International Council of Nurses (ICN) Code of Ethics for Nurses (ICN, 2000). The ICN outlines four fundamental responsibilities to nurses:

- To prevent illness
- To promote health
- To alleviate suffering
- To restore health

These four responsibilities outline the standards of ethical conduct for all nurses. The International Code of Ethics for Nursing is recommended as essential for further reading.

It may be helpful to consider the following steps of a reflective process in ethical decision making when making an ethical decision in partnership with others. This approach may help you to highlight the relevant ethical questions and the moral reasoning involved in this process.

Step one: how to decide if it's an ethical dilemma

Not all problems are ethical in nature. We have adapted Curtin and Flaherty's (1982) characteristics of a true ethical dilemma and given a list of considerations for reflection that may guide the nurse practitioner through the dilemma. If the problem cannot be resolved through a review process, speak to all involved in the ethical dilemma and gather as much information relevant to the case. It is essential to gather as much information as possible from healthcare records, literature and consultation with colleagues, family members and the person with an intellectual disability. If there is no logical solution to the problem, others may differ in their opinion. This is often the case when a solution may affect other areas of the person's life. Alternative feeding, such as a PEG tube, may impact on the person's ability to take part in social activities, such as swimming, which may be a key area of enjoyment in a person's life.

Step two: identify and examine your own views and values on the issues

Do consider that part of deciding whether the issue poses an ethical dilemma is dependent on examining your own opinion about the issue. People can reach different conclusions about the same situation and often there is no right or wrong. It is good practice for the qualified nurse to discuss the issue within a framework of clinical supervision, ideally within a multi-disciplinary setting or similarly reflective environment.

Step three: identify the problem

After the nurse has reviewed the relevant information, he or she will need to develop a clear statement about the problem in an accessible format that can be easily understood by all. This statement will form the basis for all negotiation for others. Allow time to ensure the client is involved with decision making with regards to their care.

Step four: gather all possible courses of potential actions and conflicts

The nurse should make sure that they have all the relevant information and possible actions to resolve the ethical dilemma. This can then be presented to all involved. The intellectual disability nurse's role will be to facilitate a discussion and identify with the group an agreed course of action. This may form part of a person-centred plan and also contribute to a health action plan or care programme approach.

Step five: evaluate actions taken

The nurse should ensure at all times that the person-centred actions are adapted and reviewed and that information remains in an accessible format for the individual concerned. In the care plan the nurse needs to have a clear date for a review of the agreed actions. Documentation of the decision made is imperative to record at every step within the nursing notes, health action plan summary, care programme approach minutes, person-centred plan or minutes of any meetings related to the ethical decision making process. The intellectual disability nurse should be clear in the care plan about how they will measure the success of the decision made.

Critical thinking and the nursing process

Critical thinking is central to the ethical and legal implications of care planning. This section concentrates on strategies intellectual disability nurses may draw on to aid critical thinking. Gordon (1995) has stated that critical thinking involves making conclusions, decisions, drawing inferences and reflecting. Intellectual disability nurses will use critical thinking to identify and challenge assumptions, consider what is important about a situation, explore alternatives and consider ethical principles to make an informed decision when care planning.

Critical thinking aids partnership working with people with learning disabilities and facilitates better informed choices during care planning and care delivery processes. It is more than just problem solving. One has to continually improve how one adapts and faces problems presented in a variety of health and social care settings. Critical thinking has been defined as:

> 'the active, organised, cognitive process used to carefully examine one's thinking and the thinking of others.' (Chaffee, 1994)

Critical thinking will aid in assisting the intellectual disability nurse to work within the Nursing and Midwifery Council Code of Professional Conduct (Nursing and Midwifery Council, 2004). The UKCC *Guidelines for Mental Health and Learning Disability Nursing* state:

> '... that you must not practise in a way which assumes that only you know what is best for the client. This may create dependency, hinders team work and can interfere with the client's right to choose.... Advocacy is about promoting client's rights to choose and empowering them to decide for themselves.' (UKCC, 1998, p. 14, Section 29)

Because critical thinking is complex, the following model may help to facilitate how you make clinical decision and judgements. Kataoka-Yahiro and

Box 5.3   Five components of critical thinking

Specific knowledge base

This will vary according to the intellectual disability nurse's education and post registration learning and development.

Experience

This varies in relation to an intellectual disability nurse's clinical practice experience and awareness of clinical decision making. Each experience that the nurse comes across serves as a stepping stone, building on knowledge and developing innovative thinking.

Competence

Making a decision within the nurse's own scope of professional practice based on the competencies that she or he has. Agenda for Change (Department of Health, 2003) identifies a specific key skill framework for competencies. Further information about Agenda for Change can be found on the following website: www.dh/agenda4Change.gov.uk

Attitudes

Paul (1993) has identified 11 attitudes that are a central feature of the critical thinker. These are: confidence, independence, fairness, responsibility, risk taking, discipline, perseverance, creativity, curiosity, integrity and humility. These attitudes will help intellectual disability nurses approach a problem and be successful in their critical thinking.

Standards

Paul (1993) has identified 14 intellectual standards and three professional standards. The intellectual standards are being clear, precise, specific, accurate, relevant, plausible, consistent, logical, deep, broad, complete, significant, adequate (for purpose) and fair. The professional standards are professional responsibility, ethical criteria for nursing judgement and criteria for evaluation. All of these form part of the Nursing and Midwifery Council Code of Professional Conduct: standards for conduct, performance and ethics.

Saylor (1994) have developed a critical thinking model that is based on previous work by Paul (1993) and Miller and Malcolm (1990). This model has been adapted in Box 5.3 because the authors feel it is relevant to intellectual disability nurses regardless of the nature of their employment. According to the model, any experience a nurse is faced with has five components of critical thinking that will lead them to make a safer and more effective decision. These components of critical thinking may assist you in ethical decision making. In addition, the authors would also recommend that this achieved in conjunction with the elements of the nursing process (Fig. 5.1).

The nursing process facilitates the nurse in organising and delivering appropriate nursing care. When applying the nursing process successfully nurses need to integrate elements of the critical thinking model to aid them in making judgements and taking reasoned actions. The authors consider that the

'The nursing process enables [the intellectual disability nurse]
to organise and deliver appropriate nursing care to a client. It
is a systematic approach that nurses use to gather client data,
critically examine and analyse the client's data, identify the
client's response to health problems . . .' (Potter and Perry,
2003, p. 64).

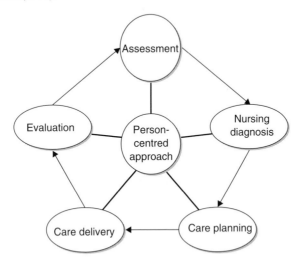

Fig. 5.1 The nursing process.

nursing process is a specific critical thinking competency that can be applied
to the care planning and care delivery process. In care planning it is paramount
that consent issues are addressed and the process for this is outlined in the
next section.

Consent

This section considers the legal and ethical dilemmas that may be involved
when individuals with intellectual disabilities cannot consent for treatment.
Intellectual disability nurses are often involved in facilitating complex decisions
involving consent. Therefore it is imperative for them to refer at all times to
existing guidance, such as *Seeking Consent: Working With People With Learning
Disabilities* (Department of Health, 2001b). These guidelines refer to consent as
'a patient's agreement for a health professional to provide care'. Under Clause
3 of the Nursing and Midwifery Council Code of Professional Conduct, nurses
are advised to think of consent as a continuing process, with the nurse giving
clear accessible and in-depth information about what is going to happen to
the person. Information should make clear any potential risks and benefits
of proposed procedures, as well as alternatives that may be available. The
Nursing and Midwifery Council has recommended that nurses obtain written

Box 5.4

Four Department of Health consent forms can be downloaded:

- Form for adults who are unable to consent to investigation and treatment
- Patient/parental agreement to investigation or treatment where consciousness is not impaired
- Patient agreement to investigation or treatment
- Parental agreement to investigation or treatment for a child or young person

Further reading
The Prodigy website (www.prodigy.nhs.uk) gives excellent examples of how this information might be presented and also has information about a wide range of chronic conditions.

The Joseph Rowntree Foundation's, *Plain Facts* magazine includes an issue on health care decision making. This can be found at www.plain-facts.org

The Department of Health has produced model consent forms for people with learning disabilities and other vulnerable groups, for example children and vulnerable adults. Website address:
www.dh.gov.uk/PolicyAndGuidelinesAndSocialCareTopics/Consent/fs/en

consent in situations where treatment is complex or high risk (Nursing and Midwifery Council, 2004). Box 5.4 provides some more useful sources of information on consent.

Seeking Consent: Working with People with Learning Disabilities (Department of Health, 2001b) guidance considers that to obtain legal consent requires the individual to be:

- Capable of taking that particular decision (competent)
- Acting voluntarily (not under pressure or duress from anyone)
- Provided with enough information to enable them to make the decision

In other words, individuals must have the capacity to give consent. The Mental Capacity Act (2005) provides a statutory framework to empower and protect vulnerable people who are unable to make their own decisions. The act is underpinned by a set of five key principles, which are:

- A presumption of capacity – every adult has the right to make his or her own decisions and must be assumed to have capacity to do so unless it is proved otherwise
- The right for individuals to be supported to make their own decisions – people must be given all appropriate help before anyone concludes that they cannot make their own decisions
- That individuals must retain the right to make what might be seen as eccentric or unwise decisions
- Best interests – anything done for or on behalf of people without capacity must be in their best interests

- Least restrictive intervention – anything done for or on behalf of people without capacity should be the least restrictive of their basic rights and freedoms

Case illustration 5.3 will guide you through a framework for consent and decision making, covering best interest and capacity issues related to Mohammed's care.

Case illustration 5.3   Mohammed

Mohammed is 54 and has severe intellectual disabilities. He lives with his father and attends a resource centre three days a week. Mohammed enjoys horse riding at the weekends, finger painting and dancing. Following a health action planning meeting, it is identified that there may be a deterioration in Mohammed's eyesight, which has lead to him falling over while dancing, holding his hands out in front of him and displaying possible difficulties with depth of perception (walking in sunlight over patio squares and uneven surfaces).

On first presenting at the ophthalmology outpatient clinic at a district general hospital, routine examinations and tests revealed that Mohammed had no sight in his left eye and a cataract was diagnosed in the right eye with recommendations from the senior house officer to operate. Mohammed, through the support of his community nurse and father, is attending the ophthalmology clinic for the second time so that the proposed operation to improve his sight can be fully explained to him.

Reader activity 5.3

Spend some time thinking about the actions that the community nurse may take in advance of the appointment in order to best prepare Mohammed. At the appointment it is clear that Mohammed requires a simple operation to remove the cataract using laser treatment.

Capacity

Mohammed's father and community nurse have explained to him what the laser treatment may involve, using pictures, videos and a trip to the day surgery unit. Mohammed is not able to understand the detail of the operation. It is deemed therefore that he lacks the capacity to decide whether to have the operation or not. This means that a decision will need to be made for Mohammed with his best interests in mind.

Best interest

The ophthalmologist has explained that if Mohammed does not have the operation in the next 9 months there is a high risk of permanent loss of sight in his right eye, which would lead to Mohammed going blind. The effect of blindness on Mohammed's quality of life may reduce his independence to self care, participation in finger painting, dancing and all his social resource activities. Most importantly the loss of the sensory experience of sight and the benefits of horse riding independently would be lost.

Reader activity 5.4

Think about the dilemma above and the steps that you might take as the community intellectual disability nurse to ensure that the best decision is made to safeguard Mohammed's health and well being.

Decision

It was agreed by all those close to Mohammed, including his father and his community nurse, that it would be in his best interests to have the operation. The reason for this decision is based on the decreased quality of life that Mohammed would be faced with if he lost his sight. Some of the key pleasures in his life are dependent on him having his eyesight and those close to him feel it is in his 'best interest' to have the operation to ensure that he can maintain these activities. The care planning process considers the best way of supporting Mohammed and reassuring him.

General points

The following seven general pointers may be useful when exploring care planning and care delivery for people with intellectual disability:

- Seek the person's permission in advance to act on their behalf and ask questions during the medical consultation. This will help in determining the clinical risks to enable you to be able to interpret what the treatment will involve, implications of not having the treatment, alternatives and practical effects on the person's life
- Provide information in a format that a person understands; for example, use pictures, symbols, simple terms, short sentences, communication visual aids, interpreters and other resources. If required, get input from a speech and language therapist as this may aid effective communication between yourself and the person being supported. The speech and language therapist may also be able to equip the person being supported with accessible

communication aids that empower them to directly communicate with health professionals

- Familiarise yourself with *Seeking Consent: Working With People With Learning Disabilities* (Department of Health, 2001b) guidance and take a copy with you to any hospital or clinic appointment. This will give guidance on the requirements from health professionals to seek informed consent from people with intellectual disabilities. This should include information about treatment to be undertaken and the benefits and risks of that treatment, including side effects and outcomes
- Ensure the person is well supported by people close to them, for example a family member, carer, friend, independent supporter, health facilitator or advocate
- Be aware that the person may withdraw their consent during treatment. If this is the case you may wish to support stopping the procedure and discuss the person's concerns. However if interrupting the procedure may put the person's life at risk the doctor may decide to continue until the risk no longer applies
- Make use of a clinical supervision session to discuss any practice issues relating to a specific or more general situation involving consent
- Ensure you are familiar with your local NHS trust or organisation's consent policy. Refer to the resources set out at the end of this chapter for website addresses

Conclusion

This chapter set out to explore issues facing intellectual disability nurses in everyday practice in relation to care planning and care delivery. The sections have drawn together some of the legal and ethical issues that may face intellectual nurses during this process, using the Nursing and Midwifery Council Code of Professional Practice (Nursing and Midwifery Council, 2004) and legal and ethical decision-making frameworks to illustrate key points. These decision making frameworks were set within the context of critical thinking and the nursing process.

It is hoped that the use of case illustrations has demonstrated how a systematic, person-centred approach may be used to problem solve in care planning. The Nursing and Midwifery Council Code of Professional Conduct (Nursing and Midwifery Council, 2004) has been used as a central thread running throughout the chapter. This is because of the significant influence that this code has on all intellectual disability nurses' professional conduct, regardless of the nature of their employment.

As highlighted in this chapter, the creativity, versatility and adaptability of the pioneering intellectual disability nurse has led this unique practitioner to be at the cutting edge of contemporary intellectual disability practice (Gates, 2002). It is impossible to include the many legal and ethical dilemmas facing intellectual disability nursing today. It is hoped, however, that this chapter has offered guidance and a range of different approaches and frameworks to stimulate further thinking. These should equip intellectual disability nurses to steer their way through the uncharted waters facing them throughout their careers working to improve the quality of life for people with intellectual disabilities.

References

Alaszewski, A., Motherby, E., Gates, B., Ayer, S. and Manthorpe, J. (2001) *Diversity and Change: the Changing Roles and Education of Learning Disability Nurses*. London: English National Board.

Beauchamp, T.L. and Childress, J. (2001) *Principles of Biomedical Ethics*. New York: Oxford University Press.

Chaffee, J. (1994) *Thinking Critically*. Boston: Houghton Mifflin.

Curtin, L. and Flaherty M.J. (1982) *Nursing Ethics: Theories and Pragmatics*. Stamford: Appleton and Lange.

Department of Health (1971) *Better Services for the Mentally Handicapped*. London: Her Majesty's Stationery Office.

Department of Health (1983) *The Mental Health Act*. London: Department of Health.

Department of Health (1995) *The Disability Discrimination Act*. London: Department of Health.

Department of Health (1998) *The Human Rights Act*. London: Department of Health.

Department of Health (2001a) *Valuing People*. London: Department of Health.

Department of Health (2001b) *Seeking Consent: Working with People with Learning Disabilities*. London: Department of Health.

Department of Health (2003) *Agenda for Change: A New System of Pay for the NHS*. London: Department of Health.

Gates, B. (2002) The new learning disability nursing: agents of inclusion for the 21st century. Guest Editorial. *Learning Disability Bulletin*. British Institute of Learning Disability.

Glaser, E. (1941) *An Experiment in the Development of Critical Thinking*. Columbia University, New York: Bureau of Publications.

Gordon, M. (1995) *Nursing Diagnosis: Process and Application*. St Louis: Mosby.

HM Government (2005) *Draft Mental Capacity Bill*. London: Stationery Office.

International Council of Nurses (2000) *The ICN Code of Ethics for Nurses*. Geneva: International Council of Nurses.

Jay, P. (1979) *The Report of the Committee of Enquiry into Mental Handicap Nursing and Care*. London: Her Majesty's Stationery Office.

Kataoka-Yahiro, M. and Saylor, C. (1994) A critical thinking model for nursing judgment. *Journal of Nursing Education* **33**, 351–6.

Mencap (2004) *Treat Me Right*. London: Mencap.

Millar, M., Babcock, D.E. (1996) *Critical Thinking Applied to Nursing*. St Louis: Mosby.

Miller, M.A. and Malcolm, N.S. (1990) Critical thinking in the nursing curriculum. *Nursing and Health Care* **11**, 67–73.

National Patient Safety Agency (2004) *Understanding the Patient Safety Issues for People with Learning Disabilities*. London: National Patient Safety Agency.

Nursing and Midwifery Council (2004) *The NMC Code of Professional Conduct: Standards for Conduct, Performance and Ethics.* London: Nursing and Midwifery Council.

Paul, R.W. (1993) *Critical Thinking: How to Prepare Students for a Rapidly Changing World.* Foundation for Critical Thinking.

Potter, P. and Perry, A. (2003) *Nursing Essentials for Practice,* 5th edn. St Louis: Mosby.

Sines, D. ed. (1995) *Community Health Care Nursing.* London: Blackwell Publishing.

Turnbull, J. ed. (2004) *Learning Disability Nursing.* London: Blackwell Publishing.

United Kingdom Central Council for Nursing Midwifery and Health Visiting (1998) *Guidelines for Mental Health and Learning Disabilities Nursing.* London: UKCC.

Further reading and resources

Department of Health (2001) *Towards Person-centred Approaches; Planning with People, Guidance for Implementation Groups.* London: Department of Health.

Department of Health (2002) *Liberating the Talents.* London: Department of Health.

Fry, S. and Johnstone, M. (2002) *Ethics in Nursing Practice. A Guide to Ethical Decision Making,* 2nd edn. Oxford: Blackwell Publishing.

Rolph, S. (1998) Ethical dilemmas in historical research with people with learning difficulties. *British Journal of Learning Disability* **26**, 135–9.

UK Clinical Ethics Network: www.ethics-network.org.uk

Chapter 6

Risk and care planning and delivery in intellectual disability nursing

Phil Boulter and Alison Pointu

Introduction

In these changing times of service delivery for people with intellectual disabilities, there is a clear emphasis on improving safety and quality of care. These have become two of the key requirements for all services providing care and support to people with intellectual disabilities. It is generally accepted that safety and quality go hand in hand.

Keeping people safe is paramount; it is vital that people with intellectual disabilities are supported to remain safe. People with intellectual disability are leading more independent lives than they have done in the past, and this means that they may be exposed to risks of day-to-day living. It is the duty of all those working with people with intellectual disability to ensure that safety is maintained; however, this does not mean eliminating risk from their lives but ensuring that there is an absence of unacceptable risks, by applying a risk management process. Everyone of us take risks each day of our lives, and although risk has a general negative connotation there is a positive view of risk; this can be demonstrated through successful risk takers, whether in exploration, business or mountaineering (Giddens, 1998).

Risk management is a wide and complex area of practice. It is a process that is ongoing, requires time and commitment and requires those planning care to ensure that the individual remains central to the plan, which should be reviewed regularly. Adoption of risk management principles should be supportive rather than a hindrance to the provision of good quality care, and signify value and opportunity, rather than control and a means of preventing harm (Tindall, 1997).

This chapter will identify ways in which nurses can support people with intellectual disabilities to live a full life whereby risk issues are recognised and managed. It will also look at issues relating to risk and risk management and, for this purpose, the authors focus on a number of key principles. Firstly the chapter reflects on the historical perspective of intellectual disability practice, then a variety of frameworks available to assess and plan for risk are discussed. A case study approach addresses some risks people with intellectual disability may encounter in their day-to-day life. Some ethical dilemmas and issues are raised, relating to individual accountability for nurses as part of the risk management process. There are also opportunities for the reader to reflect on their experiences within the chapter by completing a series of activities. The chapter will also challenge the reader to examine their practice and their organisation's approach to risk and risk management.

Key principles

The key principles for any risk management process must recognise that people with intellectual disabilities should not be restricted in their daily life because of perceived risks. Intellectual disability nurses have a responsibility to identify risks and work with others to ensure that these are planned risks that have the appropriate levels of support. People with intellectually disabilities have the same rights as anyone else; the right to experience life events and to participate fully in their community. Whilst it can be accepted that this may pose some risks to particular individuals, wrapping a person in cotton wool or being risk-averse is not an option.

A second key principle must be that person-centred approaches are an essential part of the risk management process, and risks should be discussed as part of the development of a person-centred plan. Person-centred planning is a process of planning with an individual that puts them at the centre and in control of their life. It is about supporting individuals to achieve their aspirations, shifting the power base from the professional to that of the individual (see Chapter 3). However, one cannot plan with a person and not discuss risks that may sit alongside the choices they wish to make about their lives. People with intellectual disabilities have a right to know about the risks that sit with the choices that they are making and should be supported to experience their choices safely.

The third principle recognises that all organisations have a responsibility to have procedures and guidance in place to support good risk management strategies. All nurses working within these organisations are equally accountable to ensure that they are aware of local policy guidance, and how this can support their clinical practice (see Chapter 5).

Risk

What is meant by risk? Risk has been defined in a number of ways. Alaszewski (1998) has stated that risk is the possibility that a given course of action will not achieve its desired and intended outcome but instead some undesired and undesirable situations will develop. Alberg et al. (1996) have provided a more rounded approach to the definition by describing risk as the possibility of beneficial and harmful consequences likely to occur. Risk is a much written about topic, and risk assessment is central to providing a safe and fulfilled life for people with intellectual disabilities; identification of risk will be central to the development of, for example, person-centred plans, the care programme approach and health action planning. Risk is an essential and unavoidable part of everyday life, and involves both compromise and negotiation (Titterton, 2005).

More people with intellectual disabilities are now exposed to everyday risks with the move from institution-based care to living more independently within a variety of settings, in the wider community. To understand this fully it is useful for the reader to understand the history of services for people with intellectual disabilities.

Historical background and risk

Over the past 25 years the way that people with intellectual disability receive care and support in the United Kingdom and Ireland has changed considerably. In England the White Paper, *Valuing People* (Department of Health, 2001a), has laid out four main principles in the strategy for the 21st Century; these are rights, choice, independence and inclusion. These principles are a long way from the vision held at the turn of the last century when people with intellectual disabilities were regarded by society as uneducable, and a social problem. At this time people with learning disabilities were kept in segregated settings, protecting both the society and the individual from harm. In a collection of views from the early 20th century, Bartlett and Wright (1999) have recollected how society was thought to need protecting from people who had definite criminal tendencies, or were ready to commit crimes on the instigation of others; these poor creatures, although relatively harmless, needed to be kept away to protect society from the burden caused by their non-productiveness. It is difficult to imagine that this was how society viewed people with an intellectual disability; however this demonstrates the thinking that was the foundation to institutional care in the United Kingdom. In this climate of segregated care, the theme of practice was the protection and control of a vulnerable population. People had very little independence, and neither opportunity nor choice was part of the vocabulary of the era. During the 1980s–1990s moving from controlled and restricted environments to care in the community was thought to be the key to ensuring that the principles of normalisation could be realised, and that people with learning disabilities would be given the same life opportunities as others (Wolfensberger, 1972). Initially very little thought was given to supporting people to achieve their aspirations whilst managing the risks that these new opportunities might encounter.

The culture of risk management is not isolated to services for the intellectually disabled, but can be viewed in all aspects of society. For example, within the NHS there are clear policy and procedures for the management of risk within the organisation. NHS organisations have clear responsibilities with regard to the management of risk by systematically assessing, reviewing and seeking ways to prevent its occurrence (Department of Health, 1999).

> **Box 6.1   Key definitions used within clinical governance concerning issues of risk**
>
> - Risk – the chance of something happening that will have an impact upon objectives; it is measured in terms of consequences and likelihood
> - Risk management – the culture, processes and structures that are directed towards the effective management of potential opportunities and adverse effects
> - Risk management process – the systematic application of management policies procedures, and practices to the tasks of establishing the context, identifying, analysing, evaluating, treating, monitoring and communicating risks
> - Risk identification – the process of determining what can happen, why and how
> - Risk analysis – a systematic use of available information to determine how often the specified events may occur and the magnitude of their consequences
> - Risk control – that part of risk management which involves the implementation of policies, standards, procedures and physical changes to eliminate or minimise adverse risks
> - Risk treatment – selection and implementation of appropriate options for dealing with risk
> - Risk evaluation – the process used to determine risk management priorities by comparing the level of risk against predetermined standards, target risk levels or other criteria

The advent of clinical governance brought with it a statutory duty for NHS trusts to ensure the level of services they deliver to people is satisfactory, consistent, responsive and safe. Clinical governance provides an opportunity for staff to take the lead in delivering safe care. Organisations have to meet statutory requirements in relation to providing safe care and treatment for service users and there are several external influences which impact on risk management.

In order to meet these requirements, organisations follow standards and guidance issued by the Department of Health and other agencies, for example the Health and Safety Executive, National Institute for Clinical Excellence (NICE), NHS Litigation Authority, Commission for Social Care Inspection (CSCI), the Healthcare Commission and the National Patient Safety Agency (NPSA). The Healthcare Commission is charged with assessing all organisations (public and private) in meeting the standards for better health (Department of Health, 2004). Within these standards there are core standards that must be met and these include safety and risk issues.

Risk management can be viewed as a complex process that covers a wide range of issues, as can be seen in Box 6.1.

Because of the complexity of this area of practice there have been several books published that are dedicated solely to the thinking of and management of risk within organisations. With this in mind and supporting the need to transfer academic learning to practice, the reader should undertake Reader activity 6.1.

Reader activity 6.1

Over the next few days endeavour to answer the following:

  (1) Who is your local risk manager?
  (2) Identify and read the risk policy/strategy for your organisation.
  (3) Is there a separate policy for people with intellectual disability?
  (4) How are quality and risk monitored, and which are the external bodies that influence this?
  (5) What is assessed within the standards for better health (Department of Health, 2004) and how are these being addressed within your organisation?
  (6) How are adverse events or incidents managed and supported in your organisation?
  (7) How would you report safety/risk issues?
  (8) How would you bring identified risk/safety issues to the organisation?
  (9) How are lessons learnt from incidents and accidents shared across your organisation?
 (10) Undertake a literature search on risks relating to people with intellectually disabilities, and find out if these issues are being addressed by your organisation.
 (11) Read about the functions of the NPSA Health and Safety Executive, NICE, Healthcare Commission and CSCI, NHS Litigation Authority.

Risk and people with intellectual disabilities

There are many risks that relate to everyday living; as this chapter has particular relevance to nurses and other health professionals who support people with intellectual disabilities, however, there is a deliberate emphasis on the risks that relate to an individual's health and well-being. Appropriate healthcare leads to better quality of life for individuals, and, to be effective in obtaining this healthcare, individuals must have the ability to express their health concerns and problems. People with intellectual disabilities are at a distinct disadvantage: they often do not have the communication skills that allow them to articulate their health needs, and healthcare professionals usually do not have the skills to obtain the necessary information to enable diagnoses. Mencap (2004) highlighted in their report that many of the poor experiences happened because of lack of training skills amongst healthcare staff.

As a group, individuals with intellectual disabilities have a greater variety of healthcare needs compared with individuals of the same age and sex in the general population. Research has found high rates of previously unrecognised or poorly managed co-morbidity amongst individuals with intellectual disabilities (Cohen, 2001; NHS, Scotland, 2004). Individuals with intellectual disabilities are more likely to have physical disabilities, hearing impairments,

Box 6.2   The five key areas of risk in intellectual disabilities reported by the National Patient Safety Agency (2004)

Swallowing difficulties (dysphagia)
Swallowing difficulties are common in people with learning disabilities, if not managed safely they can lead to respiratory tract infection, a leading cause of early death.

Lack of accessible information
People are unable to understand the information they are given about their illness, treatment and interventions leading to varying degrees of harm to their health.

Inappropriate use of physical interventions
Inaapropriate use of physical restraint can result in injuries and harm to the individual.

Illness or disease being mis- or undiagnosed
Access to treatment is delayed because symptoms are not diagnosed early enough, leading to undetected serious health conditions and avoidable death.

Vulnerability of people with learning disabilities in general hospital
People with learning disabilities are more at risk of things going wrong, and this can lead to various degrees of avoidable harm.

vision impairments, neurological disorders (25–50% of people with an intellectual disability have primarily epilepsy), mental health problems (up to 40% of people with a learning disability may have a mental health problem) and/or communication disorders (Prasher and Janicki, 2002). These co-existing disabilities combined with the limitations in intellectual functioning and in adaptive behaviours, make people with intellectual disabilities particularly vulnerable to health disparities, and at a greater risk of being in poor health with increased mortality (Hollins et al., 1998; Shavelle and Strauss, 1999; Patja et al., 2000).

Research also indicates that people with intellectual disabilities are exposed to a number of risks that relate to lifestyle choices. For example, Robertson et al. (2000) studied a group of 500 people living in a variety of accommodation options in the community, and found high levels of obesity, poor nutrition/diet and low rates of physical activity that were much higher than those of the general population.

The National Patient Safety Agency (NPSA) compiled a report understanding the patient safety issues for people with a learning disability (National Patient Safety Agency, 2004). The report highlighted five patient safety priorities as identified by people with intellectual disabilities (Box 6.2). The NPSA is looking in more detail at each priority area to develop solutions that address the issues identified.

We all have a part to play in this by ensuring these issues are addressed within the organisation's risk management arrangements and risk planning for individuals. It is also important that we share our local issues and practice developments with the NPSA so that we can reduce the risks for people with intellectual disabilities.

Nursing assessment and care planning

A nursing care plan is best thought of as a written reflection of the nursing process: What does the assessment show? What should be done? How, when and where should these planned interventions be carried out? What is the desired outcome? This process includes identifying existing needs, as well as recognising potential needs and risks (Gulanick et al., 2003).

The ability to assess is a key nursing skill that enables practitioners to gather relevant information about clients for the individualised planning, delivery and evaluation of care (McGee and Castledine, 2003). All the information that the nurse gathers regarding a particular client contributes to the assessment. This is done through talking to the client, talking to people who know them well, listening to the client, listening to people who know them well, and through observation. The intellectual disability nurse requires expert communication skills during this process, and should be summarising and recapping to clarify their understanding, ensuring that the assessment retains a client-centred approach.

The assessment provides a picture that enables initial decisions to be made. Without a comprehensive nursing assessment it would be haphazard as to whether one would be doing the right thing. Once this data is compiled one begins to build a holistic picture of the problem, risk or need. During this process specific areas of risk can be identified. This is when the nurse may seek particular tools, such as that used for epilepsy (O'Brien and Loughran, 2004) or sex offenders (Ferguson, 1999); these tools are available to help intellectual disability nurses through this process. However, the uniqueness of the individual and attention to the person's views can only be achieved through the adoption of a person-centred approach (Spross et al., 2000).

The findings from the nursing assessment will inform the person-centred planning and health action planning process. It is essential that risk issues are identified and addressed in a way that supports the individual to achieve their hopes and aspirations.

Registered nurses have a duty of care for their clients, the Nursing and Midwifery Council Code of Professional Conduct (Nursing and Midwifery Council, 2004) has stated that nurses are personally accountable for their practice, and that in caring for patients and clients they must act to identify and minimise risk to them. Section 1.4 of the Code states that nurses have a duty of care to patients and clients who are entitled to receive safe and competent care. Whenever care for people with intellectual disabilities is being planned, it must be person centred and nurses must also identify risk issues.

Principles of person-centred risk assessment

Good risk management is both a need and a necessity for services and for people with intellectual disabilities. Adoption of risk management principles should be supportive, rather than a hindrance to, the provision of good quality services. They should signify value rather than control, and they should not be seen as a way of protecting organisations from litigation (Saunders, 1999).

Intellectual disabilities services work with a diverse and often vulnerable group of people. Completion of risk assessments can assist with the identification of risk towards individuals and others. The ethos of risk management should be to minimise the risk for the individual, and should be instrumental in balancing safety with quality of life. Risk assessment and management are complex, dynamic and culturally defined (Douglas, 1992) and should be viewed as a process that requires time and commitment and places the individual at the centre of the process. Therefore it is essential that person-centred planning should be used as the means to identify risks and agree ways of supporting individuals to experience their choices safely.

Risk management is not in lieu of competent practice; the notice that 'if I do a risk assessment I will be alright' is not a sufficiently sophisticated model. Risk management has to be seen as an integral part of everyday practice in order to support individuals to lead as full and independent lives as possible.

To commence a process of assessing risk there must be a willingness to take appropriate risks, talk honestly about risk, be person centred in approach and to ensure that all risks are acknowledged. The individual needs to be involved as fully as possible and throughout the process there needs to be a collaborative approach to all communication that includes information from professionals, service user and relatives (Langan, 2004). When considering these issues we need to take into account the individual's vulnerability, physical health and risk of self-harm. Additionally there are other issues that may arise in relation to over-protection or paternalism.

A person-centred approach to risk assessment is key to ensuring that issues of risk to individuals which are relevant to:

- People with intellectual disabilities making their own decisions and choices
- The rights of people with intellectual disabilities to experience opportunities
- Being supported by others to do the things people with intellectual disabilities want

The risks need to be well thought out and considered from the perspective of a personal balance between 'what seems to be right' to an individual, as opposed to 'what is right' as determined by someone else; this dilemma is shown diagrammatically in Fig. 6.1.

The values that underpin a person-centred approach to risk assessment are that:

- Everyone should be supported to experience opportunities in a supportive environment

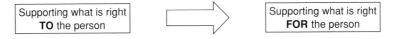

Fig. 6.1 Risk as a balance between different perspectives.

- Risk issues for people with intellectual disabilities will be considered in a person-centred and individual way
- Issues of risk for individuals will be reviewed in order to support and empower people with intellectual disabilities and not to over-protect and limit opportunities for people
- The organisation fully supports those who have been involved in supporting people to review and agree risks with individuals

The process of thinking through risks or dilemmas is a complex procedure, and the intellectual disabilities nurse is required to have the ability to understand the information provided, be clear about what the choices are, and be able to decide if the individual is able to make an informed choice/decision about whether this is something that they should or should not do. For some individuals with intellectual disability this process will be difficult and they may be unable to make an informed choice. Individuals will need to be supported by people and professionals who know them well, to ensure that they are kept central to this process.

To ensure that a person-centred approach is adopted for risk assessment the intellectual disabilities nurse will need to work through a number of steps of risk with the person in order to clarify risk issue and to plan, record and communicate what has been agreed with the person (Box 6.3).

Box 6.3   Steps for risk assessment and planning

STEP 1: Who should be involved?
- The person
- Family/friends/carers
- Those who support the person at home/other environments, now or in the future
- People who legally may need to be involved
- People who have contributed to the individual's person-centred plan

STEP 2: What is the issue that is causing the concern?

- Share and explore thoroughly what the issue is. Is it a risk or is it a general support issue?
- Be clear in the language used to enable understanding of the risk
- Clarify what the risk is and what the hazards are
- Always be respectful in discussing and recording the issue
- Identify behaviours or actions that present as a danger or potential risk to the individual

STEP 3: Find out when, where and how often the risks occur

- Don't progress further until everyone understands and agrees what the issue and associated risks are
- Plot any patterns to the risk
- Does it happen at a particular time, place or with certain people?
- Are there any regular things which happen before or after the risk?

- How often has the issue happened in the past?
- How recent was the risk experience?
- What impact does it have on the person or other people?

STEP 4: What are the consequences of the risk?

- Who is at risk: self, children, parents, support staff?
- What impact does it have on other people?
- What impact does it have on other people the person meets: general public, neighbours, family?
- What impact does it have on the people who support the person?
- How often does the behaviour occur?
- Has anyone been hurt or injured?
- Has there ever been any damage to property?
- Are there any warning signs? Consider any actions of changes that manage the risk.

STEP 5: If the issue does not happen for the person, what will the person lose out on?

- What opportunity will be lost?
- What will not happen for the person that is in their person-centred plan?
- Does the person want to carry on or start to do the issue discussed?
- What restrictions will it impose on the individual?
- Can anything in the environment be changed?

STEP 6: How can the person or others be supported more safely to do the issue discussed?

- Can the support of staff be adapted?
- Is there any training which can be introduced?
- Is there anything else we need to find out to make it safer?
- Be creative in looking at different ways to support the risk
- Can the environment, place or time be changed?

STEP 7: What do we document about the risk?

- The decision made about the issue and support
- Use clear and concise language
- Only use respectful ways to describe the person and the risk
- Record all the things which need to be done and which have been agreed to make the risk safe/safer
- What has been agreed to be introduced?
- Record all known interventions known to reduce risk plans assessments

STEP 8: Who do we communicate the risk to?

- The person
- Those responsible for supporting the person
- Those who may need to know about the risk in order to keep the person or others safe
- Not everyone who was involved in looking at the risk needs to have a copy, only if they are involved in supporting the person

---

Case illustration 6.1

John is a young man with mild intellectual disabilities; he lives independently in his own flat. John attends the local college 3 days a week, and the rest of the week he participates in a variety of community leisure pursuits. John receives outreach support for 3 hours a day; this is to help him with his general household chores and budgeting. John's parents live a couple of miles away, and John visits them at the weekends. John has a girlfriend, Chloe, who he has been seeing for some time. John has diabetes, and he manages this with support from the community intellectual disabilities nurse, who works closely with the diabetic specialist.

John and Chloe have been discussing going on a holiday to Spain together; they have never been away on their own before. Both have been on holidays, but always with their families. John's family is very concerned about the holiday that John is planning; they contact the outreach worker to say that they want him to put them off this dangerous idea, as he has diabetes and will not be able to manage. The outreach worker contacts the community nurse as he feels that he is in an awkward position, and wants to support John but feels that his knowledge about diabetes is limited. By using a person-centred approach to risk the intellectual disability nurse is able to see how John and his circle of support were able to agree a plan of action as seen in Fig. 6.2.

Arguably the case illustration of John demonstrates that there are several factors that need to be followed in managing and supporting people with intellectual disabilities. The wishes of the individual are paramount in any discussion on risk; however, involving their network of support is also crucial to the plan's success. The risk action plan must respect the rights of individuals with intellectual disabilities as citizens. Actions agreed at the meeting should be written as simply as possible in a way that is accessible to the person with an intellectual disability.

Risk plans should not create inflexible or bureaucratic duties or tasks, but should be integrated with person-centred planning, to ensure people with intellectual disabilities are continually listened to and others learn from what they say (Department of Health, 2001a).

Risk assessment and adult protection policy

It is important to tackle the issues of adult protection whilst thinking about risk assessment and care planning, as people with intellectual disability may be more vulnerable, and therefore at a greater risk of abuse compared to other groups. The Green Paper, *Independence, Wellbeing and Choice* (Department of Health, 2005), sets out a vision where adults have a greater control of their lives, and states that this will be achieved through balancing the protection of individuals and enabling people to manage their own risks. However, the need will continue for a framework for protection that ensures that people are free from harm,

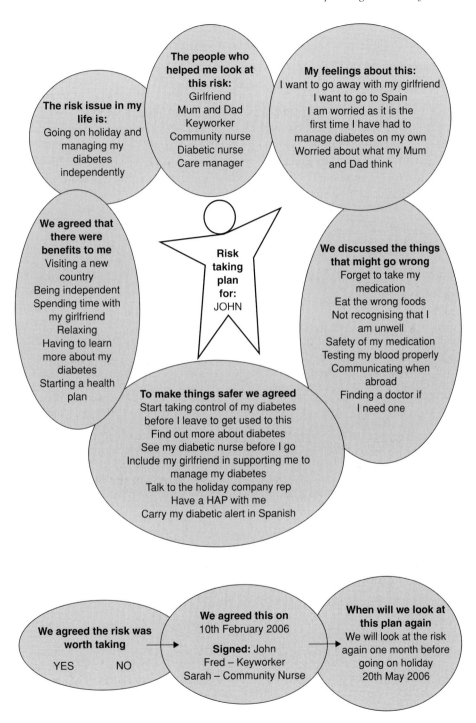

Fig. 6.2 Risk-taking plan for John.

exploitation and mistreatment. Nurses can only protect people from abuse if they have an awareness of why protection is important. Abuse can be defined as:

> 'a violation of individual human and civil rights by another person or persons.' (Department of Health, 2000)

The guidance papers, *No Secrets* (Department of Health, 2000) in England, and *In Safer Hands* (National Assembly for Wales, 2000) in Wales, offer guidance around the protection of vulnerable groups from abuse, and the detection and management of investigations. These papers categorise vulnerable adults into groupings, with intellectual disability being one. Some individuals may find themselves belonging to more than one grouping of vulnerable adults, for example the older person with intellectual disability; whether this produces increased risk of abuse is uncertain due to the limited research carried out (Jenkins, 2000). Scotland is in the process of developing proposals for improved protection for vulnerable adults; the Scottish Executive Health Department (2005) has completed a third consultation of the proposals, *Protecting Vulnerable Adults? Securing their Safety.*

The Nursing and Midwifery Council (2002) has strongly emphasised that there should be zero tolerance to abuse, and they provide clear guidance for all registered nurses. Intellectual disability nurses are in a unique position to detect and respond to abuse (Davies and Jenkins, 2004). They also have a responsibility to work with and provide information to individuals that enable them to protect themselves from abuse. By educating clients and their family/carers to ask pertinent questions, this power could effectively be transferred to clients enabling individuals and carers to feel empowered (Chadwick and Tadd, 1992). If abuse is reported to a nurse during a risk assessment process it is essential that the local adult protection policy and guidance is adhered to. To clarify local policy and practice the reader is asked to respond to questions posed in Reader activity 6.2.

Reader activity 6.2

(1) Identify who the adult protection lead is within your organisation/area.
(2) How is the adult protection policy communicated within your organisation?
(3) Identify where the adult protection guidance is located.
(4) Find out how you would report an adult protection issue.
(5) Find out if people with intellectual disabilities in your area know who to talk to, if they are victims of abuse.
(6) Think about some of the things you might observe or recognise as possible alerts to abuse.
(7) Identify the stages in alerting others of the possibility of potential abuse.

An example of a flow diagram (Barnet Multi-agency Committee, 2003) for reporting potential abuse is included at the end of this chapter (see Appendix 6.1).

Professional, ethical and legal dilemmas: balancing risk and protection

As has previously been identified in Chapter 5, nurses working with people with an intellectual disability are bound by their Code of Professional Conduct (Nursing and Midwifery Council, 2004). This code is not law, but as a registered nurse this code provides guidance on what is considered best practice (Burnard and Chapman, 1993). The code states that nurses should,

> 'act always to the best of their professional ability to safeguard their clients, and do nothing by error of commission or omission which might expose clients to harm.'

It could be argued that this code presents an ethical challenge to the nursing profession, as how can nurses encourage clients to develop skills and try new opportunities, if they involve a degree of risk? Does the code imply that nurses are then responsible if something goes wrong? Will nurses find themselves at a disciplinary hearing having to justify their actions on the basis of their professional code? When examining the legal perspective, the law states that those who take on the duty of care have a responsibility to protect their clients/patients from harm, and could be accused of negligence (Sellars, 2002). It is to be expected that the duty of care nurses display will be of a higher standard than that of those working as social care staff.

The power of the law and the professional code cannot be ignored. However, it is equally unacceptable for nurses actively to deny people with learning disabilities the opportunities to fulfil their aspirations and dreams just in case there is a repercussion on them. However, risks are inevitable if nurses are to provide people with learning disabilities the self determination the majority of the population enjoys. Self determination and opportunities are essential to personal development and are a basic human right (Baldwin and Thirkettle, 1999). Therefore, although there is potential conflict between professional conduct and law, with the promotion of choice for individual clients in practice, the answer to this dilemma lies in the whole process of assessment, care planning and evaluation of risks.

All stages of the risk process have to be clearly communicated, documented and justifiable to all concerned and to the profession at large. Although the law is frequently unclear about risk taking in the clinical environment, there is an expectation that the professionals are able to show the courts that the course of action they have taken is 'reasonable', and that other professionals in similar roles would regard the action in question acceptable. Adults with intellectual disabilities may lack the capacity to understand fully some decisions that need to be made in everyday life, yet in England and Wales no-one else is able to legally provide consent on their behalf (Department of Health, 2001b). This can result in ethical dilemmas for the nurse when supporting choices that present significant risks of harm to themselves or others. Hooren et al. (2002) have described how individuals with Prader-Willi syndrome may choose to ignore dietary advice, despite clearly defined medical risks of chronic obesity.

There could be a danger of nurses taking an approach to risk that promotes risk elimination in people's lives rather that risk management (Moore, 2004). It is perhaps worth remembering that there will always be errors in risk prediction and this in itself is a challenge to the nurse, and it is important that organisations promote a culture where there is a degree of tolerance for the inevitable error that will occur (Lindsay and Beail, 2004). A person's right to have control over their life is central to ethical thinking within nursing practice (Cox, 2002); ultimately the law is clear that adults with learning disability who have the capacity to consent, can and do make decisions, and these may not always fit with what others think is safe or right.

There is often an expectation that the nurse will be able to use their clinical judgement to predict risk. This has particular relevance to the intellectual disabilities nurse, as research has demonstrated that clinical judgement is extremely poor when applied to risk prediction (Borum, 1996; Quincey et al., 1998; Elbogen, 2002). However, nurses should not be too despondent: clinical judgement has been shown to improve significantly when there is an agreement about risk between different professionals (McNiel et al., 2000). The intellectual disability nurse is predominantly working in partnership with the individual, family members and other professionals, and working together should produce a more reliable assessment of risk.

Winchcombe (2001) has stated that practitioners need to help people identify what they need to manage their lives safely and independently, and this may involve considering risk. If this is something that nurses find difficult to take on perhaps we should ask ourselves whether we are, in fact, denying people the right to take responsibility and control in this aspect of their lives.

Conclusion

This chapter has provided an overview of a variety of processes that can be used to identify and plan for the management of risk for people with intellectual disabilities. The chapter also explored how the risk assessment process sits alongside other statutory procedures, such as adult protection and the care programme approach. Risk has been reviewed from a number of positions: that of the organisation, the professional and the individual with a learning disability. However, whichever viewpoint the intellectual disability nurse finds themselves in, there are clear accountability issues and responsibilities for them.

Intellectual disability nurses can recount stories from the press where mistakes have had a dire consequence due to poor communication, risk assessment and

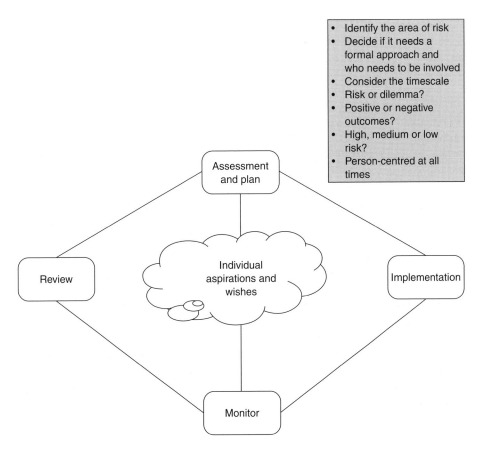

Fig. 6.3 The person-centred risk assessment process.

care planning. If good risk management skills are not applied in practice, there will be human cost. A challenge for all intellectual disability nurses is to ensure that they make all necessary information available in a format that individuals with intellectual disabilities can access and understand. People with intellectual disabilities need to be listened to as highlighted in the National Patient Safety Agency (2004) document, which clearly raises key concerns in relation to managing health risks.

It can not be overemphasised that successful risk management is central to person-centred planning, as it provides opportunities for people with intellectual disability, and enables them to take risks which are carefully planned and assessed in order for them to achieve their aspirations and lead valued lives (Fig. 6.3).

Appendix 6.1
Adult protection procedure for alerters of potential abuse (Barnet Multi-agency Committee, 2003)

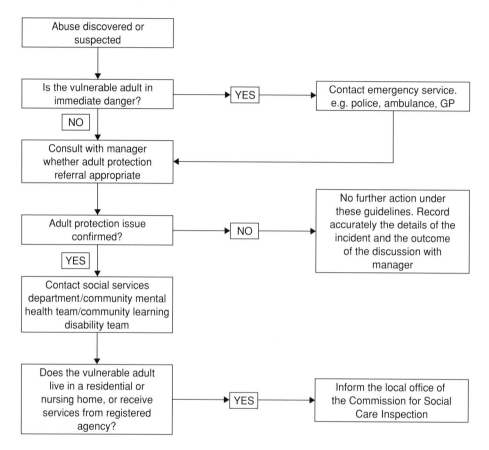

References

Alaszewski, A. (1998) The dangers of risk: professional practice and organisational policies. In: *Best Value, Risk and Regulation* (Allen, I., ed.). London: Policy Studies Institute.

Alberg, C., Bingley, W., Bowers, L., Ferguson, G., Hatfield, B., Hoban, A. and Maden, A. (1996) *Learning Materials on Mental Health Risk Assessment.* University of Manchester: Department of Health.

Baldwin, S. and Thirkettle, B. (1999) Care in the community for people with a learning disability: choice, opportunity and risk. *Mental Health Care* **21** (5), 167–9.

Barnet Multi-agency Committee (2003) *Barnet Multi-agency Adult Protection Guidance.* Barnet: Barnet Council.

Bartlett, P. and Wright, D. (ed.) (1999) *Outside the Walls of the Asylum. The History of Care in the Community 1750–2000.* Athlone Press: London.

Borum, R. (1996) Improving the clinical practice of violent risk assessment. *American Psychologist* **51**, 945–56.

Burnard, P. and Chapman, C.M. (1993) *Professional and Ethical Issues in Nursing,* 2nd edn. Middlesex: Scutari Press.

Chadwick, R. and Tadd, W. (1992) *Ethics and Nursing Practice: A Case Study Approach.* Basingstoke: Macmillan.

Cohen, J. (2001) Countries' health performance. *The Lancet* **358**, 929.

Cox, C. (2002) *Enhancing the Practice Experience.* Chichester: Nursing Praxis International.

Davies, R. and Jenkins, R. (2004) Protecting people with learning disabilities from abuse: a key role for learning disabilities nurses. *The Journal of Adult Protection* **6** (2), 31–41.

Department of Health (1999) HSC 1999/065: *Clinical Governance in the New NHS.* London: Her Majesty's Stationery Office.

Department of Health (2000) *No Secrets: Guidance on Developing And Implementing Multi-agency Policies and Procedures to Protect the Vulnerable Adult from Abuse.* London: The Stationery Office.

Department of Health (2001a) *Valuing People: A Strategy for the New Century for People with Learning Disabilities.* London: The Stationery Office.

Department of Health (2001b) *Seeking Consent: Working with People with Learning Disabilities.* London: The Stationery Office.

Department of Health (2004) *Standards for Better Health.* London: Department of Health.

Department of Health (2005) *Independence, Wellbeing and Choice.* Department of Health: London.

Douglas (1992) *Risk and Balance: Essays in Cultural Theory.* London: Routledge.

Elbogen, E.B. (2002) The process of violence risk assessment: a review of descriptive research. *Aggression and Violent Behaviour* **7**, 591–604.

Ferguson, D. (1999) Eco-maps: facilitating insight in learning disabilities sex offenders. *British Journal of Nursing* **8** (18), 1224–9.

Fox, G. (1998) Risk assessment: a systematic approach to violence. *Nursing Standard* **12** (32), 44–7.

Giddens, A. (1998) Risk society: the context of British politics. In: *Risk and Risk Taking in Health and Social Welfare* (Titterton, M., ed.). London: Jessica Kingsley.

Gulanick, M., Myers, J.L., Klopp, A., Galanes, S., Gradishar, D. and Puzas, M.K. (2003) *Nursing Care Plans,* 5th edn. St Louis: Mosby.

Hollins, S., Attard, M.T., von Fraunhofer, N., McGuigan, S. and Sedgwick, P. (1998) Mortality in people with learning disabilities: risks, causes and death certification findings in London. *Developmental Medicine and Child Neurology,* **40**, 50–6.

Hooren, R., Widdershoven, H., Van den Borne, H. and Curfs, L. (2002) Autonomy and intellectual disability: the case of prevention of obesity in Prader-Willi syndrome. *Journal of Intellectual Disability Research* **46** (7), 560–8.

Jenkins, R. (2000) The needs of older people with learning disabilities. *British Journal of Nursing* **9** (19), 2080–9.

Langan, J. (2004) *Living with Risk: Mental Health Service User Involvement in Risk Assessment and Management.* London: Policy Press.

Lindsay, W.R. and Beail, N. (2004) Risk assessment: actuarial prediction and clinical judgement of offending incidents and behaviour for intellectual disability services. *Journal of Applied Research in Intellectual Disability* **17**, 229–34.

McGee, P. and Castledine, G. (2003) *Advanced Nursing Practice,* 2nd edn. Oxford: Blackwell Publishing.

McNiel, D.E., Lamb, J.N. and Binder, R.L. (2000) Relevance of inter-rater agreement to violence risk assessment. *Journal of Consultancy in Clinical Psychology* **68**, 1111–5.

Mencap (2004) *Treat Me Right*. London: Mencap.

Moore, D. (2004) Shall we dance? *Learning Disabilities Practice* **7** (9), 39.

National Assembly for Wales (2000) *In Safer Hands: Protection of Vulnerable Adults in Wales*. Cardiff: Social Services Inspectorate for Wales.

National Health Service Executive (1999) HSC 123: *Governance in the New NHS: Controls Assurance Statements 1999/2000. Risk Management and Organisational Controls*. London: National Health Service Executive.

National Health Service Scotland (2004) *Health Needs Assessment*. Edinburgh: NHS Scotland.

National Health Service Scotland (2005) *Third Consultation Paper on the Protection of Vulnerable Adults and Related Matters. Protecting Vulnerable Adults. Securing Their Safety*. Edinburgh: NHS Scotland.

National Patient Safety Agency (2004) *Understanding the Patient Safety Issues for People with Learning Disabilities*. London: National Patient Safety Agency.

Nursing Midwifery Council (2002) *Practitioner–Client Relationship and the Prevention of Abuse*. London: Nursing and Midwifery Council.

Nursing and Midwifery Council (2004) *Code of Professional Conduct*. London: Nursing and Midwifery Council.

O'Brien, D. and Loughran, S. (2004) Risk, assessment and epilepsy. *Learning Disability Practice* **7** (3), 12–17.

Patja, K., Ivanainen, M., Vesala, H., Oksanen, H. and Ruoppila, I. (2000) Life expectancy of people with intellectual disability: a 35-year follow up study. *Journal of Intellectual Disability Research* **44**, 591–9.

Prasher, V.P. and Janicki, M.P. (2002) *Physical Health of Adults with Intellectual Disabilities*. Oxford: Blackwell Publishing.

Quincey V.L., Harris, G.T., Rice, M.E. and Cromier, C.A. (1998) *Violent Offenders: Appraising and Managing Risk*. Washington D.C.: American Psychological Association.

Robertson, J., Emerson, E., Gregory, N., Hatton, C., Turner, S., Kessissoglou, S. and Hallam, A. (2000) Lifestyle related risk factors for poor health in residential settings for people with intellectual disabilities. *Research in Developmental Disabilities* **21**, 469–86.

Saunders, M. (1999) *Managing Risk in Service for People with Learning Disabilities*. York: Association of Practitioners in Learning Disability (APLD).

Scottish Executive Health Department (2005) The Scottish Health Department. Scotland. www.scotland.gov.uk/Resource/Doc/55971/0015247.pdf

Sellars, C. (2002) *Risk Assessment in People with Learning Disabilities*. Oxford: Blackwell Publishing.

Shavelle, R. and Strauss, D. (1999) Mortality of persons with development disabilities after transfer into community care: a 1996 update. *American Journal on Mental Retardation* **104**, 143–7.

Spross, J., Clarke, E. and Beauregard, J. (2000) Expert coaching and guidance. In: *Advanced Nursing Practice: an Integrative Approach* (Hanric, A., Spross, J. and Hanson, C., eds.). Philadelphia: W.B. Saunders.

Tindall, B. (1997) People with learning difficulties: citizenship, personal development and management of risk. In: *Good Practice in Risk Assessment and Risk Management* (Kemshall, H. and Pritchard, J., eds.). London: Jessica Kingsley.

Titterton, M. (2005) *Risk and Risk Taking in Health and Social Welfare*. London: Jessica Kingsley.

Winchcombe, M. (2001) Rights and responsibilities: can we take the risk? *British Journal of Therapy and Rehabilitation* **8** (4), 125.

Wolfensberger, W. (1972) *The Principles of Normalisation in Human Services*. Toronto: National Institute of Mental Retardation.

Further reading and resources

Books

Bongar, B., Berman, A., Maris, R., Silverman, M., Harris, E. and Packman, W. (1998) *Risk Management with Suicidal Patients*. London: Guilford Press.

Haynes, K. and Thomas, M. (2005) *Clinical Risk Management in Primary Care*. Abingdon: Radcliffe.

Home Farm Trust. *Keeping Safe. Developing Skills for People with Learning Disabilities to Minimise Risk of Abuse*. Brighton: Pavilion Publishers.

Jukes, M. and Bollard, M. (2003) *Contemporary Learning Disability Practice*. Bath: Bath Press.

James, A., Worrall, A. and Kendall, T. (2005) *Clinical Governance in Mental Health and Learning Disability Services*. Trowbridge: Cromwell Press Ltd.

Lehr, D. and Brown, F. (1996) *People with Disabilities who Challenge the System*. Maryland: Paul H. Brookes Publishing Company.

Mayatt, V.L. (2004) *Tolley's Managing Risk in Healthcare. Law and Practice*. London: Lexis Nexis Tolley.

Powell, S. (2001) *Risk in Challenging Behaviour: A Good Practice Guide*. London: BILD.

Simmons, K. (2000) *Getting in Trouble: Life on the Edge*. London: Pavilion/Rowntree Foundation.

Sobsey, D. (1994) *Violence and Abuse in the Lives of People with Disabilities. The End of Silent Acceptance?* Maryland: Paul H. Brookes Publishing Company.

Turner, S. (1998) *The Assessment of Risk and Dangerousness as Applied to People with Learning Disabilities Considered at Risk of Offending. Part 1. Literature Review*. Manchester: Hester Adrian Research Centre, University of Manchester.

Turner, S. (1998) *The Assessment of Risk and Dangerousness as Applied to People with Learning Disabilities Considered at Risk of Offending. Part 2. Developing Good Practice*. Manchester: Hester Adrian Research Centre, University of Manchester.

Journals

British Journal of Learning Disabilities. Oxford: Blackwell Publishing.

Journal of Adult Protection. Brighton: Pavilion.

Tizard Learning Disability Review. Tizard, University of Kent: Pavilion.

Journal of Intellectual Disabilities. London: Sage.

Journal of Intellectual Disability Research. Oxford: Blackwell Publishing.

Journal of Intellectual and Development Disability. Australia: Australasian Society for the Study of Intellectual Disability Inc.

Useful websites

Alzheimers Society: www.alzheimers.org.uk/Facts_about_dementia/PDF/i_learningdisabilities.pdf
American Association on Mental Retardation: www.aamr.org
British Institute of Learning Disabilities: www.bild.org.uk
Disability Rights Commission: www.drc-gb.org
Intellectual Disability Research: www.intellectualdisabilityinfo/home.htm
Joseph Rowntree Foundation: www.jrf.org.uk
Mencap: www.mencap.org.uk
National Autistic Society: www.nas.org.uk
National Network for Learning Disability Nursing: www.nnldn.org.uk
People First: www.peoplefirst.org.uk
Royal College of Nursing: www.rcn.org.uk
The Foundation for People with Learning Disabilities: www.learningdisabilities.org.uk
Valuing People Support Team: www.doh.gov.uk/vpst

Chapter 7

Care planning and delivery in forensic settings for people with intellectual disabilities

Karina Hepworth and Mick Wolverson

Introduction

This chapter presents a comprehensive overview of the key aspects of care planning and delivery for individuals involved with forensic services. In order to achieve this it is necessary to discuss the care pathway relating to people involved with forensic services. Box 7.1 provides a list of the components of a forensic care pathway. The influential Reed Report (Department of Health, 1992) can be seen as an attempt to shift the focus of forensic provision of care from custodial, to less restrictive environments while placing an emphasis on individualised care plans and a care pathway that encourages diversion from custody schemes. Because of this and other contemporary developments (outlined in the chapter) there will be discussion of care planning within forensic units as well as preventative work, holistic assessment, supporting people involved with the criminal justice system and the care programme approach. The chapter will also offer an exploration of these forensic issues in relation to both youth offending and adult perspectives. The chapter will discuss the broad principles of care planning and delivery in relation to services and also, where appropriate, offer discussion of more specific assessment and care planning issues, including inappropriate sexual behaviour and arson. The chapters within this book discuss the complexities and intricacies associated with care planning and delivery across both a range of settings and a wide spectrum of needs. Care planning within forensic settings is also extremely complex and this complexity is largely attributable to the following:

- Person centeredness versus risk management
- The nature of the behaviour of clients within a forensic setting
- The dominance of the medical model
- The Mental Health Act 1983

Person centeredness versus risk management

Within the recent past there has been a cumulative paradigm shift in the configuration of intellectual disability services from the institutional to community

> **Box 7.1   Components of a forensic care pathway**
>
> - Early identification of those at risk of developing offending behaviour
> - Appropriate assessment processes
> - Provision of specialist professionals within a youth offending team
> - Provision of appropriate care planning via specialist support and robust assessment
> - Provision of appropriate adults during police interviews
> - Diversion from custody processes
> - Therapeutic components of care plans that address individual causative factors
> - Use of the Mental Health Act for assessment and treatment
> - Provision of quality treatment and assessment units
> - Provision of outreach teams
> - Robust risk assessment
> - Appropriate and individualised use of the care programme approach to include contingency planning
> - Consistent support for families and carers

based, individualised and person-centred services. Theorists, such as O'Brien and Tyne (1981), and a succession of policy initiatives, such as the Human Rights Act 1998 and, of course, the *Valuing People* (2001) White Paper, all stress the importance of the key principles that underpin person-centred care. These principles are based around the concepts of rights, inclusion, independence and choice.

There is consensus that these principles should underpin all human services, but they present a huge challenge within forensic settings. The very nature of forensic settings compromises the implementation of these key principles. This is because forensic settings are designed to treat, assess and manage people with intellectual disability who present a significant risk to themselves or to others. People in such a position will be subject to regimes of care designed to limit their potential for self-harm, or that of harming others, and this will almost inevitably create tensions between the wishes of the individual and their care plan. In ethical terms this is the tension between autonomy and paternalism. Alongside the drive towards person-centred care planning there has been a concurrent drive towards a culture of robust risk management (see Chapter 6). The policy initiatives that compel nurses to engage in risk management include *The New NHS: Modern and Dependable* (Department of Health, 1998) and the clinical governance agenda. Phillips (2004) has also discussed how an increasingly litigious culture has created risk-averse services. Whereas person-centred care planning and risk management are not mutually exclusive, they do create antagonisms, dichotomies and ambivalences that nurses within forensic settings must attempt to reconcile as part of the care planning and delivery process.

The nature of the behaviour of clients within a forensic setting

Within intellectual disability forensic settings clients will have, at some stage, displayed behaviour that has been judged harmful to themselves or others, and often this will have involved offending. Some such behaviours/offences are more prevalent within the intellectual disability client group than within other groups of people. Studies by Murphy et al. (1983) and Hayes (1991) have all suggested that sexual offences are more prevalent among individuals with learning disabilities than in other groups. Blanchard et al. (1999) have discussed that the sexual offences committed by men with intellectual disabilities are also more likely to involve children. Bradford and Dimock (1986), Raesaenen et al. (1994) and Rowe and Lopes (2003) have all discussed that arson is more prevalent amoung people with intellectual disabilities than in other groups of people. Assaultive behaviour is also indicated to be a common reason for people with intellectual disabilities to be admitted to forensic settings (Musker, 2001). Less commonly, damage to property can also be another reason for admittance to forensic settings (Musker, 2001). Priest and Gibbs (2004) have discussed how mental ill health is more common in intellectual disabilities than in other groups and that people with this 'dual diagnosis' of intellectual disability and a mental health problem may receive care in forensic settings. Self-harm is also a significant issue in intellectual disability forensic settings (Phillips, 2004). From this brief overview it is evident that people with intellectual disabilities within forensic settings do not comprise a homogenous group. Their behaviours and reasons for admission are disparate, and therefore it is imperative that care planning and delivery reflect the complexity of each individual's history, propensity to offend and reasons for admission.

The dominance of the medical model

Mason and Mercer (1998) have suggested that forensic settings are characterised by hierarchical structures and that they tend to be dominated by the medical model of care. It is often the case that consultant psychiatrists are in powerful positions in relation to planning the care of individuals. It may be the case that the medical domination of a service mitigates against person-centred care planning and reinforces the antagonisms between it and risk management. As part of the care planning process, nurses working within specialist forensic settings should attempt to encourage holistic and person-centred approaches to care planning. It is acknowledged that this may be difficult within forensic settings. The discussion of the differing categories of offending behaviour will offer some ideas for person-centred care planning.

The Mental Health Act 1983

The Mental Health Act 1983 provides a legislative framework for the treatment and assessment of people with learning disabilities associated with forensic settings. The structure of the Act and its stipulations can mitigate against person-centred care planning and delivery. This is because it can inevitably create antagonisms between the wishes of clients and care plans that result from requirements of the Act that may involve some degree of control over an individual's free will. Such situations may require that individual consent be not necessarily sought for treatment as part of the care planning and delivery process, depending upon which section of the Act is applied to the individual. Nurses working within forensic services will need a working knowledge of the Act. Briefly, those sections of the Act that allow for assessment are sections 2, 4, 5, 135 and 136 (these sections are outlined in Appendix 7.1). Sections 3 and 7 (outlined in Appendix 7.2) provide for both assessment and treatment. Those associated with criminal proceedings are sections 35–37, 41 and 47–49 (outlined in Appendix 7.3). Section 117 (outlined in Appendix 7.4) is involved with after care. It is very important that intellectual disability nurses supporting individuals who are involved with forensic services be very familiar with these sections of the Mental Health Act as part of the care planning process.

The reform of the Mental Health Act 1983 (the Draft Mental Health Bill)

In November 1999 the Government published a Green Paper entitled *Reform of the Mental Health Act 1983: Proposals for Consultation*. The rationale for the proposals within this document was to reflect main changes in mental healthcare since the introduction of the Mental Health Act 1983 which has been the shift from institutionalised to community care. In 2002 the Government published a draft bill that set out proposals to reform current legislation. Whereas there was broad agreement that legislation relating to mental health needed to be reformed, there was widespread criticism of some of the proposals contained within the bill. The key proposals of the bill were that:

- There should be single broad definition of 'mental disorder'
- A mental health tribunal should be developed with powers to make orders for compulsory assessment and treatment
- Obligatory care plans should be drawn up for all people subject to compulsory treatment, without which they cannot be treated
- Compulsory treatment lasting more than 28 days should be scrutinised by an independent tribunal informed by independent expert reports
- Independent mental health advocacy services would be made available to everyone treated under the Act

- People treated under the Act can choose nominated people to speak for them
- People can be compulsorily treated in the community as well as in hospital
- The Bill should align the new Mental Health Act with recent human rights legislation

In response to this draft bill the Government received over 2000 consultation responses from service users, carers and professionals that were largely critical of the proposals and expressed fears that the bill could be used to persecute and stigmatise further people experiencing mental ill health. The most controversial proposal was the compulsory treatment of people in the community, which critics claim can lead to coercion, control of behaviour that is arbitrarily deemed to be deviant and conflict between professionals and clients (McIvor, 2001; The Mental Health Foundation, 2004). On 8 September 2004 the Government published a new draft of the bill which was meant to have addressed some of the concerns expressed in relation to the 2002 version; however, this too met with widespread criticism as it was seen to be little different from the 2002 version (Mind, 2005). A joint House of Commons and House of Lords Committee reported on the development of the Bill on 23 March 2005 and broadly concurred with existing criticisms. The Committee Chairman, Lord Carlisle of Berriew, was reported to have said that the Bill was:

'Fundamentally flawed and it is too heavily focused on compulsion and currently there are neither the resources nor the workforce to implement it.' (BBC News Online, 23 March 2005)

The Committee went on to state that legislation could be used as a form of social control. The Committee also feared that the proposals for compulsory treatment could be used as a mental health anti-social behaviour order, enforcing treatment on those who might be a nuisance, but do not actually pose a real threat. The Committee has also suggested that the wide definition of treatment could result in some people with intellectual disability being detained for safety reasons rather than to benefit their health.

Clearly there is much discussion still to take place before the bill becomes law; however, in relation to the care planning and delivery for people with intellectual disabilities and who are involved with forensic services, the key proposals from the bill could compromise the care planning process. This would mainly be due to issues of consent in relation to compulsory community treatment and how this may compromise the nurse's ability to develop mutually agreed care plans. The draft bill does acknowledge that the issue of consent can be a significant problem when working with some people with intellectual disability and it states that the bill should be integrated with the Mental Capacity Act 2005. The Mental Capacity Act 2005 offers a statutory framework to protect and empower vulnerable people.

The key principles that should underpin care planning and care delivery in relation to people with intellectual disabilities in forensic settings are identified

---

Box 7.2   The five key principles of the Mental Capacity Act 2005

- A presumption of capacity – every adult has the right to make his or her own decisions and must be assumed to have capacity to do so unless it is proved otherwise
- The right for individuals to be supported to make decisions – people must be given all appropriate help before anyone concludes that they cannot make their own decisions
- That individuals must retain the right to make what might be seen as eccentric or unwise decisions
- Best interests – anything done for or on behalf of people without capacity must be in their best interests
- Least restrictive intervention – anything done for or on behalf of people without capacity should be least restrictive of their basic rights and freedoms (Department of Health, 2005)

---

in Box 7.2. They are particularly relevant in care planning and delivery where there is a perceived conflict between the views of professionals and those of people with intellectual disabilities themselves.

Problems with terminology and definitions of intellectual disability

Intellectual disability is defined as a significant impairment of intelligence measured by an IQ of 70 or below, coupled with deficits in adaptive behaviour (World Health Organization, 1992; American Psychiatric Association, 1994). In terms of research studies in relation to young people and adults who offend, the definition is less arbitrary due to the nature of offending definitions and classifications internationally; much of the research undertaken is inclusive of people with milder disabilities (Winter et al., 1997; Holland et al., 2002; Siegal, 2003). The cut-off point of IQ 70 appears to be clear from a diagnostic perspective, but, in practice, arbitrary definitions pose problems from a research point of view, in that prevalence is then difficult to assess accurately and young people and adults with milder disabilities have difficulties in accessing help and support for their needs. There are accompanying issues of challenging behaviour, mental health issues and substance use, and many individuals fail to fit into services' eligibility criteria and subsequently find that there is little service provision to offer help and support to them and their families.

   Failure to recognise intellectual disability through early years services and education predispose to the likelihood of entering the criminal justice system with return and reconviction if needs are not identified and addressed (Hayes, 2002; Audit Commission, 2004). Lack of recognition is more likely due to lack of attendance, exclusions and behaviour problems in school, and the person is often seen as difficult or disruptive; but the underlying reasons for their behaviour are not investigated. Young people and adults with intellectual disabilities become very skilled in hiding their difficulties by using their behaviour to escape difficult or complex situations or tasks. Hence consideration of how to ensure early identification of need and early support and intervention are fundamental requirements of care planning and delivery. These young people and adults are highly vulnerable and at risk of being involved in crime. Whilst there are practical problems in ascertaining numbers who do not present at services and ethical concerns in seeking them out, it is incumbent on all professionals, whatever their agency, to use their skills to assess if they are at all concerned and look at the reasons behind the presenting issues.

Prevalence

It is generally considered that prevalence rates for offenders with intellectual disabilities may be higher than in the general population. Research study results vary from between less than 1% (Winter et al., 1997) and 8% (Gudjonsson et al., 1993). This wide variation in prevalence rate is influenced by several factors including difficulties in terminology, the criteria of intellectual disability applied, the types of methods of test used, the rigour with which the methods are applied and the characteristics of the population (Hayes, 1997; Murphy and Mason, 1999; Simpson and Hogg, 2001).

Prevalence is, therefore, almost impossible to assess given the available information. The inclusion of people with borderline intellectual disability in studies biases findings and can give an inaccurate picture if intellectual disability is defined as having an IQ of below 70. Several studies have taken their results from impression and staff report rather than formal assessment of intellectual functioning (Hall, 2000). More recently researchers have begun to question the usefulness of the studies to date and suggest that ascertaining numbers is of less importance than investigating the processes that determine movement in and/or out of the criminal justice system and developing appropriate care planning process for this client group (McBrien, 2003).

Care planning and delivery for young people with learning disabilities with forensic services and the criminal justice system

This section of the chapter will explore forensic care planning and delivery in relation to young people with intellectual disabilities. Although most of the issues discussed relate to young people, some also apply to adults and many of the concepts discussed also relate to care planning and delivery for adults.

Young people and adults with intellectual disabilities pose significant ethical, moral and practical dilemmas due to several factors. Firstly, as already discussed, recognition of need and getting help and support can result in the person not being able to access services given their eligibility criteria. Secondly, making the distinction between difficult and/or challenging behaviour and offending is also significant (Holland et al., 2002). When does challenging behaviour become anti-social behaviour or criminal behaviour? Is it only criminal behaviour when a report has been given to the police and a charge is made?

There appear to be distinct differences in how a young person is dealt with through the criminal justice system and what happens to an adult going through the same process. The ability of the criminal justice system to recognise people with intellectual disabilities who offend and to provide appropriate diversion, assessment and intervention, has yet to be adequately studied (Barron et al., 2002). The Reed Report (Department of Health, 1992) made it clear that offenders with a 'mental disorder' should be diverted from prison. However, there is evidence to show that recognition rates are low (Hall, 2000; Hayes, 2002), and there is often inappropriate support in police interview and disposal of the offence in court. The development of skills in education staff, school nurses, health visitors and Sure Start will also help to ensure a more consistent way of identifying intellectual disabilities and offer opportunities for engagement in the care planning and delivery process. This sharing information and co-operation between agencies would ensure a more cohesive pathway through services, helping to improve delivery and tackle inequality (Department of Health, 2003; Department for Education and Skills, 2003; Audit Commission, 2004).

There are two distinct groups of young people with intellectual disability who offend. Firstly there is a group already known to specialist services and secondly, a group of people who are unknown to specialist services, and have a history of impulsivity, problems with adaptive behaviour, exclusion from education, risk taking, substance abuse and social exclusion (see Box 7.3 for a

---

Box 7.3   Characteristics of young people whose needs have yet to be identified

- Lack of attendance at school
- Behaviour problems in school
- Struggling with school work
- Three in five (60%) of young people excluded from school have offended (MORI, 2004)
- Substance misuse, e.g. aerosols, alcohol, smoking cannabis and amphetamines
- Physical health – not up to date with immunisation, not registered with a GP
- Mental health problems
- Age – the peak age for youth offending is 14 (this is younger than in previous years (MORI, 2004)
- Homelessness
- Parents separated
- Other family members are offenders
- Deprivation, e.g. low income and poor housing

list of characteristics of this group). Developing evidence suggests that these people have received some form of special education support in school, but the majority have received little help up to leaving education (Audit Commission, 2002). Another characteristic of this group is that it is very difficult for families to access support; many have failed to gain assistance with problems with behaviour and the problems have escalated over time (Ball and Connolly, 2000; Hayes, 2002). The reality for families is that few receive appropriate comprehensive or consistent guidance and they question why their son or daughter had had to offend to have some assessment of their needs and at last receive support that they have been requesting for some time.

The youth offending team

Youth offending teams (Fig. 7.1) are defined under Section 39 of the Crime and Disorder Act 1998, and attempt to achieve a balance between the welfare of

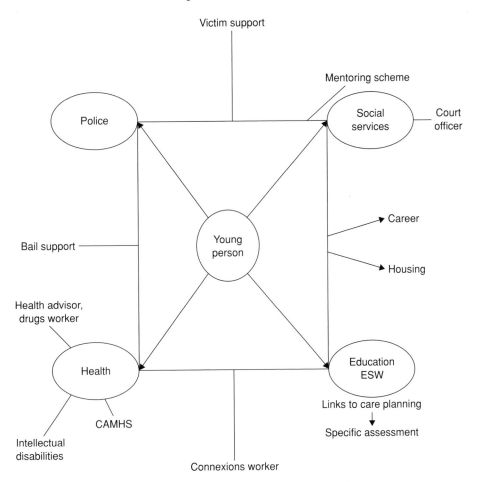

Fig. 7.1   The youth offending team.

Box 7.4   Asset assessment profile

- Offending behaviour
- Living arrangements
- Family and personal relationships
- Statutory education
- Employment, training and education
- Neighbourhood
- Lifestyle
- Substance use
- Physical health
- Emotional and mental health
- Perception of self and others
- Thinking and behaviour
- Attitudes to offending
- Motivation to change
- Positive factors
- Indicators of vulnerability

---

the young person and justice to the victim and the local community, with the principle aim being the prevention of offending.

Young people are assessed using the asset assessment profile (Box 7.4) so that an appropriate care plan can be put in place to address offending, vulnerability and ensure appropriate referrals for support to the specialist workers in the team.

The role of the intellectual disability nurse in ensuring effective, evidence-based practice

Rapport

A journey through the criminal justice system is an anxiety-provoking experience for anyone and, for someone with an intellectual disability, police interviews, an appearance in court and subsequent intervention through the youth offending team or probation, must be highly stressful and frightening. The role of the nurse, therefore, must initially be one of building a relationship, developing trust, being non-judgmental and, of utmost importance, adhering to codes of confidentiality. Many of those young people and adults on orders from court will not previously have had their needs identified and will not be in receipt of services.

Through the asset assessment profile, issues will be raised that the youth offending team officer is concerned about, with a subsequent referral to the nurse. It is vital to bear in mind that the nurse may not be dealing with an already identified need and so vigilance, observation and listening skills are crucial. Young people very often present initially as being very 'streetwise', in control of themselves and their emotions. Underneath this veneer is usually a person who has learnt to get by through developing coping strategies. Many have learnt phrases designed to make professionals think they know more than they do; many use their behaviour to guarantee a situation ends if they find it too difficult or do not understand it, and rely on their peers to help them through. Trust between the person and the nurse has to be built on over time, allowing the person to see that the nurse is supportive and may be able to help.

Assessment

As in all areas of intellectual disability nursing practice, assessment is imperative if interventions are to be successful. General health assessment is needed, as many people with learning disabilities in the criminal justice system are not registered with a GP and may have failed to access healthcare over several years. School exclusion and truancy have often led to a lack of health screening and take up of immunisation. Substance misuse and emotional and mental health are also key factors in the explanation of crime (Audit Commission, 2004). The complex needs of young people are often such that the work of reducing the risk of offending has to be based on a balance of tackling the risk factors whilst addressing the offending behaviour. Ultimately, unless those risk factors are reduced, the possibility of reconviction and recidivism appears to be inevitable. Hence, to ensure appropriate delivery of care it is essential, through screening, to assess for possible intellectual disability.

The Hayes Ability Screening Index (HASI) has been developed to determine those people in the criminal justice system who may have an intellectual disability and need to be referred on for further assessment; the HASI can be administrated by any staff provided that training is given. It can be used for young people and adults and can be completed within 20 minutes. The HASI is quick and easy to score with clear indicators of whether further assessment is required or not. If the screening indicates further assessment is needed the intellectual disability nurse must consider how to gather further evidence. There are two distinct paths that can be followed:

- Complete further assessment in relation to looking at a person's overall level of ability and adaptive behaviour in relation to their peers, using a rating scale. This in turn will influence how the person's offending behaviour programme is delivered
- Complete further assessment work but utilise the information, not only to plan for offending behaviour work, but also to refer to appropriate agencies for further investigative work with a view to on-going support and intervention

Careful consideration is needed along with the person with intellectual disabilities to decide which route to follow. Young people and adults do not want to be viewed as being different and being labelled as having any form of disability is not acceptable to them. The nurse must discuss the options available and consider what support the person will be in receipt of on completion of their order. Many professionals' first consideration is to refer on to what they feel is a more appropriate service. There are no panaceas or 'cures' and it is essential that intellectual disability nurses consider what they can do within their practice to support the care planning and delivery of care for those involved with forensic services.

Planning and intervention

Multi-agency working is the embodiment of the effective delivery of care for people with intellectual disability (Department of Health, 2001, 2003, 2004). Within the criminal justice system and the delicate balance between welfare and justice, it is imperative that at every stage of a person's journey, services work together to address predictors of future offending and on-going support needs. The results of the assessment will have identified the person's strengths and needs. Dependent on individual need, planning and intervention will include a range of factors.

Motivation to change

Understanding how a person views aspects of their behaviour and their attitude to wanting to change, along with who will be there to support them, helps in the care planning process.

Offending behaviour work

How can the person's offending behaviour be understood and what interventions are more likely to ensure the behaviour will not happen again? Gathering information with the person's consent through discussion with the key figures in school, work, residential setting, the GP, and viewing any relevant case notes will provide a background and set the scene.

Analysis of the behaviour will need to account for the what, when, why and how of the behaviour, with a view to developing a formulation or summary of the available information. This will consider how the behaviours are maintained, give a hypothesis for the behaviour and offer a way forward and rationale for intervention to include family/carers (Clare and Murphy, 1998).

Tailoring of standard offending behaviour programmes is essential to ensure appropriate delivery in terms of the person having an understanding of the impact of the offence on the victim and the wider community. This means refining programmes so that work can be delivered at the level and pace of understanding of the individual. Failing to do so can alienate a person from the worker and the work itself. Many use their behaviour as a communicative act and if they are finding the situation difficult, will use their behaviour to escape and guarantee the situation ends.

Health

Prescribed medication and its effects, known diagnoses, awareness of mental and emotional health and substance use, will need to be borne in mind in planning and executing an intervention. Liaison with health professionals in secure facilities will be necessary to give and receive appropriate information for the delivery of the person's care. Signposting to, or liaison with, adult or child and adolescent mental health services may be needed, based on the original assessment and subsequent work with the person.

Case illustration 7.1

John is aged 12 years and lives with his mother and older sister. He has been permanently excluded from his mainstream school and for the last 18 months has been at home. There has been involvement from Social Services who have been unable to suggest ways of helping and supporting the family. John is verbally abusive to his mother, physically threatens her to obtain money, refuses to look at or speak to anyone other than his friends and stays out until the early hours of the morning. John's mother finds coping with John's behaviour extremely difficult, resulting in her having anxiety attacks and feeling generally unwell; she also reports incidents of John taking cycles, aerosols, toys and furniture to pieces and reports that he goes into the cellar and urinates in bottles.

John is arrested for three offences of arson, one where John has set fire to a tent with two people inside. Whilst on police bail it is crucial to try to build rapport and trust with John and succeed in managing to complete an assessment. It becomes clear that John has great difficulties with verbal and written communication, understanding of numbers and time, undertaking personal care and is at great risk when in the community, as he is unable to understand the risks around him or the consequences of his actions for himself and others. John is given a detention and training order where he serves 3 months in custody in a secure provision far away from his family. While in custody he is assessed by the educational psychologist and the community paediatrician, who feel that he has significant learning and communication difficulties; he has an IQ of 55. John misses his family and begins to realise how his behaviour has had an effect on himself and his family.

Preparation for John's return home has several facets:

- Working with education to put together a statement of special educational needs and a home tutor initially to help to prepare John for returning to school
- Taking photographs of the boundaries that John will need to adhere to when he leaves custody as part of his licence/order from court. The youth offending team spend time with John in custody, preparing him for this using the photographs

---

Cont.

- Preparing a volunteer mentor to support John in developing leisure activities
- Support the mother in her application for Disability Living Allowance
- Draw up a plan of how to support the mother in dealing with behavioural issues using positive strategies, developing a routine through caring for his reptiles which ensures preparation for getting up to go to school
- Work with the youth offending team office to look at how work on offending behaviour can be delivered, especially in relation to victim awareness and consequences of actions
- Liaise with the community learning disability service to ensure on-going support at the end of John's order

John took several weeks to adjust to being back at home and become almost reclusive; over several months the care plan put in place saw John slowly begin to develop his trust in those supporting him. Eighteen months later, he is back in school, the family are supported by the learning disability service and there have been no further incidents of offending.

Case illustration 7.2

Matthew, aged 17 years, lived with his parents and younger brother. Mathew's mother has reported long-standing difficulties in dealing with behavioural issues. Matthew rarely played as a young child; he had few friendships and was always on the move. Sleep patterns were disrupted and Matthew would shout out every night in his sleep. Matthew seemed to be fixated on certain foods and would become very upset if there was any change in his daily routine.

Mathew's parents became increasingly concerned as Matthew grew up, as he began to pose increasing risk to the family through setting fire to his stereo, hitting family members, throwing the computer and throwing a brick at the living room window. On one occasion Mum found over 20 lighters in his bedroom. Matthew attended mainstream school up to leaving at 16 years, but had a history of always being on report at school. Staff felt that they did not understand Matthew's behaviour and, towards the end of his school life, felt at a loss as to how to approach Matthew. The youth offending team became involved following a conviction for burglary. Assessment, using the Adaptive Behaviour Scale S:2 (Nihira et al., 1993), revealed deficits in social skills, responsibility, motivation and in areas of adaptive behaviour, such as lack of ability to conform to rules, rigidity in thoughts and actions and concerning interpersonal behaviour.

Work focused on enabling Matthew to develop insight and understanding into his needs and why he feels as he does. The offending behaviour work completed by his youth offending team officer was tailored and modified to ensure that delivery was meaningful. Each section of the programme of work was carefully reviewed to ensure the best delivery possible.

Contributing to the report for the court enabled the magistrates to have a clearer view of the needs of Matthew and how his needs impacted on the way he behaves. Matthew has now left the family home and is living with informal carers. A period of work in a factory went well initially as the work was routine and Matthew felt able to cope. Things began to change when Matthew started to be late for work; then he began to take days off until he was given his notice. A marked deterioration followed with missed youth offending team appointments, poor self-care, increased substance use, behavioural issues, feelings of persecution, worries that people were watching him, and an increased feeling of apathy and worthlessness.

Further offences were committed and consisted of two assaults on other young people. Despite requests for advice from the child and family service, he was deemed too old for their service. A subsequent referral was made to the learning disabilities service for advice as to appropriate support and intervention but again was not felt to be appropriate. A referral was made to the consultant psychologist. Whilst waiting for an appointment, a further offence of assault took place and Matthew was put on remand in a young offenders institution. Liaison with the health team proved to be crucial in Matthew receiving appropriate support on his arrival and continuing detention. Matthew has been seen by a psychiatrist and forensic psychologist with an initial report suggesting an autistic spectrum disorder. Psychological reports are being requested for court in order to plan for disposal of the offences.

The principles of care planning in adult forensic services

Chapter 1 of this book discussed the key components of care planning and delivery in intellectual disabilities. The good practice discussed in Chapter 1 should inform and underpin care planning and delivery within forensic settings; however some specific core values are highly relevant within forensic settings and they contribute to appropriate care planning and delivery as follows:

- Respect for the individual as a human being irrespective of their offending behaviour
- Care planning and delivery should be predicated on as much background information as is possible. This should include childhood experiences, family issues, education and contact with services
- Being non-judgemental
- Maintaining confidentiality
- A necessity to understand the causation of the behaviour(s) so that care plans can offer appropriate treatment
- The application of equally high quality care to all clients

It is imperative that the care planning and delivery for people with intellectual disabilities within a forensic setting is based on thorough assessment. As discussed earlier, clients within a forensic setting will have been admitted for a variety of reasons and, therefore, each client should be assessed on an individual basis. It is good practice in care planning initially to use a generic assessment tool that covers all the psychological, physical, social, environmental and emotional domains of an individual's life. The assessment process should also be predicated on as much personal 'history' as is feasible. Assessment should also take into account any potential causative factors that may have created the 'setting' conditions in which offending behaviour may have occurred. Such an eclectic basis for assessment can comprehensively inform subsequent care planning and delivery and ensure that plans are devised aimed at meeting all aspects of a person's life.

So that care plans can reflect the individual nature of a person's pattern of behaviour, further assessment should be undertaken that assesses specific areas of concern. The assessment process should be conducted within a multi-disciplinary/multi-agency context and it should be co-ordinated by a designated individual. Ideally care planning and delivery should involve the client in the planning process and, wherever possible, consent should be sought.

Specific forensic issues

The text on page 127 of this chapter offered an overview of the range and nature of the behaviours associated with clients within forensic settings. The chapter will now focus on two of these behaviours in more detail. It should be noted that the key elements, care planning and delivery, covered in the following discussion of inappropriate sexual behaviour and arson are generalisable to other offending behaviours.

Inappropriate sexual behaviour

It has been suggested from research findings that the potential causation for inappropriate sexual behaviour is multifactorial (O'Conner and Rose, 1998). An appropriate care plan for a client with a history of sexually inappropriate behaviour should be informed by an assessment of the potential causation(s) of the behaviour. This is extremely important, as subsequent care planning and delivery can therefore include measures that will attempt to address the causative factors that contributed to the development and maintenance of the behaviour. Research literature in this area has suggested that inappropriate sexual behaviour may not have a sexual motive but could serve a communicative function. This is particularly so for people with poor verbal skills who may use sexually inappropriate behaviour to gain attention, 'escape' from difficult situations, control people or situations, provide self-stimulation or in an attempt to reveal abuse. Sexually inappropriate behaviour may also be attributable to a lack of knowledge regarding appropriate sexual behaviour, a lack of appropriate role models or a lack of encouragement to adopt appropriate behaviour (Brown and Barret, 1994; Rushton, 1994 and 1995). Hayes (1991) discussed that sexual offenders with an intellectual disability have poor peer relationships, lack sexual knowledge and personal power and have negative formative sexual experiences. Rowe and Lopes (2003) have also suggested that some sexually inappropriate behaviour relating to children may arise through some people with intellectual disabilities feeling an 'emotional congruence' with children.

This brief overview demonstrates that inappropriate sexual behaviour in intellectual disabilities is extremely complex. The accurate and thorough assessment of it is therefore crucial so that care planning and delivery can help address these underlying factors. A good specific assessment tool and aid to care planning and delivery in relation to sexually inappropriate behaviour in intellectual disabilities is *Sex and the 3 Rs* (McCarthy and Thompson, 1994). Brown and Barret (1994) and LaVigna and Donnellan (1986) have recommended that care plans and subsequent care delivery that need to address sexually inappropriate behaviour should be designed so that they do not include 'punishment' for the behaviour but, rather, should instead work towards encouraging appropriate rather than inappropriate behaviour. This can be achieved if individual care plans include some provision for:

- Increasing sexual knowledge and competence (McCarthy and Thompson, 1994)
- Cognitive behavioural therapy (Clare, 1993)
- The individual's motivation to develop appropriate sexual behaviour (Clare, 1994; Mann and Rollnick, 1996)
- Decreasing inappropriate arousal and increasing appropriate arousal (O'Conner and Rose, 1998)
- Treating sexual dysfunction
- Anger/anxiety management and relapse prevention (Murphy, 1997)
- Medication can be used to lower libido (Myers, 1991; Cooper, 1995); however, gaining consent for this from an individual with an intellectual disability could be difficult and this treatment may have damaging side effects and so is ethically questionable

All care planning and delivery relating to individuals in contact with forensic settings must include a risk assessment designed to safeguard the individual and anyone they may harm. Care plans will need to identify which option(s) should be pursued. The chosen components of a care plan should be based on the assessment process and their intention should be to offer constructive interventions that target identified causative factors. Care plans should identify how interventions will be conducted and who will be responsible for their implementation and evaluation. The processes discussed here constitute good practice in care planning in forensic settings and they can be equally applied to other specific offending behaviours such as arson.

Arson

Rowe and Lopes (2003) have discussed that the offence of arson may serve a variety of functions for the perpetrator. White and Dalby (2000) have also discussed that arson may arise due to a combination of causative factors. Those committing arson may do so as they may seek the sensational impacts that come from the fire and they may have fantasies about being involved in the fire fighting. They may also seek sexual pleasure from starting fires. Arson is also strongly associated with impulsivity and personality disorder. Rowe and Lopes (2003) report that people who commit arson may also be more likely than others to commit other criminal offences and that those convicted for arson for a second time are extremely likely to re-offend. It is evident that arson is a complex phenomenon and therefore the care planning process should take into account this complexity and dangerousness by considering the following:

- Risk assessment and subsequent care planning and delivery will need to take into account that the individual may commit offences other than arson. Assessment and subsequent care planning and delivery take into account underlying mental ill health and any personality disorder
- Observation and security measures as outlined under 'care planning and the forensic environment'
- Individual history and personal characteristics. This is important, as arsonists who have an intellectual disability commonly have a disrupted home background and a history of long-term behavioural problems. They also differ from other offenders in that they present as being passive with a history of destructiveness to property rather than aggression towards people
- Cognitive approaches that emphasise victim empathy and the risks associated with re-offending

Risk management

Risk assessment was discussed in detail in Chapter 6, but the importance of this subject for forensic services warrants some further discussion. The care planning process and care delivery for people who are involved with forensic services must include a risk management component. The risk assessment and subsequent care plan must clearly identify both the risks to the individual and others and explicit mechanisms for managing these risks. The preceding discussion of sexually inappropriate behaviour and arson highlighted that the gathering of background information and individual histories is of paramount importance in understanding factors that contribute to and maintain these behaviours. Risk assessment, and its management within care plans, must similarly focus on these factors so that treatment can be offered in a constructive way. Individual services may well have developed their own risk assessment tools and care plans that include risk management as integral component

---

Box 7.5   The components of robust risk management in care planning

- Clear identification of the behaviour(s) likely to pose a risk to self or others
- Consideration of immediate, short-term and long-term risk
- The collating of as much background information as possible
- Awareness of probable sources of error
- The identification of and inclusion of specialists, multi-disciplinary and multi-agency team members
- Planning for key interventions
- Apportioning responsibility for components of the care plan
- Client involvement
- Prediction of factors likely to increase or decrease future risk
- Contingency options
- Consideration of the balance between the frequency, imminence and potential dangerousness of the behaviour(s)
- Identification and management of factors likely to trigger dangerous behaviour
- Prioritising areas of concern so that treatment can be focused
- Provision for regular evaluation and alteration of the care plan as required

---

of them. Many such assessments are derived from the Sainsbury Centre Risk Management Tool (Morgan, 2000). Those wishing to explore this subject further should access this document for further reading.

Risk management within care planning in forensic services must be consistently integrated throughout an individual's care plan. The care programme approach (which is discussed next) offers a systematic process for the management of risk as part of an individual's care plan. The care programme approach, The Sainsbury Centre Tool and other risk management plans share some common themes that are listed in Box 7.5. The reader is advised to refer to Chapter 6 for a full discussion of risk assessment in relation to care planning and delivery for people with intellectual disabilities.

The care programme approach

The care programme approach offers a systematic and comprehensive guide to integrated care planning as applied to people who have contact with forensic services. It can also be used as a significant part of a forensic care pathway. The guide was initially introduced in 1991 as a mechanism for ensuring the integrated and appropriate care of those who require assessment and treatment of their mental health needs. The major components of the care programme approach can be seen in Box 7.6. The major components of the care programme approach are based on the principles of best practice as discussed within this and other chapters of the book. The care programme approach was significantly strengthened and modernised in 2001 and this included the introduction of two levels of the care programme approach: standard and

---

Box 7.6   Components of the care programme approach

- Systematic arrangements for assessing the health and social needs of people involved with specialist mental health services
- The formation of a written care plan, risk assessment, risk management guidelines and a crisis contingency plan that covers both health and social needs
- The appointment of a named care co-ordinator (formerly key worker) to monitor, coordinate care and involve the service user in the care planning process
- A process of regular review and care planning update within a multi-disciplinary/multi-agency context

---

Box 7.7   Characteristics of people on the enhanced care programme approach

- They are only willing to co-operate with one professional/agency but have multiple care needs
- They are likely to have mental health problems co-existing with other problems, such as substance misuse, neurological, developmental and personality disorders
- They are more likely to be at risk of harming themselves or others and of displaying offending behaviour
- They may be in contact with a number of agencies, including the criminal justice system, and they are likely to require more frequent and intensive interventions
- They have multiple care needs that require multi-disciplinary/multi-agency input
- They often display poor co-operation with treatment, lack insight and disengage from services
- They have poor social and family support networks and may have been abused or neglected

---

enhanced. It is likely that the enhanced level of care programme approach (see Box 7.7) will apply to those people with intellectual disability and in contact with forensic services. Nurses working within care programme approach guidelines are, therefore, adhering to best practice in relation to care planning and will also be able to use the care programme approach alongside other specific areas of individual assessment and care planning as previously discussed.

Priest and Gibbs (2004) have reported that there is a substantial body of evidence indicating that categories of mental ill health are common in intellectual disabilities and in most instances higher than within the general population. Because of this strong association between mental ill health and intellectual disabilities, the care programme approach provides a very important component of the care planning process. Box 7.7 lists the characteristics of people with intellectual disabilities receiving care under the enhanced care programme approach. As can be seen from these common characteristics they are often also associated with those in contact with forensic intellectual disability services and this demonstrates that the care programme approach is hugely influential in the care planning and delivery process. Nurses working within this field of intellectual disability nursing should familiarise themselves with the care programme approach; however the concepts and good practice associated with it are applicable to other areas of nursing.

Care planning and delivery within the forensic environment

As previously discussed clients within a forensic setting can be at risk of self harm or they may present a risk to others. The care planning process should allow for this on an individual basis and also in relation to the safe management of the environment. Phillips (2004) has discussed how forensic environments manage risk by having the following characteristics:

- Secure fences
- Locked doors
- Restriction on window openings
- 'High risk' areas, such as kitchens, being locked
- Reinforced glass
- Property checks
- Restriction of flammable materials

Although most forensic units will have some or all of these features, care plans can offer some, albeit limited, flexibility in relation to how they affect individuals. As part of a person's care plan it is possible, for example, to allow clients access to some areas within the building and for them not to have property checks if assessments have demonstrated that this will not present a risk.

Conclusion

This chapter has offered a summary of some of the key issues associated with care planning and delivery for people with intellectual disabilities who are involved with forensic services. A main aim of this chapter has been to demonstrate that the development of behaviours likely to result in contact with forensic services are complex and multifactorial and that thorough assessment of these factors is a prerequisite of good care planning and delivery. Some specific forensic manifestations, such as youth offending, sexually inappropriate behaviour and arson, and the care planning approach relating to them, have been outlined to highlight the complexity and intricacy of forensic issues. It is acknowledged that this chapter provides a brief overview of the main issues associated with care planning in forensic services. To develop a greater understanding, readers should consult the further reading and resources guide supplied at the end of the chapter.

Appendix 7.1
Sections of the Mental Health Act that allow for assessment

Section 2: Admission for assessment

Summary: This section allows for a person to be detained in hospital for assessment. It is based on two medical representations.

Duration: This section can last for up to 28 days. This period should allow time for an assessment to be made. If it is felt that a person requires to be detained further it is customary to do so by using section 3. This section is often used when an individual is detained for the first time or if there have been considerable gaps between admissions.

Circumstances: An application can be made if the following are felt:

- That an individual is suffering from a mental disorder of a degree that warrants detention in a hospital for assessment, or for assessment followed by medical treatment for at least a limited period
- That the individual should be detained in the interests of their own health and safety or in order to protect others

Section 4: Emergency admission for assessment

Summary: This section requires only one medical representation. It is intended to be used for emergency admissions; section 2 would be used if it were not for the urgency of the situation.

Duration: Up to 72 hours. During this period a second medical representation can be obtained and this converts the section 4 into a section 2.

Circumstances: As for section 2 and additionally it must be stated that:

- It is an urgent necessity that the individual be admitted and detained under section 2; and
- The section 2 requirement of obtaining a second medical representation would involve an undesirable delay

Section 5(2): Detention of an in-patient

This section allows for an approved doctor to detain an informal patient for up to 72 hours by reporting to hospital managers. Before this time period elapses an application can be made for a section 2 or 3 to be applied or the individual can revert to informal status.

Section 5(4): Nurse's holding power

This section allows for the registered learning [intellectual] disability nurse or registered mental nurse to prevent informal persons from leaving an in-patient environment if it is considered to be in their best interest or that of others. This holding power can last up to 6 hours. As soon as it commences a doctor with the authority to detain the individual must be alerted. The holding power will cease as soon as the doctor arrives and completes an assessment of the individual.

Section 135: Power to enter premises and take a person to a place of safety

Summary: This section allows for an approved social worker to seek a warrant from a justice of the peace (JP) that will give permission to a police officer to enter premises (if necessary by force) to search for a person with mental health problems and take them to a place of safety. The police officer, with this authority, must be accompanied by an approved social worker and a doctor. It is not an admission section but one that allows for assessment to be undertaken in a place of safety. The assessment will consider whether a section 2 or other admission section will need to be implemented. The section can last up to 72 hours from when the person arrives at the place of safety. This section also allows for a police officer (accompanied by an approved social worker) to enter premises to 're-take' an already sectioned person who is absent without leave.

Circumstances: The grounds for the warrant are that it appears to the JP that there is reasonable cause to suspect that, at a place within the JP's jurisdiction, a person with a mental disorder is:

- Being (or has been) ill-treated, neglected, or not kept 'under proper control'; or
- Is living alone and unable to care for themselves

Section 136: Removal of people from public places

Summary: This section allows for a police officer to remove someone from a public place and take them to a place of safety. As with section 135 its purpose is to allow for an assessment in a place of safety and to consider if a section 2 or any other admission section is required. Its duration is for up to 72 hours from when the person arrives at the place of safety.

Circumstances: The police officer must find that:

- The person is in a place to which the public have access; and
- The person must appear (to the police officer) to have a mental disorder and be in need of immediate need of care or control; and

- It is necessary to take the person to the place of safety in the best interest of the person or the protection of others

Appendix 7.2
Sections of the Mental Health Act concerned with both assessment and treatment

Section 3: Admission for treatment

Summary: This section enables a person to be detained in hospital for treatment. It is often used to follow a section 2 and when an individual and their mental health history are well known. It requires the recommendation of two doctors.

Duration: Initially for up to 6 months, after which it can be renewed for another 6 months and then annually.

Circumstances: The doctors must confirm that the individual is:

- Suffering from one of the following four categories – mental illness, severe mental impairment, psychopathic disorder or mental impairment. In addition to this the mental disorder must be of such a degree that it is appropriate for the individual to receive treatment in hospital
- In relation to psychopathic disorder or mental impairment the treatment is likely to alleviate or prevent a deterioration in the condition of the individual
- The treatment is necessary for the health and safety of the individual or the protection of others and that the treatment cannot be provided unless the individual is detained under this section

Section 7: Guardianship

Summary: This section allows a person to be cared for under guardianship. It requires the recommendation of two doctors that need to be accepted by the local social services authority. The guardian can be the local social services authority or a person deemed appropriate to be so by the authority.

Duration: As with section 3 guardianship can initially last for up to 6 months. It can be renewed for a further 6 months and then annually.

Circumstances: The individual must be deemed have one of the four specified categories of mental disorder listed in the act (see the conditions for section 3). It is also a requirement that guardianship is in the interests of the welfare of the individual and the protection of others. The guardian has the power to:

- Require that the individual reside at a place specified by the authority or the person named as the guardian
- Require that the individual attend at places and times specified for treatment, occupation, education or training

- Require that the individual can be seen at the place they are residing by any registered practitioner, approved social worker or other specified persons

Appendix 7.3
Sections of the Mental Health Act associated with criminal proceedings

Section 35: Remand to hospital by the courts

Summary: This section allows a court to send a person to hospital rather than prison so that a report can be prepared on their mental condition. People subject to this section cannot be made to accept treatment, as the consent to treatment issues stipulated in sections 57 and 58 do not apply.

Duration: Initially for up to 28 days. This can be extended by the court for not more than 28 days at a time to a maximum of 6 weeks.

Circumstances: The person must have been charged with an offence that could lead to imprisonment (including an accusation of murder) and the person:

- Is before a crown court but has not been tried, convicted, sentenced or dealt with in any other way
- Has been convicted by a magistrates court; or
- Will be before a magistrates court and has not been convicted and either the court is satisfied that the person has done what they have been accused of, or the person agrees to the section 35 being made

The court must be satisfied that:

- There is reason to suspect that the person has at least one of the four categories of mental disorder listed within the Mental Health Act. The evidence of this mental disorder is supplied by one doctor
- A report could not be made if person were allowed bail
- A specified hospital can admit the person within 7 days

Section 36: Remand to hospital by the courts for treatment

Summary: Unlike section 35 this section allows for compulsory treatment (if deemed necessary) in hospital rather than remanding the individual to prison.

Duration: As for section 35.

Circumstances: The person must be before a crown court facing a charge that could lead to imprisonment. This is unless the person has been either accused or convicted of murder when a sentence of life imprisonment must be imposed. The court must be satisfied that:

- The person has mental illness or mental impairment based on evidence supplied by two doctors
- A specified hospital is available to admit the person within 7 days

Section 37: Hospital orders made by the courts

Summary: This section enables a court to send an individual to hospital for treatment or make them subject to guardianship rather than commit them to prison.

Duration: Initially for 6 months. It can then be renewed for a further 6 months and then annually.

Circumstances: The section can apply if the person:

- Has been convicted of a crime by a crown court (or magistrates court) which could have resulted in imprisonment (apart from murder where a life sentence is mandatory)
- Has not yet been convicted but may be before a magistrates court charged with an offence that could lead to imprisonment

Without making a conviction the court can make a hospital order using section 37 if the individual has mental illness or mental disorder and that the Court is convinced that the person did what they are accused of.

Other conditions: The court must be satisfied that:

- The person has at least one of the four categories of mental disorder listed in the Act based on two doctors agreeing on at least one of these categories
- The mental disorder is of such a degree that it is appropriate for the person to be admitted to hospital for treatment and, in the case of mental impairment or psychopathic disorder, that treatment will alleviate or prevent a deterioration in the condition
- Using section 37 is the most appropriate method of dealing with the person
- That a specified hospital can admit the person within 28 days

Section 41: Restriction orders

Summary: If a crown court decides to impose a section 37 it may also impose a section 41. This section (along with section 37) is commonly applied to people with intellectual disabilities with a forensic history who are deemed to be in need of care in hospital. It increases the limitations associated with section 37 and imposes the following restrictions:

- Leave of section can be granted only by the Secretary of State for the Home Office; also the responsible medical officer can recall a person from leave of section

- Any transfer of the person between units requires the agreement of the Home Office
- Similarly discharge requires the agreement of the Home Office

Duration: The imposition of sections 37/41 allows for a person to remain under section for an indefinite period. There is a requirement for the responsible medical officer to provide a progress report each year (as requested by the Home Office).

Circumstances: The individual will have been convicted of an offence that could have resulted in a prison sentence and the court must be in agreement that section 41 is necessary for the protection of the public from serious harm in relation to:

- The individual's history of offending
- The risk of re-offending if set free
- The nature of the offending behaviour

Sections 47/48/49: Transfer from prison to hospital

Summary: These three sections of the Mental Health Act are concerned with the transfer of prisoners from prison to hospital for treatment.

Section 47: People serving prison sentences

The Home Office is able to make a transfer direction if the following conditions apply:

- The person is diagnosed (on the basis of reports from two doctors) with at least one of the four types of mental disorder defined with the Mental Health Act
- The mental disorder is of such a degree that it is appropriate for the person to receive treatment in hospital
- If the person is diagnosed as having a psychopathic disorder or mental impairment and treatment can alleviate or prevent deterioration in the condition
- The Home Office believes treatment in hospital is in the public interest

Duration: As for section 37, if section 47 is used alone It is more likely that section 49 (restriction direction) conditions will apply (see below). The transfer direction can come to an end 2 weeks after it was imposed if the transfer did not take place, or as for section 37, if a section 49 is not applied.

Section 48: People not serving prison sentences

Summary: This section allows for people not yet convicted of a crime to be admitted to hospital for treatment.

Circumstances:

- The person is diagnosed with mental illness or mental impairment
- The person is in urgent need of treatment

Duration: The transfer direction ends when the court makes a final decision about the case.

Section 49: Restriction directions

Summary: This section is used to prevent discharge under section 23. It is often used in conjunction with sections 47 and 48.

Appendix 7.4
The Mental Health Act and aftercare

Section 117: Aftercare arrangements

Summary: This section of the Mental Health Act is of great importance to nurses working with people with intellectual disabilities. Along with section 5.4 it is likely that intellectual disability nurses (particularly those working in the community) will be actively involved with aftercare arrangements under section 117. This section is also clearly linked to aspects of care planning and delivery to which nurses can contribute. Section 117 is also linked to the care programme approach, and again this aspect of care planning and delivery is an increasingly important aspect of the role of the intellectual disability nurse. Section 117 places a statutory duty on health and social authorities to plan the aftercare of people who have been detained under sections 3, 37 and 47 or 48. Whereas it is a statutory obligation to provide aftercare services, people subject to it are under no obligation to accept it.

The role of the nurse in relation to section 117 aftercare

As an integral member of the multidisciplinary team that is involved with the planning and delivery of aftercare, the nurse could be involved in the assessment of the person during their time in hospital and the planning for successful aftercare. The nurse (particularly the community nurse) may be involved with the monitoring of support arrangements under section 117, including the potential gaps in services that may exacerbate the clinical symptoms that warranted admission to hospital originally. This is skilled work involving the preparation of and presentation of regular progress reports. Aftercare arrangements are ended when the relevant social and health authorities are satisfied that they are no longer required. Nurses may well be in a position where their views are sought as to whether aftercare arrangements should end.

References

American Psychiatric Association (1994) *Diagnostic and Statistical Manual of Mental Disorders (DSM-IV)*, 4th edn. Washington, DC: American Psychiatric Association.

Audit Commission (2002) *Special Educational Needs: A Mainstream Issue*. London: Audit Commission Publications.

Audit Commission (2004) *Youth Justice 2004: A Review of the Reformed Youth Justice System*. London: Audit Commission Publications.

Ball, C. and Connolly, J. (2000) Educationally disaffected young offenders. *British Journal of Criminology* **40**, 594–616.

Barron, P., Hassiotis, A. and Banes, J. (2002) Offenders with intellectual disability: the size of the problem and therapeutic outcomes. *Journal of Intellectual Disability Research* **46** (6), 454–63.

Blanchard, R., Watson, M. and Choy, A. (1999) Paedophiles: mental retardation, maternal age and sexual orientation. *The Archives of Sexual Behavior* **28** (2), 111–27.

Bradford, J. and Dimock, J. (1986) A comparative study of adolescents and adults who wilfully set fires. *Psychiatric Journal of the University of Ottawa* **11**, 228–34.

Brown, H. and Barret, S. (1994) Understanding and responding to difficult sexual behaviour. In: *Practice Issues in Sexuality and Learning Disability* (Craft, A., ed.). London: Routledge.

Clare, I. (1993) Issues in the assessment and treatment of male sex offenders with mild learning disabilities. *Sexual and Marital Therapy* **8** (2), 167–80.

Clare, I. (1994) Treatment of men with learning disabilities who are perpetrators of sexual abuse: motivational difficulties and effects on practitioners. *National Association for the Protection from Sexual Abuse of Adults and Children with Learning Disabilities (NAPSAC) Newsletter* **8**, 3–6.

Clare, I. and Murphy, G. (1998) Working with offenders or alleged offenders with intellectual disabilities. In: *Clinical Psychology and People with Intellectual Disabilities* (Emerson, E., Hatton, C., Bromley, J. and Caine, A., eds.). Chichester: Wiley.

Cooper, A.J. (1995) Review of the role of two antilibidinal drugs in the treatment of sex offenders with mental retardation. *Mental Retardation* **33** (1), 42–8.

Department for Education and Skills (2003) *Together from the Start – Practical Guidance for Professionals Working with Disabled Children (Birth to Third Birthday) and Their Families*. London: Department for Education and Skills Publications.

Department of Health (1992) *Reed Report: Review of Mental Health and Social Services for Mentally Disordered Offenders and Others Requiring Similar Services: Vol. 1: Final Summary Report*. (Cm. 2088). London: Her Majesty's Stationery Office.

Department of Health (1994) *Guidance on the Discharge of Mentally Disordered People and their Continuing Care in the Community*. London: Her Majesty's Stationery Office.

Department of Health (1998) *The New NHS: Modern and Dependable. A National Framework for Assessing Performance*. London: Her Majesty's Stationery Office.

Department of Health (1999) *Reform of The Mental Health Act 1983: Proposals for Consultation. Cm 4480*. London: Her Majesty's Stationery Office.

Department of Health (2001) *Valuing People: A New Strategy for Learning Disability for the 21st Century*. London: Stationery Office.

Department of Health (2002) *Draft Mental Health Bill: Consultation Document*. London: Stationery Office.

Department of Health (2003) *Getting the Right Start: National Service Framework for Children*. London: Stationery Office.

Department of Health (2004) *Draft Mental Health Bill*. London: Stationery Office.

Department of Health (2005) *Mental Capacity Act*. London: Stationery Office.

Department of Information Service (2001) *Health Evidence Bulletins Learning Disabilities, Wales*. Cardiff : Department of Information Service.

Gudjonsson G.H., Clare, I., Rutter, S. and Pearce, J. (1993) *Persons at Risk During Interview in Police Custody: The Identification of Vulnerabilities*. Research Study No 12. The Royal Commission on Criminal Justice. London: Her Majesty's Stationery Office.

Hall, I. (2000) Young Offenders with a Learning Disability. *Advances in Psychiatric Treatment* **6** (4), 278–85.

Hayes, S. (1991) Sex Offenders. *Australia and New Zealand Journal of Developmental Disabilities* **17** (2), 221–7.

Hayes, S. (1997) Learning and intellectual disabilities and juvenile crime. In: *Juvenile Crime, Juvenile Justice and Juvenile Corrections* (Borowski, A. and O'Connor, I., eds.). Cheshire: Longman Publications.

Hayes, S. (2002) Early intervention or early incarceration using a screening test for intellectual disability in the criminal justice system. *Journal of Applied Research in Intellectual Disability* **15** (2), 120–8.

Holland, T., Clare, I. and Mukhopadhyay, T. (2002) Prevalence of 'criminal offending' by men and women with intellectual disability and the characteristics of 'offenders': Implications for research and service development. *Journal of Intellectual Disability Research* **46** Suppl 1, 6–20.

Home Office and Department of Health (1994) *Reviewing Health and Social Services for Mentally Disordered Offenders and Others Requiring Similar Services, Volume 7: People with Learning Disabilities (Mental Handicap) or with Autism*. London: Her Majesty's Stationery Office.

Jahoda, A. (2000) Offenders with a learning disability: the evidence for better services? *Journal of Applied Research in Intellectual Disabilities* **15** (2), 175–8.

LaVigna, G. and Donnellan, A. (1986) *Alternatives to Punishment: Solving Problems with Non-aversive Strategies*. New York: Irvington.

Mann, R. and Rollnick, S. (1996) Motivational interviewing with a sex offender who believed he was innocent. *Behavioural Psychotherapy* **24** (2), 129–35.

Mason, T. and Mercer, D. (1998) Introduction: the silent scream. In: *Critical Perspectives in Forensic Care* (Mason, T. and Mercer, D., eds.). Basingstoke: MacMillan Press.

McBrien, J. (2003) The intellectually disabled offender: methodological problems in identification. *Journal of Applied Research in Intellectual Disabilities* **1** (11), 95–105.

McCarthy, M. and Thompson, D. (1994) *Sex and the 3 Rs Rights, Responsibilities and Risks: A Sex Education Package For People Working With People With Learning Disabilities*. Brighton: Pavilion.

McCarthy, M. and Thompson, D. (1997) A prevalence study of sexual abuse of adults with intellectual disabilities referred for sex education. *Journal of Applied Research in Intellectual Disabilities* **10** (2), 105–24.

McIvor, R. (2001) Care and compulsion in community psychiatric treatment. *Psychiatric Bulletin* **25**, 369–70.

Mental Health Foundation (2004) *Draft Mental Health Bill: Memorandum from the Mental Health Foundation and the Foundation for People with Learning Disabilities*. London: The Mental Health Foundation.

Milne, R. (2001) Interviewing witnesses with learning disabilities for legal purposes. *British Journal of Learning Disabilities* **29** (3), 93–7.

Mind (2005) Mind: News policy and campaigns (online). Available at: www.mind.org.uk/
News+policy+and+cmpaigns/press/govtresponsetopls.htm

Morgan, S. (2000) *Clinical Risk Management*. London: The Sainsbury Centre for Mental
Health.

MORI (2004) *Youth Survey 2004*. London: Youth Justice Board for England and Wales.

Murphy, G. (1997) Working with offenders: assessment and intervention. In: *There are
No Easy Answers* (Churchill, J., Brown, H., Craft, A. and Horrocks, C., eds.). Chester-
field/Nottingham: ARC/National Association for the Protection from Sexual Abuse
of Adults and Children with Learning Disabilities (NAPSAC).

Murphy, G. and Mason, J. (1999) People with developmental disability who offend. In:
Psychiatric and Behavioural Disorders in Developmental Disabilities and Mental Retardation
(Bouras, N., ed.). Cambridge: Cambridge University Press.

Murphy, W.D., Coleman, E.M. and Haynes, M.R. (1983) Treatment and evaluation issues
with the mentally retarded sex offender. In: *The Sexual Aggressor: Current Perspectives
on Treatment* (Greer, J.G. and Stuart, I.R., eds.). New York: Van Nostrand.

Musker, M. (2001) Learning disability. In: *Forensic Mental Health: Issues in Practice* (Dale,
C., Thompson, T. and Woods, P., eds.). London: Bailliere Tindall.

Myers, B. (1991) Treatment of sexual offences by persons with developmental disabilities. *American Journal on Mental Retardation* **95** (5), 563–9.

Nihira, K., Leland, H. and Lambert, N. (1993) *AAMR Adaptive Behaviour Scales –
Residential and Community*, 2nd edn. Austin, Texas: American Association on Mental
Retardation.

O'Brien, J. and Tyne, A. (1981) *The Principle of Normalisation: A Foundation for Effective
Services*. London: Campaign for the Mentally Handicapped.

O'Conner, C.R., Rose, J. (1998) Sexual offending and abuse perpetrated by men with
learning disabilities: an integration of current research concerning assessment and
treatment. *Journal of Learning Disabilities for Nursing and Social Care* **2** (1), 31–8.

Phillips, J. (2004) Risk assessment and management of suicide and self harm within a
forensic setting. *Learning Disability Practice* **7** (2), 12–18.

Priest, H. and Gibbs, M. (2004) *Mental Health Care for People with Learning Disabilities*.
London: Churchill Livingstone.

Raesaenen, P., Hirvenoja, R., Hakko, H. and Vaeisaenen, E. (1994) Cognitive functioning ability of arsonists. *Journal of Forensic Psychiatry* **5**, 615–20.

Rowe, D. and Lopes, O. (2003) People with learning disabilities who have offended in
law. In: *Learning Disabilities: Toward Inclusion*, 4th edn, (Gates, B., ed.). Edinburgh:
Churchill Livingstone.

Rushton, J. (1994) Learning together. *Nursing Times* **90** (9), 44–6.

Rushton, J. (1995) Learning capers. *Nursing Times* **91** (16), 42–3.

Siegal, L. (2003) IQ – discrepancy definitions and the diagnosis of learning disability.
Journal of Learning Disabilities **36** (1), 2–3.

Simpson, M.K. and Hogg, J. (2001) Patterns of offending among people with intellectual
disability: a systematic review. Part 1: methodology and prevalence data. *Journal of
Intellectual Disability Research* **45** (5), 384–96.

White, J. and Dalby, J.D. (2000) Arson. In: *Forensic Mental Health Care* (Mercer, D.,
Mason, T., McKeown, M. and McCann, G., eds.). London: Churchill Livingstone.

Winter, N., Holland, A. and Collins, S. (1997) Factors predisposing to suspected offending by adults with self-reported learning disabilities. *Psychological Medicine* **27** (3),
595–607.

World Health Organization (1992) *The ICD–10 Classification of Mental And Behavioural Disorders*. Geneva: World Health Organization.

Further reading and resources

Two extremely useful documents from the Audit Commission. The first puts into context the developments within the youth justice system, what seems to be working well and what needs to be done to build on the reforms. The second document looks at how well the system of education meets the needs of children with special educational needs and considers their experience in four key stages: identifying needs, presence in mainstream school, participation and achievement.

Audit Commission (2002) *Special Educational Needs: A Mainstream Issue*. London: Audit Commission Publications.
Audit Commission (2004) *Youth Justice 2004, a Review of the Reformed Youth Justice System*. London: Audit Commission Publication. www.audit-commisson.gov.uk

Susan Hayes has completed extensive work in relation to people with intellectual disabilities who offend in the Criminal Justice System in New South Wales. Details of the Hayes Ability Screening Index can be found at www.usyd.edu.au/su/bsim/hasi

Hayes, S. (2001) Early intervention or early incarceration? Using a screening test for intellectual disability in the criminal justice system. *Journal of Applied Research in Intellectual Disabilities* **15**, 120–8.

Indicative reading for an independent view of the youth justice system can be found in the following: Goldson, B. (2000) *The New Youth Justice*. Dorset: Russell House Publishing.

Useful contacts

Adaptive Behaviour Scale: RC:2 (Adult), SC:2 (School), www.proedinc.com
Considers level of ability across daily living spectrum in relation to peers and adaptive behaviour.

Audit Commission: www.audit-commission.gov.uk
This independent public body has produced reports which relate to youth justice and special educational needs.

Children Now Magazine: www.childrennow.co.uk

Home Office Crime Statistics: www.crimereduction.gov.uk/statsindex.htm

NACRO, the crime reduction charity: www.nacro.org.uk
Independent voluntary organisation working to prevent crime. Useful website offering information in terms of news/publications and services.

National Association for Youth Justice (NAYJ): www.nayj.org.uk
Promoting the rights of, and justice for, children in trouble.

National Family and Parenting Institute: www.njpi.org.uk

reSearchWeb: researchweb.org.uk/challsex/cs4.html
This site supports social work in Scotland and provides a comprehensive literature review of all aspects of forensic issues relating to intellectual disabilities.

Young People Now Magazine: www.ypnmagazine.com

Youth Justice Board: www.youthjusticeboard.gov.uk
Provides a comprehensive overview of all aspects relating to youth justice, including legislation, research and available publications.

Youth Justice Trust: www.youth-justice-trust/org.uk
The Trust was set up in 1994 with Home Office funding. Its role is to act as a catalyst in bringing agencies together to tackle youth offending. Youth Justice Trust, 4th Floor, Cheetwood House, 21 Newton Street, Manchester M1 1FZ, UK.

0–19: www.zero2nineteen.co.uk
Publication for all who work with children and young people.

Chapter 8

Care planning in mental health settings

Laurence Taggart and Eamonn Slevin

Introduction

Mental illness is a distressing condition; it can disintegrate the personality or descend on one's life like a dark cloud and overshadow all aspects of one's personhood. If a person has an intellectual disability and a co-morbid mental illness or mental health problem, then this can compound the detrimental impact of these co-existing conditions. In this chapter we detail the pertinent issues associated with planning and delivering care for people with intellectual disabilities who have mental health problems. We begin with an initial discussion on key principles that guide the chapter; relevant aspects related to defining mental illness, its prevalence in the intellectually disabled population and other aspects of concern are then discussed. Following on from this, we offer guidance on the care planning process that will have value for intellectual disability nurses and other care staff who may work with this client group.

Key principles

A number of key principles have informed this chapter. Firstly, intellectual disability nurses, like all nurses, provide care through a process that involves five interrelated aspects, as detailed in Fig. 8.1. Second, some view a care plan as something that follows an assessment; here, however, care planning involves all five of these aspects, from assessment, identification of care needs, the planning and implementation of the care plan through to the evaluation (and reassessment, as and when required). The third key principle is that the plan of care aspires to a 'person-centred' approach (as can be seen in Fig. 8.1) i.e. the 'person' is at the centre; carers are partners. The focus is on what is important for the person and requirements to achieve this; it is about 'life' planning, and it involves openness, learning and future action (for further information on person-centred and life planning see Sanderson, 2003). Fourth, we do not present any one model or framework to guide the planning and delivery of care here as it is our belief, in keeping with the view of Aldridge (2004), that the nature of intellectual disability is so dynamic and multi-dimensional that

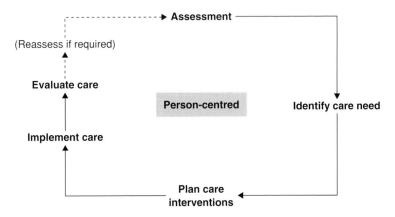

Fig. 8.1 The process of nursing.

no one theory or model can 'fit all' care. We therefore present several frameworks that have value when used eclectically in care delivery: this eclectic perspective is in recognition of the need for a multi-disciplinary care. Finally, we present a number of systematic frameworks for assessment and care planning, emphasising that a 'humanist' approach is essential and that 'therapeutic care' should be the cornerstone of nurses who work with people who have mental health problems. Watkins (2001) has stated:

> 'a phenomenological view of man does not try to impose any theoretical construct . . . but seeks to make sense of distressing and disturbing behaviour . . . in so doing it unshackles differentness from pathology.' (p. 5)

Definition of mental illness

There are many definitions of 'mental illness' or 'mental disorder' or 'psychiatric disorder', but a universal definition of 'mental illness' uses 'clinically recognisable patterns of psychological symptoms or behaviours causing acute or chronic ill health, personal distress or distress to others' (World Health Organization, 1996).

Similarly, there is also difficulty in obtaining an agreed term for 'mental illness' in people with intellectual disabilities. Bouras (1999b) has suggested that the term 'mental health problem' is more acceptable among the intellectually disabled community. A contemporary view envisages the co-morbidity of intellectual disabilities and mental health problems within the context of a 'bio-psycho-social' model (Fig. 8.2). This model acknowledges 'the complex interaction between biological, environmental, cultural and behavioural factors' (IASSID, 2001, p. 4). In this chapter the term 'mental health problems' is used, although depending on the context, the term 'psychiatric disorders' may also be employed where appropriate. Alongside this, the term 'dual diagnosis' is

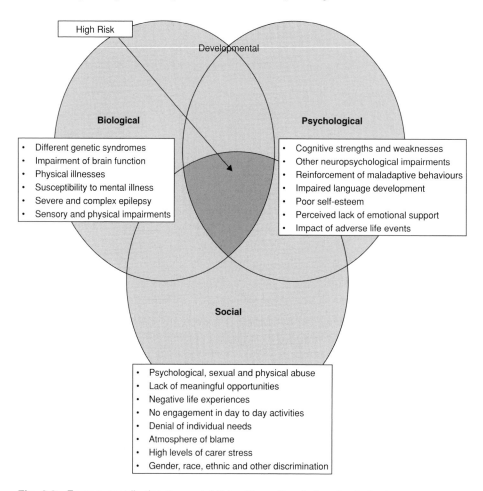

Fig. 8.2 Factors contributing to mental ill health and/or challenging behaviours (predisposing, precipitating and maintaining) (adapted from a report by the Mental Health Special Interest Research Group of the International Association for the Scientific Study of Intellectual Disabilities to the World Health Organization, 2001).

used to describe the co-morbidity of an intellectual disability and a mental health problem.

Aetiology of dual diagnosis

Understanding the factors that predispose, precipitate and/or maintain mental health problems in the population of people with intellectual disabilities is crucially important to the possible prevention, and overall care of people with these conditions. Fig. 8.2 shows that a dynamic interaction of biological, psychological, developmental and social factors may contribute to the development of a mental health problem in this population (Lowery and Sovner,

1992; Gardner and Sovner, 1994; IASSID, 2001). In the next section of this chapter a range of explanations that may predispose this population to develop a mental health problem will be explored.

Biological explanations

Several known causes of intellectual disabilities have been found to be linked to chromosomal/genetic abnormalities that may predispose the person to develop a specific mental health problem. The most obvious of these is people with Down's syndrome and its association with Alzheimer's disease. The Foundation for People with Intellectual Disabilities (2001) in the UK reported that prevalence rates of Alzheimer's disease in adults with Down's syndrome, between the ages of 50–59 years, were 36% compared with that of 5% for the general population. Organic brain damage, genetic abnormalities, cognitive deficits, communication problems and delayed development have also been identified as factors attributed to the development of a mental health problem in this population. It is also widely reported that a relationship exists between specific mental health problems, challenging behaviours and genetic disorders (for example Fragile X syndrome, Prader–Willi syndrome, Lesch–Nyan syndrome) (Clarke et al., 1995; Berney, 1997; State et al., 1997).

Psychosocial factors

Impaired intelligence concurrent with a low level of social ability may increase the risk of developing a mental health problem, particularly in a population that already has a limited range of coping behaviours to buffer the negative effects of daily life and stress. Limited communication skills and comprehension may further lead to difficulties in understanding or being understood. This can manifest itself in frustration and loss of motivation; such deficits may leave many people with an intellectual disability vulnerable to a range of psychosocial stresses that can lead to mental health problems.

It has been suggested that substantial numbers of people with an intellectual disability have experienced a range of negative life events (Russell, 1997). Such events include institutionalisation, labelling, stigmatisation, being bullied, frustration (i.e. lack of choice, inability to communicate), several separations and loss of carers, inadequacy in keeping up with peers and repeated failures in academic tasks. As a consequence of these negative life events Russell (1997) has further reported that many people with a mild intellectual disability experience feelings of worthlessness and low self-esteem.

Epidemiology of dual diagnosis

There is growing recognition that individuals with a borderline, mild and possibly a moderate intellectual disability do experience a similar range of neurotic and affective disorders as the general population. Psychotic disorders (e.g. schizophrenia) and personality disorders are also experienced, with more recent studies finding that a small number of persons with intellectual disability has a substance abuse disorder (Sturmey et al., 2003). For people with a severe/profound intellectual disability, higher rates of autism and challenging behaviours compared to the non-intellectual disabled population have been reported. It is clear from the literature that depression has received the greatest level of research interest.

Reader activity 8.1

How many people with intellectual disabilities do you work with that:

- Have a diagnosed 'mental health problem'?

or

- You suspect to have a 'mental health problem'?

There is a wide variation in the reported prevalence rates of people who have a dual diagnosis. Discrepancies centre upon methodological problems related to what is meant by a 'mental health problem', the method employed (that is, service user reports, family reports, staff reports), the type of classification system used to diagnose a mental health problem, whether 'behavioural disorders' are included within the diagnosis and the location of where the study took place (i.e. community or hospital samples). For the purpose of comparison Box 8.1 provides a summary of various prevalence rate studies of dual diagnosis. As can be seen, even in those studies that used samples of people with intellectual disabilities living in the community, prevalence rates were found to vary from between 39% and 49% (Reiss, 1990; Cooper and Bailey, 2001). Evidence suggests that people with intellectual disabilities are more likely to have a mental health problem than non-disabled people (Turkistani, 2003).

Reasons why mental health problems in people with intellectual disabilities are not recognised

Despite such alarming figures identified above, mental health problems in people with intellectual disabilities continue to go unnoticed and undetected. A number of explanations have been forwarded to explain this under-reporting and these are discussed below.

Diagnostic overshadowing

Historically, many health personnel believed that people with intellectual disabilities could not develop a mental health problem due to their cognitive and

Box 8.1 Prevalence rate studies of mental health problems in people with intellectual disabilities

Study	N	Sample characteristics	Prevalence
Corbett (1979)	402 (>14 yrs)	Population sample, based in London	46% prevalence (using ICD-8)
Jacobson (1982)	27 023 adults	New York: case records (66% aged 21–64 years)	12.4% of adults with a psychiatric disorder
Eaton and Menolascino (1982)	798 adults	Sample referred to community psychiatrists	14% received a psychiatric diagnosis
Lund (1985)	302 adults	Danish population based sample	28% (using modified version of DSM-3)
Iverson and Fox (1989)	165 adults	Community sample in the Midwestern USA	54% prevalence rate (using PIMRA)
Reiss (1990)	205 adults	Community based, day centre	39% prevalence rate (using Reiss Scale)
Borthwick-Duffy and Eyman (1990)	78 603 adults	Community sample in California (case records)	10% prevalence rate
Bouras and Drummond (1992)	318 adults	Community sample referred to a psychiatrist	41% prevalence rate (using DSM-3-R)
Hurst et al. (1994)	157 adults	Learning disability hospital in England	66% prevalence rate (using DSM-3-R)
Roy et al. (1997)	127 adults	Consecutive sample using case register	33% prevalence rate (PAS-ADD Checklist)
Cooper (1997)	73 adults	Population based In one area in the UK	43.8% prevalence rate (using PPS-LD)
Gustafsson (1997)	36 adults	Swedish based hospital sample	75% prevalence rate (using DSM-3)
Trower et al. (1998)	117 adults	Learning disability hospital in England	76.1% prevalence rate (using ICD-10)
Raitasuo et al. (1999)	40 adults	Swedish psychiatric hospital	100% prevalence rate (using ICD-10)
Cooper and Bailey (2001)	207 adults	Community sample in Leicestershire, England	49.2% prevalence rate using the PPS-LD
Deb et al. (2001a)	90 adults	A Welsh community sample	14.4% prevalence rate (using Mini PAS-ADD)
Taggart (2003)	154 adults	Northern Ireland Hospital Sample	65.6% prevalence rate (using DC-LD)
Taylor et al. (2004)	1155 adults	Community sample in north-east England	20.1% prevalence rate (PAS-ADD Checklist)

PAS-ADD = psychiatric assessment schedule for adults with developmental disabilities; DSM-3-R = diagnostic and statistical manual, 3rd edition – revised; PIMRA = psychopathology instrument for mentally retarded adults; PPS-LD = present psychiatric state for adults with learning disabilities.

emotional deficits associated with the 'organic' intellectual disability (Mason and Scior, 2004). Therefore, many felt that such mental health symptoms were associated with the person's intellectual disability rather than a separate psychiatric condition. Reiss et al. (1982) have called this 'diagnostic overshadowing'.

Presentation of 'atypical' symptomology

Schizophrenia symptomology may be similar to organic brain disorder or a pervasive developmental disorder (e.g. ritualistic behaviours, repetitive speech); nurses, therefore, need to be aware of this. Behaviours that are part of the person's disability may be mistaken as symptoms of a mental health problem, such as talking to self, solitary fantasy play, stereotypical movements, bizarre language, poor social skills and withdrawal; these are all symptoms that can be associated with schizophrenia. Clarke (1999) has indicated that these 'atypical' behaviours could lead to 'diagnostic confusion' and the rejection of a mental health problem existing at all.

Co-morbidity between challenging behaviours and mental health problems

Emerson et al. (1999) have highlighted that the presence of challenging behaviours can pose major difficulties in detecting mental health problems in people with intellectual disabilities. Despite such complexities in distinguishing between these co-existing problems other studies have established suggestive links between the presence of challenging behaviours and mental health problems (Lowery and Sovner, 1992; Reiss and Rojahn, 1993). Furthermore, studies have found a range of 'challenging behaviours' exhibited by people with intellectual disabilities, such as aggression, self-injurious behaviour, screaming, stereotypy and spontaneous crying, to be a secondary atypical feature of a psychiatric disorder among this population (Meins, 1995; Marston et al., 1997; Emerson et al., 1999).

Lack of education and training

Intellectual disability nurses are arguably in the best position to identify the early signs of deterioration in a person's mental health. However, it has been suggested that many nurses lack the skills and competence to recognise such conditions (Day, 1999; O'Dwyer, 2000). Gilbert et al. (1998) have also argued that although intellectual disability nurses have a key role to play in the detection, prevention and management of this population, the profession 'presently operates without a clear model of mental health' (p. 1151). Despite such criticisms, a number of advancements have occurred regarding training material and courses for nurses and other health personnel in the area of mental health problems in people with intellectual disabilities (see Resources at the end of this chapter).

Box 8.2   Aims of an assessment

- To identify the underlying reason(s) for a person's behaviours
- To identify patterns of normative behaviours and the changes in these normative behaviours (baseline distortion)
- To describe clearly the person's explicit behaviours in terms of quality of life, life events, gender and social mores
- To exclude any other explanations for the presenting behaviours, thereby formulating a 'working hypothesis' or suspected reasons for the behaviour(s)
- To develop a socially valid and effective intervention programme
- To determine whether a person is eligible for particular supports and who will provide these supports
- To provide a basis so the implemented care can be evaluated/re-assessed

Assessment

Assessing the mental health needs of people with intellectual disabilities is a core role of the intellectual disability nurse. Assessments are necessary for a number of key reasons (see Box 8.2). However, given the complexities regarding the cause of such problems and lack of training by many health staff, it is clear that other factors in the individual's wider intra- and inter-ecological context will have to be considered in order to assess accurately the mental health needs of the person.

Reader activity 8.2

How would you describe to a doctor that you feel sad because your mother has died, and that you do not want to go to the day-centre, if you have no verbal communication skills?

Reader activity 8.3

How would you describe the concepts of self-esteem and guilt? You might find this challenging, even when you have good verbal communication skills. Now imagine someone with intellectual disabilities undertaking the same exercise.

The diagnosis of the majority of psychiatric disorders primarily relies upon the ability of the 'patient' to communicate their own experiences to a psychiatrist or psychologist, but this ability may be impaired or absent altogether, given the associated cognitive deficits and communication problems inherent in this population. However, as highlighted by Barker (2004), psychiatrists draw significantly on reports from nurses in making a diagnosis. This being so, it is crucial that nurses are skilled in accurately and validly reporting manifestations of mental health problems. Nursing assessments can be difficult and the nurse assessing such individuals will often have to rely strongly upon behavioural observations, as many clients are unable to describe their inner world and feelings.

For those individuals who have a mild intellectual disability, a number of other linguistic barriers may be present but go unnoticed. For example, the type of questions employed in psychiatric classification systems may be too abstract for an individual to understand (for example the concept of self-esteem or guilt). Similarly, sentence structure can be quite complex and lengthy. Studies show that persons with an intellectual disability are more likely to 'acquiesce' or 'agree' to what they believe the interviewer wants to hear. Moss (1999) has concluded that the interviewing of people with an intellectual disability about their mental state is difficult. It is fundamental that nurses and other health professionals can recognise, and report, the signs and symptoms exhibited by the individual early on, therefore making a more prompt referral to appropriate specialists for a comprehensive assessment.

Emerson et al. (1998) have indicated that a wider framework is required for the provision of an accurate assessment, a clinical diagnosis and the development of 'socially valid efficacious interventions'. Two standardised assessment frameworks have been developed using the 'bio-psycho-social' model (see Fig. 8.2) as advocated by IASSID (2001) to guide nurses to make a comprehensive assessment:

- An expert panel of psychiatrists and psychologists reported a number of preferred methods for the assessment of psychiatric disorders and behavioural problems in this population in the *American Journal on Mental Retardation* (May 2000) (Aman et al., 2000)
- The European Association for Mental Health in Mental Retardation (see Deb et al., 2001) have published guidelines on the assessment and diagnosis of dual diagnosis

Both these practice guidelines indicate that a systematic and wide-ranging approach is necessary to provide an accurate diagnosis of this population's holistic needs (Box 8.3).

Advances in the assessment and detection of dual diagnosis

In the last decade there have been considerable advances made in the recognition, detection and classification of mental health problems in people with intellectual disabilities. Given the difficulties with diagnosis of this population, mainstream psychiatric classification systems (ICD-10 or DSM-4) are limited in detecting problems and a number of authors have argued that caution is required if such systems are used as part of a diagnosis process (Sturmey and Bertman, 1995; Moss, 1999).

Box 8.3   Structured assessment frameworks

Aman et al. (2000)

- Interview with carers
- Direct observation
- A medical history and physical examination
- Functional/behavioural analysis
- Medication and side-effects investigation (i.e. scales)
- Unstructured psychiatric interview
- Standardised rating scales
- Laboratory tests (i.e. blood levels of medication, toxicology)

Deb et al. (2001)

- Family history
- Personal history
- Developmental history
- Medical history
- Psychiatric history
- Social history
- Drug history
- Forensic history
- History of presenting complaint

DC-LD: diagnostic criteria for psychiatric disorders

A more recent development has seen the publication of the DC-LD: diagnostic criteria for psychiatric disorders for use with adults with intellectual disabilities/ mental retardation, by the Penrose Society (the UK's intellectual disabilities research group for medical doctors) and The Royal College of Psychiatrists (2001). The aim of this classification system is 'to improve upon existing general population psychiatric diagnostic classificatory systems' for the intellectual disability population (p. 2). The DC-LD system reflects current practice within both the UK and the Republic of Ireland (Box 8.4). A special supplement of the *Journal of Intellectual Disability Research* (September 2003, Vol. 47(1), 1–83) provided a series of research papers that examined the use of DC-LD with this population. This offers readers a valuable insight into methods of diagnosing dual diagnosis.

Screening tools

In order to provide a comprehensive diagnostic assessment, it is important that nurses gather information from a range of relevant sources. One such method that can be employed is the use of behavioural rating scales and early screening tools (see Box 8.5). The Department of Health has recently published 'good practice' guidelines in relation to the use of screening tools for the early recognition and detection of mental health problems in this population (*Signposts for Success*, Department of Health, 1998). These guidelines emphasise that the utilisation of such instruments may avoid the need for crisis management and prevent placement breakdown from occurring, therefore nurses can obtain a more prompt referral to the appropriate specialists for a comprehensive assessment. Saunders (2001) has stated that the 'early screening of people

Box 8.4   A hierarchical approach to diagnosis (DC-LD)

Axis	Disorder
Axis 1	Severity of intellectual disabilities (i.e. mild, moderate, profound)
Axis 2	Cause of intellectual disabilities (i.e. infectious and metabolic diseases, chromosomal abnormalities and injurious)
Axis 3	Psychiatric disorders
DC-LD level A	Developmental disorders (i.e. autism)
DC-LD level B	Psychiatric illness (i.e. dementia, psychotic, affective, stress related, adjustment, eating and hyperkinetic disorders)
DC-LD level C	Personality disorders (i.e. paranoid, dissocial, emotionally unstable, histrionic and anankastic personality disorders)
DC-LD level D	Problem behaviours (i.e. verbally and physically aggressive, destructive, self-injurious, sexually inappropriate and opposition behaviours)
DC-LD level E	Other disorders (i.e. mental and behavioural disorders due to alcohol, drugs, non-organic sleep disorders, sexual dysfunction, habit and impulse distress, gender identity disorders)

Box 8.5   Behavioural rating scales for challenging behaviour and mental health problems

Aman et al. (2000)

- Adaptive behaviour scale (Nihja et al., 1993)
- Aberrant behaviour scale (Aman and Singh, 1986): 'gold standard'
- Conner's parent and teacher rating scale
- Vineland adaptive behaviour scale Pt2
- Child behaviour checklist
- Reiss screen for maladaptive behaviour
- Psychopathology inventory for mentally retarded adults (PIMRA)
- Diagnostic assessment of severely handicapped (DASH-11)
- Reiss scale for children's dual diagnosis
- Behavioural and emotional rating scale (BeERS)

Deb et al. (2001)

- CANDID – a needs assessment tool (Xentiditis et al., 2000)
- DASH – a scale for severely LD (Matson et al., 1991)
- Mental retardation depression scale (Meins, 1993, 1996)
- Self-report depression questionnaire (Reynolds and Baker, 1988)
- Yale-Brown OCD Scale (Feurer et al., 1998)
- Dementia scale for DS (Deb and Braganza, 1999)
- PIMRA (Matson et al., 1984)
- REISS (Reiss, 1988)
- PAS-ADD Checklist (Moss, 2002)
- Mini PAS-ADD Interview (Moss, 2002)

who have a intellectual disability has the potential to become one of the most contentious issues of the new millennium' due to the 'cost and benefits' that health screening can lead to (p. 37).

Challenging behaviour rating scales

Emerson et al. (1999) have reported that since a close relationship exists between challenging behaviours and mental health problems it is important to identify clearly and describe the challenging behaviours exhibited. A number of scales have been developed to describe the frequency of challenging behaviours in this population (see Box 8.5). An expert panel of psychiatrists and psychosocial experts in the USA (Aman et al., 2000) identified the aberrant behaviour checklist (ABC) (Aman and Singh, 1986) as the 'goldstar' of rating scales for assessing behavioural, and also psychiatric problems in this population.

Mental health screening tools

Several mental health screening instruments have been published regarding screening for general and specific mental health symptoms in people with intellectual disabilities. Among these are the following American instruments:

- The psychopathology instrument for mentally retarded adults (PIMRA) (Matson et al., 1984)
- The REISS Screen (Reiss, 1988)
- The diagnostic assessment for the severely handicapped (DASH) (Matson et al., 1991)

Although used on both sides of the Atlantic (Deb et al., 2001), these scales have been criticised as they are based upon the explicit behaviours presented rather than specific mental health symptomology (Sturmey and Bertman, 1995).

PAS-ADD schedules

Within the UK, the PAS-ADD schedules (psychiatric assessment schedule for adults with development disabilities) have been developed (see Box 8.6). The PAS-ADD checklist (revised) (Moss, 2002) is a 27-item screening instrument examining three broad psychiatric disorders: affective/neurotic disorders, organic conditions and psychotic disorders. This is an efficient tool that can identify and monitor those most at risk. If a mental health problem has been detected within the PAS-ADD checklist then a mini PAS-ADD interview should be conducted.

The mini PAS-ADD interview (Moss, 2002) probes a wider range of mental health symptoms and behaviours than the PAS-ADD checklist. The format involves the nurse, after training, interviewing the person's key informant (for example, the carer, day-care worker, residential worker) about the person's behaviours over approximately the previous 4-week period. Alternatively, the interview can also be self-completed by the nurse if no key informant is

---

Box 8.6   Example items within the PAS-ADD schedules

Mini PAS-ADD interview

Item 14. Is N happy?
Probes: Does N ever feel depressed? How does he/she show it? What does he/she do? Does he/she cry? Can he/she snap out of it? How often is he/she depressed?

Item 25. Does N get very anxious in special places or situations?
Probes: On the bus? When out alone? When there are dogs or spiders?

Item 42. What can you tell me about the voices?
Probes: How many voices are there? Do you know who the voices are? Do they talk to each other? What do they say? How often do you hear them? Do you hear them at a particular time?

PAS-ADD 10 interview

Item W 3. When you get anxious, do you feel anything in your body?
Probes: Heart pounding, sweating, hot or cold flushes, trembling hands, churning stomach, can't get a breath.

Item AH 1: Do you hear voices?
Probes: Do you hear them during the day? Do you hear them at night? Do you hear them when you are waking up? Do you hear them any other times? When?

TD2: Do people read your thoughts?
Probes: Can someone know what you are thinking even if you say nothing? How does this happen? Do people know from the look on your face?

---

available. Using 66 questions the mini PAS-ADD interview investigates seven key areas of potential mental health problems; these include depression, anxiety and phobias, hypomania, obsessive–compulsive disorder, psychosis, unspecified (dementia) and developmental disorders. Furthermore, the mini PAS-ADD interview can also be used to monitor the impact of a treatment upon the persons' health to examine if the intervention(s) has been successful.

During the interview, the nurse uses an interview score sheet and a clinical glossary that provides questions, definitions, probes and indicates how to rate the severity of each symptom (see Box 8.6). Like the PAS-ADD checklist, the mini PAS-ADD interview also uses the scores of each item to tally the different psychiatric disorders. When these are obtained then the scores can be compared against 'threshold' scores that indicate whether a potential psychiatric disorder is present or not. It is, however, important to note that both the checklist and the mini PAS-ADD interview do not provide an actual psychiatric diagnosis but rather the necessity for a further detailed psychiatric assessment by a psychiatrist or psychologist. One such possible method for diagnosing a psychiatric disorder is to interview the person using the PAS-ADD 10 interview.

The PAS-ADD 10 interview (Moss, 2002) has been shown to be a reliable and valid method for interviewing people with intellectual disabilities (Moss et al., 1993). The questions asked in this semi-structured interview are flexible, less complicated and allow for a number of probes to be used (see Box 8.6). Moss (2002) has described the PAS-ADD 10 interview as the 'gold standard' of clinical interviewing of people with intellectual disabilities.

Nursing models

Nurses can use a combination of instruments to undertake assessments of the mental health needs of clients. Some of the above instruments may be usefully integrated with an appropriate nursing model to guide nursing assessments, or nurses may use the outcomes from such assessments within a multi-disciplinary co-ordinated person-centred approach. As stated at the beginning of this chapter, no one specific model is advocated, as there is a number of models to choose from, and in practice a combination of suitable models may be useful rather than using one model for all clients. Examples of nursing models that may be of use for this client group are listed in Box 8.7.

Some of these models are useful and could be used by intellectual disability nurses to frame assessments and subsequent care delivery. For example, Peplau's (1991) theory focuses on psychodynamic aspects and provides a model particularly suited to the care of people with mental health problems. Also, the value of King's (1981) model, as can be seen in Box 8.7, guides the assessor to consider aspects within three systems, personal, interpersonal and social. This allows for a comprehensive assessment to focus on the individual and

---

Box 8.7   Examples of some nursing models that may be useful in practice

Author	Focus	Who it might benefit
Peplau (1991) (1952 original publication)	Psychodynamic and focus is on: • Development of therapeutic relationship • Esteem building • Education and helping • Cooperation in care • Counselling and interaction • Surrogate/advocacy • Clinical Phases in nurse-patient relationship • Orientation to the illness/need • Identification of assessed need • Exploitation capturing care relationships to heal • Resolution letting go recovery, or acceptance of life change	People with learning disabilities who have a mental illness requiring psychodynamic care. People with 'unmet need, incomplete life skill development, frustration and opposing goals giving rise to conflict, aggression, and anxiety' (Meleis, 1997, p. 191)

King (1981)	Interaction and goal realisation focus is on:		People with learning disabilities who have a mental illness that is amenable to: nursing interactions, family support, community participation enhancement, environmental change
	• Growth and development • Perceptions of self/others	personal system	
	• Communication • Life role • Interaction • Transaction	interpersonal system	
	• Stress • Community/society • Decision-making/ power	social systems	
Orem (1991)	Self-care or self-care deficit focus is on: • Universal self-care needs • Self-care need alternations due to health • Self-care needs due to developmental problems		Self-care may be limited due to person's intellectual disability but has value in guiding care towards promoting the person's optimum self-care ability and identification of aspects requiring support
Paterson and Zderad (1988)	Philosophical and existential focus is on: • Presence and relating to others with humility • Authentic caring • Openness to the other person • Knowing the other person intuitively • Reality in caring situations which are objective, subjective and intersubjective		People who have lost (or never had) a sense of 'belonging', or who require affirmation as a person and that as a human being they are valued

what personal factors may or may not be contributing to their health need; what interpersonal aspects such as interactions with others (or lack of) are relevant; and social systems such as environment, the community the person lives in and wider societal aspects. This model has value across a range of settings and has a lot to offer the intellectual disability nurse when working with people with dual diagnosis. (For further detail on King's model see Frey and Sieloff, 1995.)

Orem's (1991) self-care deficit model, which focuses on self-care ability, is another model that is useful from two perspectives. First, it can guide the person towards regaining, or developing, whatever degree of self-care is viable given their intellectual disability. Second, it can be used to identify those areas in which the person has a self-care deficit and thus allow for supportive care to be directed towards this. Despite this model's broad application across a variety of mental health settings, nurses have rarely applied this model to people with intellectual disabilities. Nevertheless, Horan et al. (2004a, b) have reported upon a number of anecdotal examples of how this model is being successfully applied to this client group and how this model promotes those philosophical goals of normalisation, social role valorisation and community integration that have underpinned recent service developments. This model acknowledges the dynamic interplay between the physical, psychological, environmental and social worlds of the person thereby providing greater meaning in understanding the person's behaviours: that is both their challenging behaviours and/or mental health problems. Such components equate to the model that IASSID (2001) proposed to the World Health Organization (see Fig. 8.2) regarding the factors that may predispose, precipitate and/or maintain challenging behaviours and mental health problems in this client group. One of the strengths of this holistic model is that it focuses upon supporting and educating the person to manage their current and potential problems. Although optimistic, this model will have to be tested with this population of people.

Referring to Paterson and Zderad's (1988) model, Kirby (1999, p. 418) has stated it has relevance to 'psycho-therapy that involves a cognitive or existential approach'. Their model is one of a number that fall within the rubric of 'humanistic nursing'. While abstract, as guidance such approaches have value in instilling in nurses ways to think about and relate to clients. Cognitive and existential approaches may only have value to people with the cognitive ability to self-negotiate. But, we suggest 'humanistic nursing' has immense value even for people with more severe disability as it opens up areas such as presence, therapeutic touch, reaching the other at a spiritual level, using the senses, valuing personhood and not merely focusing on 'ability' or 'disability'. These issues are so important to mental health that they should be considered in all assessments of this client group. Kirby (2003, p. 531) has stated 'the nursing voice speaks in the name of humanity; the human heart opens and responds in a caring-healing presence'.

Identification of care need

Within the process of nurse care planning and delivery the essential aspect of 'identification of need', which follows assessment, is often not given the attention it merits. With people who have, or are suspected of having, a dual diagnosis the outcome of an assessment should be stated, bearing in mind the following considerations:

- We use the term 'identification of need', as the outcome to an assessment as this may not always be considered as a 'problem'. When stated as a 'problem' it can also be portrayed as a negative way of viewing people with intellectual disabilities. Although if a clear 'problem' is identified then this should be stated in precise terms. Gates (2003, p. 226) has stated 'imprecise terminology [can lead to] some distressing conditions [being] to some extent trivialised'. Many needs that are identified following an assessment will relate to a requirement to focus on a person's positive aspects; and, as discussed above, for some it may be the need to be valued as a 'human being'

- Regarding a nursing assessment 'identification of need' will usually be stated in terms of relatively objective behaviours, for example: 'John isolates himself from others by not leaving his room'
- Subjective views are limiting in the care of this client group but 'patterns' of relating behaviours, history of life events, or ecological aspects can lead to a 'hypothesis' of the care need (which should be varied by further assessments and evaluations), for example: 'John has potentially a neurotic illness related to his recent displacement from his own home to a group living environment.' This potential mental health need would then be verified, or not, by a co-ordinated multi-disciplinary assessment
- The client and family should be at the centre of the care plan, and whenever this is possible should jointly agree the care need. For some clients the mental health problem or intellectual disability may limit their insight and in such cases the nurse will use the family, the multi-disciplinary team, advocacy systems and human rights considerations to empower the person to their optimum level. Being able to contribute at some level can be empowering and affirming for people who are undervalued. The following comment should be kept in mind: 'the person who can't presumably could if something wasn't stopping him.' (Barker, 2004, p. 205)

The plan of care

Following assessment and need identification, a structured systematic plan of interventions should be constructed. A dilemma exists with structured written care plans and this relates to the legal requirements to document care on the one hand, and on the other the view that many written plans usually lead to routine interventions (Carpenito, 1999). Indeed the time spent on administration of written plans can impinge on the nurse's time to provide 'hands on' interventions. Carpenito further poses the question: 'What does the nurse need to know to provide, responsible competent care to an individual?' Some general principles are outlined here with actual interventions being detailed in the next section. The authors suggest that the aspects listed in Box 8.8 are the main elements that are required in most care plans for dually diagnosed people. However, any plan needs to be dynamic to allow flexibility to changing circumstances in care encounters. Local policy issues will influence such things as:

Box 8.8 Outline of what should be contained within a nursing care plan

History and assessments

- Relevant history of the person
- Relevant conditions related to health, mental health, social and life skills
- Significant other people for the person
- Results of assessments undertaken
- Person's abilities and disabilities

Identified needs

- Clear statements of care needs (at this time)
- Concurrent needs that may impact on care

Planned care

- Statement of goals to be achieved
- Sub-goals if required
- Parameters of care, time-limiting, prolonged without limit, life-long
- User involvement and person at centre
- Who will provide what aspects
- Review and evaluation dates

Interventions

- Therapeutic interventions
- Education interventions/health promotion
- Biopsychsocial interventions
- Humanistic spiritual/relational interventions
- Environmental change
- Clinical interventions
- Provide leadership and co-ordinate other care agencies as required

Evaluations

- Methods of evaluation
- Process/continual evaluation
- Periodic evaluation
- Set reviews

For each of the above:

- Who will undertake (team/individual)
- Who will co-ordinate
- When will it be undertaken
- How is care to be recorded
- Client and service user involvement
- Are referrals required
- Is active discharge from care provider/team planned

- Do individual professional groups maintain separate care plans?
- Are care plans integrated within central multi-disciplinary core documentation?
- Whether or not plans are hand written or computerised
- If plans espouse to 'person-centeredness', are they client/service user held?

Implementation of care strategies

The neglect of the mental health needs of people with intellectual disabilities over the last century can clearly be observed in the corresponding lack of developments in the provision of eclectic interventions and services. Historically, the only treatment that was afforded to people with a dual diagnosis was containment within locked wards in the institutions/intellectual disability hospitals, or chemical restraint by medication. However, from undertaking a comprehensive holistic assessment a multi-modal plan of care that may include behavioural approaches, other psychological interventions, changes in the person's environment, improving communication, social skills training and medications (if required), can be implemented. In addition, the humanistic ways of relating to people already alluded to, have potential value to counter the reductionist medical and deficit psychiatric models that may disenfranchise the humanity of this population, thereby providing a more holistic and pro-active approach to care planning and delivery for this client group.

The following section discusses the evidence of the successes, along with the limitations, of such bio-psycho-social interventions that can be incorporated into the care plan that forms the nature of the delivery of care. As no one factor can be fully attributed to the possible cause of the mental health problem, or of challenging behaviours, then to no one intervention can be used: care planning and delivery should embed this bio-psycho-social approach.

Behavioural interventions

The main use of behavioural interventions is the reduction/eradication of challenging behaviours and the development of a broad array of new social competencies, through the application of operant conditioning principles, otherwise known as 'behaviour modification' or 'behaviour therapy'. These include:

- Behavioural parent and teacher/staff training
- Behaviour-accelerating procedures (that is, differential reinforcement of alternative behaviour (DRO) or incompatible behaviour (DRI) and social skills and communication training)
- Behaviour-decelerating techniques (i.e. extinction, over-correction, response cost, response interruption and prevention, non-exclusionary time-out, exclusionary time-out). Some of these methods are considered aversive and increasingly, based on La Vigna and Donnellan (1986) and others, such strategies are being rejected in favour of non-aversive techniques

In terms of using behavioural interventions to address specific mental health problems, techniques like systematic desensitisation and exposure therapy that use cognitive reasoning processes and graduated involvement in anxiety-inducing events, have been reported to be effective in treating anxiety-related disorders and extinguishing phobic disorders in the non-disabled population. However, no methodologically robust studies have been conducted to examine the efficacy of these types of behavioural therapies in people with intellectual disabilities. A small number of single-case studies do exist that suggest such strategies can be effective in reducing simple phobias. Similarly, behavioural treatment of depression in people with intellectual disabilities has focused upon verbal statements, self-management, modelling, self-evaluation, self-reinforcement and social interaction. Despite the advances in these behavioural interventions, Emerson et al. (2000) have purported that many people with severe challenging behaviours and mental health problems are unlikely to receive effective behavioural support in the UK.

Psychotherapy

Access to psychotherapy[1] and counselling[2] for this population is limited, despite the fact that this individual group may have additional emotional needs compared to the non-disabled population. Psychotherapists have queried this population's intellectual and cognitive abilities relating to their abstract thought processes, and the necessity of communication skills, for the individual to successfully participate in this therapy. Freud stated that psychotherapy was not suitable for 'those patients who do not possess a reasonable degree of education and a fairly reliable character' (1953, p. 263). Since then, Tyson and Sandler (1971) have indicated that many therapists have strictly adhered to this principle. How much of this is due to belief of efficacy of such therapies with this population and how much to prejudice is questionable. However, Beail (2003) has suggested that by using a more directive and flexible approach, psychotherapy could be used for people with a mild to moderate intellectual disability.

Counselling

Mencap (1999), in a large national survey on 'The NHS: Health for All?' across England, Wales and Northern Ireland, reported that the availability of counselling services for people with intellectual disabilities was low, particularly in relation to bereavement. One possible explanation for this finding may be the limited number of care staff with training in counselling skills. Hassiotis (1999) has stated that psychotherapy and counselling within the UK is:

---

[1] Dawson and Morgan (1997) indicated that 'psychotherapy' covers a wide range of approaches; however 'psychotherapy' in this context will be defined as psychodynamic therapy.
[2] The AJMR (Aman et al., 2000) defines counselling or 'supportive counselling' in the field of intellectual disabilities as advice, providing a friendly relationship, affirming the individual's worth. This can be provided in a group or individual format.

'hardly ever available in standard practice ... and adult psychotherapy departments refuse to see such patients or supervise staff who are willing to engage in this work, claiming a lack of knowledge of intellectual disabilities.' (p. 106)

Cognitive behaviour therapy

Hollins and Sinason (2000) have indicated that people with intellectual disabilities rarely receive cognitive behaviour therapy in the UK. A number of explanations have been forwarded to account for this. One problem which is common to cognitive behaviour therapy, psychotherapy and counselling, is that these 'talk therapies' for people with intellectual disabilities involve 'a certain kind of intimacy. ... over a long period of time' (Bender, 1993, p. 11). Bender adds that some professionals might have negative attitudes towards the application of talk therapies with intellectually disabled individuals. A second and fundamental problem is that the rationale underpinning cognitive behaviour therapy is that psychological dysfunction is mainly due to cognitive distortions, therefore the individual must verbally express their inner thoughts (that is, self-report) (Young and Beck, 1982). However, for many individuals with an intellectual disability there is a number of associated cognitive deficits and communication difficulties that may hinder this, such as incomprehension, memory problems, acquiescence, dependency, recency effects, social desirability and anxiety; these question the reliability and validity of such self-reports. Thirdly, Hassiotis (1999) has indicated that there is a serious shortage of trained practitioners in the use of cognitive behaviour therapy, psychotherapy and counselling in the UK for people with intellectual disabilities.

Despite criticism, a number of clinicians are starting to use cognitive behaviour therapy for people with intellectual disabilities and have found that they can successfully enter into a therapeutic relationship/alliance (Stenfert Kroese et al., 1997). The intellectual and linguistic barriers experienced by this population are now being overcome with the development of alternative self-report techniques. For example, Kabzems (1985) and Helsel and Matson (1988) have used pictorial and multiple choice options in adjunct to auditory presentations. Jahoda et al. (1989) indicated that the therapist should spend time with the individual prior to the interview, therefore diminishing the effects of social desirability, anxiety and incomprehension.

Promoting a caring therapeutic environment

Collins (1999) has found that mental health problems in people with intellectual disabilities rarely existed in isolation, and that such problems are almost invariably associated with the individual's psychosocial environment. Within the behavioural perspective, environmental antecedents and consequences have been shown largely to affect challenging behaviours, particularly with the employment of a 'functional analysis'. In addition, several other approaches have been found to affect indirectly whether individuals exhibit disruptive and psychiatric behaviours. These include enriching the environment, changing the nature of preceding activities and changing the context of activities that elicit challenging behaviour (Saunders and Spradlin, 1991; Horner et al., 1996). These approaches have been found to bring about significant and rapid reductions in challenging behaviour and have also been found feasible to implement and sustain over time (Emerson et al., 1998).

Reese and Leeder (1990) have examined the 'ecobehavioural settings' of residential facilities for people with intellectual disabilities. The authors indicated that a number of environmental conditions (group size, population density, staff ratio, noise level, room temperature and location in the community) may affect the frequency and intensity of behavioural and psychiatric symptoms.

Psychopharmacology

Psycho-active medications have been universally prescribed to manage aggression, self-injurious behaviour, stereotypic behaviours and hyperactivity in people with intellectual disabilities. However, Brylewski and Duggan (1999), in a systematic review of the effectiveness of these medications, reported that there was inconclusive evidence to support their use. More alarmingly, these drug regimes were mainly employed for their sedative and calming properties. Duggan and Brylewski (1999) have questioned the efficacy of these drugs in treating schizophrenia in people with intellectual disabilities. It appears that psycho-active drug regimes are often used for sedentary and calming effects rather than therapeutic properties.

Nonetheless medication has a role to play in the treatment of mental illness in dually diagnosed people. Despite the warnings alluded to above, Aman et al. (2000) have highlighted that medication remains the first line of defence in managing both challenging behaviours and psychiatric disorders in persons with an intellectual disability. However, as Fleisher (1999) has stated:

> 'the use of medication must be a therapeutic treatment element that is part of a larger plan, and not a tool to create a convenient respite for medical personnel or for caregivers.' (p. 317)

Medication, when used, should be considered to be part of the overall integrated care plan and should be regularly reviewed and used for a minimum period of time.

Expert consensus on clinical interventions

As noted earlier in this chapter, an expert panel of psychiatrists and psychologists in the USA developed guidelines regarding the 'treatment of psychiatric and behavioural problems' for people with intellectual disabilities (Aman et al., 2000). The guidelines provide a bridge between the current scientific

---

Box 8.9   Guidelines on psychosocial interventions

- Individual and/or family education: helping individuals/family/carers to understand more about the behavioural and mental health problems that may accompany the intellectual disability and how to manage these problems
- Applied behaviour analysis: techniques that are based on the principles and methods of behaviour analysis and are intended to build appropriate, functional skills and reduce problem behaviour
- Managing the environment: reducing problem behaviours by rearranging the physical/social conditions that seem to provoke them, for example changes in each person's activities, work, social groupings, physical environment (i.e. noise, crowding) and/or enrichment of the environment through social or sensory stimulation
- Cognitive behaviour therapy: techniques that focus upon the underlying thought processes, perceptions and unrealistic expectations, attitudes and emotions (that is, anger management, conflict resolution and assertiveness training)
- Supportive counselling: advice, providing a friendly relationship, affirming the individual's worth
- Classical behavioural therapy: techniques that are primarily based upon classical conditioning principles, for example, vivo exposure (flooding), imaginary exposure, systematic desensitisation, progressive relaxation and biofeedback
- Psychotherapy: problem solving, promoting self-understanding, allowing emotional release

---

research on treatment efficacy and also clinical practice. These guidelines are based upon the most recent clinical and research evidence; they are targeted not only at clinicians, but also at policy planners, service providers and managers.

In addition to indicating that medication was the first line of defence in the treatment of a psychiatric disorder, the panel also identified seven 'psychosocial interventions' that they recommended across a variety of circumstances alongside medication (see Box 8.9). These circumstances included children, adolescents and adults; mild, moderate to severe/profound intellectual disabilities; from mild to persistent problem behaviours and for a wide variety of mental health problems. From these seven psychosocial interventions in Box 8.9 the panel uniformly agreed upon three interventions that 'were the most highly recommended in almost every situation': applied behaviour analysis, managing the environment, and individual and/or family education (Aman et al., 2000, p. 171).

Humanistic nursing care

The intellectual disability nurse will incorporate a range of the above interventions in care-planning and delivery, or co-ordinate others who are skilled in these approaches as required. Humanistic care is therapeutic and has an obvious central role in interventions such as counselling or psychotherapy (Kirby, 1999).

It should also impact on all that nurses do in their work with this client group. In their day-to-day caring work, nurses need to reach out to people with a dual diagnosis and touch them with therapeutic connections, thereby developing this therapeutic alliance and rapport, which has been purported to be an important part in any therapeutic success. For example, empathetic understanding, being attuned to the person's passive communication signals including their non-verbal cues, and supporting the person by journeying with them in their pain by ensuring 'unconditional positive regard, empathy and a genuineness' for them and their situation (Rogers, 1951). Long (2003) has stated that:

'therapeutic connecting is one of the key interaction constructs in effective human-with-human relationships.' (p. 755)

This is done by how the nurse relates to the other person, by listening, showing kindness, understanding and affirming the uniqueness of the individual. It is done by unconditional acceptance of the client as an authentic person who has needs for love, self-expression, honesty, trust and compassion.

When clients were surveyed about what they needed when distressed due to mental illness many of their responses mirrored the humanistic care called for here. Examples of these include (Mental Health Foundation, 1997):

- Someone to listen to me and whom I can talk to
- Help with feelings and emotions
- Spiritual care
- Help with social coping and acceptance
- A place to be safe and to relax
- Privacy and peace
- Easier access to psychiatric care when unwell

These reported needs were from people with mental health distress who did not have an intellectual disability, but we argue that the need for 'humanistic care' is universal and it transcends age, ability and condition and should be a core role of all nurses:

'The call I hear is for nursing. It is the call for humanity to maintain the humanness in the healthcare system which is becoming increasingly sophisticated in technology, increasingly concerned with cost containment, and increasingly less aware and concerned with the patient as a human being.' (Kleiman, 1993, p. 45)

Evaluation

The final stage in the care planning and delivery process presented here is evaluation. But, we again emphasise that the overall process of care is cyclic in nature (see Fig. 8.1) and thus evaluation takes place throughout the process and at set times (see Box 8.8). First, this will involve what we refer to here as 'process evaluation'. By this we mean that care is evaluated during the process of implementing the overall plan. Secondly, evaluation takes place at agreed dates for goal attainment. This we refer to as 'goal achievement evaluations' and times will be in accordance with agreed and realistic time periods (agreed with the service users). Finally, there will be long-term evaluations (typically called reviews) but which we refer to here as 'life-goal evaluation planning'. These evaluations focus on recovery, rehabilitation or adaptation to live life to the person's optimum ability for those who have an enduring mental illness. Evaluation methods will involve:

- Repeating assessments and comparing with baselines
- Direct observation of mood/behaviour change over time (or not)
- Data collection by various means from the client/family
- Multi-disciplinary conferences and regular meetings
- Impact assessments on client's life and others close to him/her
- Altering targets/goals for care as needed
- Being open to change of primary nurse/key worker if required

Before concluding the chapter a short Case illustration is presented which is followed by Reader activity 8.4 that relates to this illustration.

Case illustration 8.1

Mary is a 46-year-old lady with a mild/moderate learning disability. She has fairly good communication skills. Up until recently, Mary lived in her family home with her mother. During the past year Mary's mother (her sole carer) died. As a result Mary's sister Anne has taken over the caring responsibilities.

Prior to her mother's death, Mary was an activate member of the local day centre, enjoying many of the activities there. She also attended the local Gateway Club and always accompanied her mother on numerous shop outings. Mary was generally a friendly person but on occasions she would become upset if her routine was changed in the day centre. This resulted in her becoming unco-operative, emotional and clingy to staff, rocking and continually repeating questions.

Over the past few months Anne has found Mary's behaviour difficult to cope with. On many mornings Mary now refuses to get up out of bed; her appetite has declined and at times she will not eat at all. Anne hears Mary in the middle of the night moving furniture around, and talking to herself profusely about her mother's death; she also hears Mary rocking excessively and talking repetitively about different people to herself in her bedroom. Mary used to spend most of her time in the living room or around the house, but now she spends most of her time on her own in her bedroom and does not want to come out of it; in fact if Anne asks her to come out she often refuses.

The day centre staff reported that Mary now prefers to be left out of group activities. Mary indicates that she hates going out of the day centre and when staff encourage her she becomes upset, rocking, becoming very flushed and blaming others for causing her to become upset. She has got into a number of arguments in relation to other members of the day centre moving her personal belongings. Yesterday, Mary was verbally and physically abusive to a member of staff whom she claimed was 'staring at her'.

When asked about how Mary feels about her Mother's death Anne stated that she really does not like to raise this with Mary at all as she is afraid it may upset her even more.

Reader activity 8.4   Self-assessment on case illustration

Read Case illustration 8.1 and, after studying the information provided and drawing on what you have gained from this chapter, undertake the short self-assessment exercise below.

Mary has been referred to you and based on the information provided about her you must construct a care plan with her to meet her needs. We realise that there will be lots of questions that you do not have answers to in this situation but you can improvise and be imaginative. Within the overall care plan use the following questions/statements to guide your plan:

- What aspects are significant in your initial assessment history of Mary?
- From this description of Mary, can you formulate a 'working hypothesis' of her initial care needs?
- From this initial 'working hypothesis', can you identify methods that you would use to undertake a more comprehensive assessment with Mary?
- Identify and briefly list some realistic and achievable goals for Mary to work towards.
- Construct a plan of care for Mary in which you list planned interventions.
- List how and when you might evaluate Mary's care.

This is an exercise for your personal evaluation (but it could be done with colleagues if you wish). Write the plan in whatever format you wish. When you have completed the exercise you can turn to Appendix 8.1 where we provide an example care plan for Mary. You might care to compare the two care plans and account for and discuss similarities and differences between the two plans.

Conclusion

In the past, people with intellectual disabilities have not been considered, by some, capable of developing a mental illness. Barker (2004) provided an account of:

'an eminent psychiatrist proclaiming that people with intellectual impairments never suffered from proper psychiatric disorders because they were not bright enough.' (p. 298)

This is a view that many others may have heard expressed. There is now, of course, an ever increasing body of knowledge that such people not only suffer the distress of mental illness, but that higher numbers of this client group develop mental health problems than do members of the general population. In this chapter we have detailed some of this growing evidence. In the face of this evidence there is a need to provide plans of care and to deliver care that addresses the mental health needs of this dually diagnosed population. We have presented a range of evidence-based instruments that can usefully be added to the repertoire of nurses and others who work with this client group.

The chapter has detailed the process of nursing care for dually diagnosed people, asserting the requirement for a person-centred approach. Nursing theories that may have utility in guiding care for this client population are presented. Such theories do have the potential to influence care which can enhance the life quality of people who receive nursing inputs (McKenna, 1997; Meleis, 1997). Finally, we have referred to evidence-based instruments, behavioural technologies, the use of medication and psycho-social-educational elements that fall within an empirical knowledge on which to base practice. We do not question the value of these, but suggest nurses who work with dually diagnosed people should also underpin client/person–nurse encounters with 'humanistic caring' values. Watson's (1997) words portray a potent message of this:

'The artistry of caring draws from the same source as life itself; from human encounter, engaging with indelible stories of people, of caring moments or connecting through eyes, touch, sound, space, spirit itself. Such engaging moments of caring touch the human soul and provide a reflection into human existence.' (p. 59)

Appendix 8.1
Example care plan

HISTORY

What aspects are significant in your initial assessment history of Mary?
It appears that Mary's current behaviours may be a response to her mother's death.
 	
From the description of Mary a 'working hypothesis' of her initial care needs might be:
(1) That Mary may have 'a reactive depression caused by the death of her mother'.
(2) Other areas that require further investigation include:
     (a) What is the dynamic relationship between Mary and her sister Anne within their home?
     (b) What changes, if any, have occurred in Mary's day centre?
     (c) Have any physical changes occurred with Mary recently (e.g. menopause)?

(Within the history would be included the main aspects about Mary as detailed in the case illustration. Other initial relevant detail would be collected about her, e.g. any co-existing medical aspects or disabilities; medications; history of any mental illness, etc.)

ASSESSMENT	
Psychodynamics	• Changes in Mary's mood and expressed feelings? • Any risk of self-harm – any expressions of this nature? • Stress or distress evident? • Expressed fears by any means (communicated or behavioural)? • Thought processes – can Mary express these in any way? • Use the PAS-ADD checklist to examine whether Mary's behaviour over the last four weeks falls above any of the three thresholds. If the PAS-ADD checklist identifies a potential mental health problem, then a mini PAS-ADD interview with Mary's sister Anne, and also her day-care worker, would be beneficial. Similarly, if the mini PAS-ADD interview(s) identifies scores above some of the thresholds (e.g. depression or other areas), referral can be made to a psychiatrist for a more comprehensive psychiatric assessment
Behaviour	• Observed changes in behaviour (staying in room, etc.)? • Any self-harm behaviours? • Sleep and activity alterations? • When did behaviours manifest first (i.e. in relation to mothers death)? • Aberrant behaviour checklist (ABC) for specific overt behaviours and intensity (ABC will also help in evaluating Mary's treatment package) • Interview Mary's sister Anne to identify her presenting complaint in greater detail • Interviews with Mary's day-care worker and other health and social staff who are involved in working with Mary • Anne and Mary's day-care worker to observe and record behaviours both at home and day centre in an attempt to identify some of the antecedents of her behaviours
Social/role	• Avoidance of social situations (out of keeping with Mary's normal behaviour)? • Changes in Mary's life roles? • Does Mary need and has she access to an advocate?

Cont.

	• Any indication of adverse effects of social systems e.g. attitudes; exclusion; discrimination? • Adaptive behaviour scale completed (using this will help evaluate the effectiveness of the treatment package later)
Clinical/physical	• Collect information from Mary's GP about any previous medical conditions and ask GP to investigate Mary's hormonal levels to rule this out • Check any medication and side-effects of current medication. Monitor and arrange follow-up if required • Collect information, if appropriate, from Mary's psychiatrist (or GP) regarding any previous mental health history and treatments • Diet – investigate Mary's reduced appetite and follow up • Physical activity – Mary is found to stay in her room and does little or no activity
Human relations/spiritual	• Has Mary spiritual beliefs of any kind (religious or other)? • Has Mary a close relationship with anyone? • Has Mary had an open, close discussion about her mother's death? • Has she had opportunity to mourn the death of her mother, i.e. attend the funeral, visit the grave? • Is there anyone who Mary knows who has had a bereavement who could share experiences with her?
Communication/openness	• Can Mary communicate her needs well? • Will she need help to communicate her needs? • Are inappropriate behaviours being used to communicate? • Assess Mary's assertiveness? • How empowered does Mary feel about her life? • Consider May's verbal communication: pitch; resonance; rate; turn taking. • Consider May's non-verbal communication: posture; gestures; social distance; eye contact; response to touch; facial expression; activity (fidgety, etc.) • Is Mary normally an open person or reserved?
Perceptions self/other	• Talk to Mary to identify her perceptions and reasons of her current behaviours. Consider: (a) Her degree of self-awareness (b) How she feels others view her
Developmental	• Any relevant aspects due to intellectual disability? (clinical psychologist assessment) • Signs of regression in development functions?

IDENTIFIED CARE NEEDS

For the purpose of this example we will assume that Mary's main care need is 'the development of a depressive episode that is a reaction to the death of her mother'.

PLAN OF CARE – GOALS

(1) For Mary to accept and come to terms with the death of her mother
(2) For Mary's depressive symptoms to subside and to return to her normal levels of interest in her home and day centre (and related aspects such as appetite, sleep, activity etc. to return to normal)
(3) For Mary's sister Anne to take on a surrogate role to help Mary come to terms with the loss of her mother and to develop trusting friendships

PLAN OF CARE – INTERVENTIONS

Goal 1
- Mary will undertake a period of time in bereavement counselling
- A member of day-care staff who also lost her mother agrees to take Mary to the cemetery weekly where they spend time and place flowers on the graves (Anne continues this)
- Mary attends psychodrama where she is encouraged to act out and release her emotions
- Assertive training is provided so Mary will learn to express her emotions, frustrations and fears to prevent future crises

Goal 2
- Mary will attend gym as physical activity useful for mild depression
- Mary will return to the Gateway Club for short periods that will be progressively increased
- Social skills enhancement education will be provided
- Therapist will provide weekly progressive muscular relaxation sessions
- Mary is introduced to art therapy as a means of personal expression
- Cognitive behaviour therapy is provided by a specialist nurse in this area
- Reflexology and therapeutic massage is provided

Goal 3
- Anne is developing a closer bonding relationship with Mary by being a 'friend'
- Mary's primary nurse calls regularly and together all three review progress
- A local voluntary group that organises a 'buddy' system arranges a buddy friend for Mary
- The nurse makes available home respite for Anne due to the emotional labour she experiences as a carer

EVALUATION

- Regular ongoing evaluations take place involving Mary, Anne and the multidisciplinary team.
- Prescribing a course of anti-depressants for a short period of time and closely monitoring is an option, but all agree this should only be prescribed if Mary fails to respond to the above interventions within 2–3 months, or if she deteriorates.

Cont.

- Family therapy is an option but this is not required. Evaluations indicate Mary is responding well and as Mary and Anne have been central to planning her care they have developed coping strategies that should be life-long.
- Physical aspects related to the depressive episode, such as sleep disturbance, loss of appetite, etc., return to normal for Mary.
- Mary and Anne are provided with education on early recognition of depression for the future and what to do and where to seek help should Mary have a relapse.

Note: This example care plan is a model only and not meant to be all-inclusive. In the 'real world' things are not always as straightforward and plans frequently require change due to the dynamics of mental illness.

References

Aldridge, J. (2004) Learning disability nursing: a model for practice. In: *Learning Disability Nursing* (Turnbull, J., ed.). Oxford: Blackwell Publishing, 169–87.

Aman, M.G. and Singh, N.N. (1986) *Aberrant Behaviour Checklist Manual*. New York: Slossom Publications.

Aman, M.G., Alvarez, N., Benefield, W., Green, G., King, B.H., Reiss, S., Rojahn, J. and Szymanski, L. (2000) Special issue. Expert consensus guideline series: Treatment of psychiatric and behavioural problems in mental retardation. *American Journal on Mental Retardation* **105** (3), 159–227.

Barker, P.J. (2004) *Assessment in Psychiatric and Mental Health Nursing*. Cheltenham: Nelson Thornes.

Beail, N. (2003) What works for people with mental retardation? Critical commentary on cognitive-behavioral and psychodynamic psychotherapy research. *Mental Retardation* **41** (6), 468–72.

Bender, M. (1993) The un-offered chair. The history of therapeutic disdain towards people with a learning disability. *Clinical Psychology Forum* 54, 7–12.

Berney, T. (1997) Behavioural phenotypes. In: *The Psychiatry of Learning Disabilities* (Russell, O., ed.). London: The Royal College of Psychiatrists, Gaskell.

Bicknell, J. (1985) Educational programmes for general practitioners and clinical assistants in the mental handicap service. *Bulletin of the Royal College of Psychiatrists* **8**, 154–5.

Borthwick-Duffy, S.A. and Eyman, R.K. (1990) Who are the dually diagnosed? *American Journal on Mental Retardation* **94**, 586–95.

Bouras, N. (1999a) *Psychiatric and Behavioural Disorders in Development Disabilities and Mental Retardation*. Cambridge: Cambridge University Press.

Bouras, N. (1999b) Mental health and learning disabilities: planning and service developments. *Tizard Learning Disability Review* **4** (2), 3–5.

Bouras, N. and Drummond, C. (1992) Behaviour and psychiatric disorders of people with mental handicaps living in the community. *Journal of Intellectual Disability Research* **36**, 349–57.

Brylewski, J. and Duggan, L. (1999) Anti-psychotic medication for challenging behaviour in people with intellectual disability: a systematic review of randomised controlled trials. *Journal of Intellectual Disability Research* **43** (5), 360–71.

Carpenito, L.J. (1999) *Nursing Care Plans and Documentation Nursing Diagnosis and Collaborative Problems.* Philadelphia: Lippincott.

Clarke, D. (1999) Functional psychoses in people with mental retardation. In: *Psychiatric and Behavioural Disorders in Development Disabilities and Mental Retardation* (Bouras, N., ed.). Cambridge: Cambridge University Press.

Clarke, D.J., Boer, H. and Webb, T. (1995) Genetic and behavioural aspects of Prader-Willi syndrome. *Mental Handicap Research* **8** (1), 38–53.

Collins, S. (1999) Treatment and therapeutic interventions: psychological approaches. *Tizard Learning Disability Review* **4** (2), 20–27.

Cooper, S.A. (1997) Epidemiology of psychiatric disorders in elderly compared with younger adults with learning disabilities. *British Journal of Psychiatry* **170**, 375–80.

Cooper, S.A. and Bailey, N.M. (2001) Psychiatric disorders amongst adults with learning disabilities: prevalence and relationship to ability. *Irish Journal of Psychiatric Medicine* **18** (2), 45–53.

Corbett, J.A. (1979) Psychiatric morbidity and mental retardation. In: *Psychiatric Illness and Mental Handicap* (James, F.E. and Snaith, R.P., eds.). London: Gaskell.

Dawson, C. and Morgan, P. (1997) Learning disabilities and mental illness. Birmingham: Pepar Publications.

Day, K. (1999) Professional training in the psychiatry of mental retardation in the UK. In: *Psychiatric and Behavioural Disorders in Development Disabilities and Mental Retardation* (Bouras, N., ed.). Cambridge: Cambridge University Press.

Deb, S. and Braganza, J. (1999) Comparison of rating scales for dementia in adults with Down Syndrome. *Journal of Intellectual and Developmental Disability* **43** (5), 400–7.

Deb, S., Mathews, T., Holt, G. and Bouras, N. (2001) Practice guidelines for the assessment and diagnosis of mental health problems in adults with intellectual disability. Mental Health in Mental Retardation (MH-MR). Brighton: Pavillion.

Deb, S., Thomas, M. and Bright, C. (2001a) Mental disorders in adults who have an intellectual disability, 1: prevalence of functional psychiatric illness among a 16–64 year old community-based population. *Journal of Intellectual Disability Research* **45** (6), 506–14.

Department of Health (1998) *Signposts for Success.* London: NHS Executive.

Department of Health (2001) *Valuing People: a New Strategy for Learning Disability for the 21st Century.* London: Stationery Office.

Duggan, L. and Brylewski, J. (1999) Effectiveness of anti-psychotic medication in people with intellectual disability and schizophrenia: a systematic review. *Journal of Intellectual Disability Research* **43** (2), 94–104.

Eaton, L.F. and Menolascino, F.J. (1982) Psychiatric disorders in the mentally retarded: types, problems and challenges. *American Journal of Psychiatry* **139**, 660–7.

Emerson, E., Mc Gill, P. and Mansell, J. (1994) Severe learning disabilities and challenging behaviour designing high quality services. London: Chapman and Hall Publishers.

Emerson, E., Hatton, C., Bromley, J. and Caine, A. (1998) *Clinical Psychology and People with Intellectual Disabilities.* Chichester: John Wiley and Sons.

Emerson, E. Moss, S. and Kiernan, C. (1999) The relationship between challenging behaviours and psychiatric disorders in people with severe developmental disabilities. In: *Psychiatric and Behavioural Disorders in Development Disabilities and Mental Retardation* (Bouras, N., ed.). Cambridge: Cambridge University Press.

Emerson, E., Robertson, J., Gregory, N., Hatton, C., Kessissoglou, S., Hallam, A. and Hillery, J. (2000) Treatment and management of challenging behaviours in residential settings. Journal *of Applied Research in Intellectual Disabilities* **13** (3), 197–215.

Feurer, I.D., Dimitropoulos, A., Stone, W.L., Roof, E., Butler, M.G. and Thompson, T. (1998) The latent variable structure of the Compulsive Behaviour Checklist in people with Prader-Willi syndrome. *Journal of Intellectual Disability Research* **42** (6), 472–80.

Fleisher, M. (1999) The psychopharmacology in developmental disabilities. In: *Psychiatric and Behavioural Disorders in Development Disabilities and Mental Retardation* (Bouras, N., ed.). Cambridge: Cambridge University Press.

Foundation for People with Learning Disabilities (2001) *Learning Disability: the Fundamental Facts*. London: The Mental Health Foundation.

Freud, S. (1893, reprinted 1953) The psychical mechanism of hysterical phenomena. In: *Standard Edition of the Complete Psychological Works of Sigmund Freud* (Strachey, J., trans. and ed.). London: Hogarth Press.

Frey, M.A. and Sieloff, C.L. (1995) *Advancing King's Systems Framework and Theory of Nursing*. London: Sage Publications.

Gardner, W.I. and Sovner, R. (1994) *Self-injurious Behaviours: A Functional Approach*. Willow St, PA: Vida Press.

Gates, B. (2003) Self-injurious behaviour. In: *Learning Disabilities: Toward Inclusion*, 4th edn, (Gates, B., ed.). Edinburgh: Churchill Livingstone.

Gilbert, T., Todd, M. and Jackson, N. (1998) People with learning disabilities who also have mental health problems: practice issues and directions for learning disability nursing. *Journal of Advanced Nursing* **27**, 1151–7.

Gustafsson, C. (1997) The prevalence of people with intellectual disability admitted to general hospital psychiatric units: level of handicap, psychiatric diagnoses and care utilization. *Journal of Intellectual Disability Research* **41** (6), 519–26.

Hassiotis, A. (1999) Psychodynamic psychotherapy in learning disability: theory and practice revisited. *Journal of Learning Disabilities for Nursing, Health and School Health Care* **3** (2), 106–9.

Helsel, W.J. and Matson, J.L. (1988) The relationship of depression to social skills and intellectual functioning in mentally handicapped adults. *Journal of Mental Deficiency Research* **32** (5), 411–18.

Hollins, S. and Sinason, V. (2000) Psychotherapy, learning disabilities and trauma: new perspectives. *British Journal of Psychiatry* **176**, 32–36.

Horan, P., Doran, A. and Timmins, F. (2004a) Exploring Orem's self-care deficit nursing theory in learning disability nursing: philosophical parity paper: part 1. *Learning Disability Practice* **7** (4), 28–33.

Horan, P., Doran, A. and Timmins, F. (2004b) Exploring Orem's self-care deficit nursing theory in learning disability nursing: practical application paper: part 2. *Learning Disability Practice* **7** (4), 33–37.

Horner, R.H., Vaughn, B.J., Day, M. and Narde, W.R. (1996) The relationship between setting events and problem behaviour: expanding our understanding of behavioural support. In: *Positive Behavioural Support: Including People with Difficult Behaviour in the Community* (Koegel, L.K., Koegel, R.L. and Dunlap, G., eds.). London: Paul H. Brookes.

Hurst, J., Nadarajah, J. and Cumella, S. (1994) Inpatient care for people with a learning disability and a mental illness. *Psychiatric Bulletin* **18**, 29–31.

International Association for the Scientific Study of Intellectual Disabilities (IASSID) (2001) *Mental health and intellectual disabilities: addressing the mental health needs of people with intellectual disabilities*. Report by the Mental Health Special Interest Research Group of IASSID to the World Health Organization.

Iverson, J.C. and Fox, R.A. (1989) Prevalence of psychopathology among mentally retarded adults. *Research in Developmental Disabilities* **10**, 77–83.

Jacobson, J.W. (1982) Problem behaviour and psychiatric impairment within a developmentally disabled population 1: Behaviour frequency. *Applied Research in Mental Retardation* **3**, 112–13.

Jahoda, A., Cattermole, M. and Markova, I. (1989) Moving out: an opportunity for friendship and broadening social horizons? *Journal of Mental Deficiency Research* **34** (2), 127–41.

Kabzems, V. (1985) The use of self-report measures with mentally retarded individuals. *The Mental Retardation and Learning Disability Bulletin* **13** (2), 106–14.

King, I.M. (1981) *A Theory of Nursing: Systems Concepts and Process*. New York: John Wiley.

Kirby, C. (1999) The therapeutic relationship. In: *Theory and Practice of Nursing* (Basford, L. and Slevin, O., eds.). Cheltenham: Stanley Thornes.

Kirby, C. (2003) The therapeutic relationship. In: *Theory and Practice of Nursing*, 2nd edn (Basford, L. and Slevin, O., eds.). Cheltenham: Stanley Thornes.

Kleiman, S. (1993) Clinical applications of the humanistic nursing theory. In: *Patterns of Nursing Theories in Practice* (Parker, M., ed.). New York: National League for Nursing Press.

La Vigna, G.W. and Donnellan, A.M. (1986) *Alternatives to Punishment: Solving Behaviour Problems with Non-Aversive Strategies*. New York: Irvington Publishers.

Long, A. (2003) Mental health nursing. In: *Theory and Practice of Nursing*, 2nd edn (Basford, L. and Slevin, O., eds.). Cheltenham: Stanley Thornes.

Lowery, M.A. and Sovner, R. (1992) Severe behaviour problems associated with rapid cycling bipolar disorder in two adults with profound mental retardation. *American Journal on Mental Retardation* **36** (3), 269–281.

Lund, J. (1985) The prevalence of psychotic morbidity in mentally retarded adults. *Acta Psychiatry Scandinavica* **72**, 563–70.

Marston, G.M., Perry, W.D. and Roy, A. (1997) Manifestations of depression in people with intellectual disabilities. *Journal of Intellectual Disability Research* **41**, 476–80.

Mason, J. and Scior, K. (2004) 'Diagnostic overshadowing' amongst clinicians working with people with intellectual disabilities in the UK. *Journal of Applied Research in Intellectual Disabilities* **17** (2), 85–90.

Matson, J.L., Kazdin, A.E. and Senatore, V. (1984) Psychometric properties of the psychopathology instrument for mental retarded adults (PIMRA). *American Journal on Mental Retardation* **5**, 881–889.

Matson, J.L., Gardner, W.I., Coe, D.A. and Sovner, R.R. (1991) A scale for evaluating emotional disorders in severely and profoundly mentally retarded persons: development of the Diagnostic Assessment for the Severely Handicapped (DASH) scale. *British Journal of Psychiatry* **159**, 404–409.

McKenna, H. (1997) *Nursing Theories and Models*. London: Routledge.

Meins, W. (1993) Prevalence and risk factors for depressive disorders in adults with developmental disabilities. *Australian and New Zealand Journal of Developmental Disabilities* **18**, 147–56.

Meins, W. (1995) Symptoms of major depression in mentally retarded adults. *Journal of Intellectual Disability Research* **39** (1), 41–5.

Meins, W. (1996) Are depressive mood disturbances early signs of dementia. *Journal of Nervous and Mental Diseases* **183**, 633–44.

Meleis, A.I. (1997) *Theoretical Nursing Development and Progress.* Philadelphia: JB Lippincott Company.

Mencap (1999) *The NHS: Health for All? People with Learning Disabilities and Health Care.* London: Mencap.

Mental Health Foundation (1997) *Knowing our Own Minds. Survey of How People in Emotional Distress Take Control of Their Lives.* London: Mental Health Foundation.

Moss, S. (1999) Assessment and conceptual issues. In: *Psychiatric and Behavioural Disorders in Development Disabilities and Mental Retardation* (Bouras, N., ed.). Cambridge: Cambridge University Press.

Moss, S. (2002) *PAS-ADD Schedules.* Brighton: Pavilion Publishers.

Moss, S.C., Patel, P., Prosser, H., Goldberg, D.P., Simpson, N., Rowe, S. and Lucchino, R. (1993) Psychiatric morbidity in older people with moderate and severe learning disability (mental retardation). Part 1. Development and reliability of the patient interview (the PAS-ADD). *British Journal of Psychiatry* **163**, 471–480.

Nihja, K., Leland, H. and Lambert, N. (1993) *AAMR Adaptive Behaviour Scale,* 2nd edn. New York: Harcourt Brace and Co.

O'Dwyer, J.M. (2000) Learning disability psychiatry: the future of services. *Psychiatric Bulletin* **24**, 247–50.

Orem, D.E. (1991) *Nursing: Concepts of Practice.* St Louis: Mosby Year Book.

Paterson, J.G. and Zderad, L.T. (1988) *Humanistic Nursing.* New York: National League for Nursing.

Peplau, H. (1991) *Interpersonal Relationships in Nursing: A Conceptual Frame of Reference.* New York *(Original publication 1952)*: Springer.

Raitasuo, S., Taiminen, T. and Salokangas, R.K.R. (1999) Characteristics of people with intellectual disability admitted for psychiatric inpatient treatment. *Journal of Intellectual Disability Research* **43** (2), 112–18.

Reese, R.M. and Leeder, D. (1990) An ecobehavioural setting event analysis of residential facilities for people with mental retardation. In: *Ecobehavioural Analysis and Developmental Disabilities: The Twenty-First Century* (Schroeder, S.R., ed.). New York: Springer-Verlag.

Reiss, S. (1988) *Reiss Screen for Maladaptive Behaviours.* Worthington, OH: IDS.

Reiss, S. (1990) Prevalence of dual diagnosis in community based day programmes in the Chicago metropolitan area. *American Journal on Mental Retardation* **94** (6), 578–85.

Reiss, S. and Aman, M. (1998) *Psychotropic Medications and Developmental Disabilities. The International Consensus Handbook.* Columbus, OH: The Ohio State University Nisonger Centre.

Reiss, S. and Rojahn, J. (1993) Joint occurrence of depression and aggression in children and adults with mental retardation. *Journal of Intellectual Disability Research* **37** (3), 287–94.

Reiss, S., Levitan, G. and Szyszko, J. (1982) Emotional disturbance and mental retardation: diagnostic overshadowing. *American Journal of Mental Deficiency* **86**, 567–74.

Reynolds, W.K. and Baker, J.A. (1988) Assessment of depression in people with mental retardation. *American Journal of Mental Retardation* **93**, 93–103.

Rogers, C. (1951) *Client-centered Therapy.* Boston: Houghton Mifflin.

Roper, N., Logan, W.W. and Tierney, A. (1996) *The Elements of Nursing: A Model for Nursing Based on a Model for Living.* London: Churchill Livingstone Publishers.

Roy, A., Martin, D.M. and Wells, M.B. (1997) Health gain through screening mental health: developing primary health care services for people with an intellectual disability. *Journal of Intellectual and Developmental Disability* **22** (4), 227–39.

Royal College of Psychiatrists (2001) *DC-LD: Diagnostic Criteria for Psychiatric Disorders for Use with Adults with Learning Disabilities/Mental Retardation.* London: Gaskell.

Russell, O. (1997) *The Psychiatry of Learning Disabilities.* Glasgow: Royal College of Psychiatrists, Gaskell.

Sanderson, H. (2003) Person-centred planning. In: *Learning Disabilities: Toward Inclusion,* 4th edn, (Gates, B., ed.). Edinburgh: Churchill Livingstone.

Saunders, M. (2001) Concepts of Health and Disability. In: *Meeting the Health Needs of People who have a Learning Disability* (Thompson J. and Pickering S., ed.). London: Baillière Tindall.

Saunders, R.R. and Spradlin, J.E. (1991) A supported routine approach to active treatment for enhancing dependence, competence and self-worth. *Behavioural Residential Treatment* **6**, 1–37.

State, M.W., King, B.H. and Dykens, E. (1997) Mental retardation: a review of the past 10 years; Part 2. *Journal of the American Academy of Child and Adolescent Psychiatry* **36** (12), 1664–71.

Stenfert Kroese, B., Dagan, D. and Loumidis, K. (eds.) (1997) *Cognitive Behaviour Therapy for People with Learning Disabilities.* London: Routledge Press.

Sturmey, P. (1995) DSM 3R and persons with dual diagnoses: conceptual issues and strategies for future research. *Journal of Intellectual Disability Research* **39** (5), 357–64.

Sturmey, P. and Bertman, L.P. (1995) The validity of the REISS scale for maladaptive behaviour. *American Journal of Mental Retardation* **99**, 201–6.

Sturmey, P., Reyer, H., Lee, R. and Robek, A. (2003) *Substance Related Disorders in Persons with Mental Retardation.* Kingston, NY: NADD.

Taggart, L. (2003) Service Provision for People with Learning Disabilities and Mental Health Problems Living in Northern Ireland. Unpublished PhD thesis: University of Ulster, Northern Ireland.

Taylor, J.L., Hatton, C., Dixon, L. and Douglas, C. (2004) Screening for psychiatric symptoms using the PAS-ADD checklist in adults with intellectual disabilities. *Journal of Intellectual Disability Research* **48** (1), 37–41.

Trower, T., Treadwell, L. and Bhaumik, S. (1998) Acute in-patient treatment for adults with learning disabilities and mental health problems in a specialized admission unit. *British Journal of Developmental Disabilities* **86**, 20–9.

Turkistani, I. (2003) Mental ill health in learning disabilities. In: *Learning Disabilities: Toward Inclusion,* 4th edn, (Gates, B., ed.). Edinburgh: Churchill Livingstone.

Tyson, R.L. and Sandler, J. (1971) Problems in the selection of patients for psychoanalysis. Comments on the application of 'indicators', suitability and 'analysability'. *British Journal of Medical Psychology* **44**, 211–28.

Watkins, P. (2001) *Mental Health Nursing: The Art of Compassionate Care.* Oxford: Butterworth Heinemann.

Watson, J. (1997) Artistry of caring: heart and soul of nursing. In: *Reconstructing Nursing Beyond Art and Science* (Marks-Maran, D. and Rose, P., eds.). London: Baillière Tindall.

World Health Organization (1996) *International Classification of Diseases,* 10th edn (ICD-10). Salt Lake City, UT: Medicode, Inc.

Xentiditis, K., Thorncroft, G., Leese, L. and Slade, M. (2000) Reliability and validity of the CANDID – a needs assessment instrument for adults with learning disabilities and mental health problems. *British Journal of Psychiatry* **176**, 473–8.

Young, J.E. and Beck, A.T. (1982) Cognitive therapy: clinical applications. In: *Short-term Psychotherapies for Depression* (Rush, A.J., ed.). New York: Guild Press.

Resources

European Association for Mental Health in Mental Retardation (EA-MHMR)
Mental Health in Learning Disabilities Nurses Forum: A UK-based forum where intellectual disability nurses who support people who have mental health problems can exchange knowledge and information, examine the skills needed to provide effective nursing care, develop a support network and examine the evidence base in this area.
National Association for the Dually Diagnosed (NADD): www.thenadd.org

Useful websites

British Psychological Society: www.bps.org.uk
Department of Health Learning Disabilities: www.doh.gov.uk/learningdisabilities
Department of Health Mental Health: www.doh.gov.uk/mentalhealth
Foundation for People with Learning Disabilities: www.learningdisabilities.org.uk
Institute of Psychiatry: www.iop.kcl.ac.uk/IoP/home.shtml
Kings College London: www.kcl.ac.uk
Learning Disabilities UK: www.learningdisabilitiesuk.org.uk
MENCAP: www.mencap.org.uk
National Association for the Dually Diagnosed (NADD): www.thenadd.org
National Network for Learning Disability Nurses: www.nnldn.org.uk
Pavilion Publishing: www.pavpub.com
Royal College of Nursing: www.rcn.org.uk
Royal College of Psychiatrists: www.rcpsych.ac.uk
South London and Maudsley NHS Trust: www.slam.nhs.uk
Tizard Centre: www.ukc.ac.uk/tizard
Valuing People Support Team: www.doh.gov.uk/vpst
World Psychiatric Association: www.wpanet.org

Chapter 9

Care planning in palliative care for people with intellectual disabilities

Sue Read and David Elliott

Introduction

People with intellectual disabilities are living longer, and will doubtless experience a range of ill health and disease, and require the same healthcare, as the general population. Palliative care, in particular, for people with intellectual disabilities is becoming increasingly important as professionals are presented with individuals who have palliative conditions in a variety of differing care contexts. This population is often vulnerable at the end of life, and integrating the general principles of holistic, palliative care remains a crucial feature in service development and care delivery (Read, 2005b). Issues surrounding loss, preparing for death, pain and symptom assessment and management, ethical dilemmas and breaking difficult news prior to death, and bereavement support following death, require sensitive exploration and explanations within the palliative care context. The development of care planning and care pathways will provide constructive and practical opportunities for professional carers that will ensure equity and parity of palliative care for people with intellectual disabilities, and promote the accessibility and delivery of services for this marginalised population, at a time when they need it most. Costello (2004) has recognised that death is much more than just an outcome of dying, and remains:

'the single most important social factor of human existence.' (p. 178)

Death rarely occurs in a vacuum, but in a variety of differing social contexts, and the context may have a significant effect upon the social process of dying and its attitudinal shaping within society (Ahmed et al., 2004; Costello, 2004). Dying people may be perceived as being vulnerable, and, if the person also has an intellectual disability, that vulnerability may be significantly increased as a consequence of practical, philosophical, attitudinal and ideological factors (Read and Elliott, 2003).

The aims of this chapter are threefold: to identify the challenges presented when a person with an intellectual disability is diagnosed with a palliative condition; to integrate general palliative care principles into good practice for people with intellectual disabilities; and to explore the concepts of care planning

195

in the effort of ensuring equity and parity of care delivery and accessibility. Initially definitions of palliative care and intellectual disabilities will be offered to clarify understanding; a contextual background of palliative care in relation to people with intellectual disabilities will be presented; and a holistic approach to palliative care will be explored from a practical orientation. A model of good practice will be subsequently introduced and explored, as a basis for developing an integrated, consistent, planned approach to holistic palliative care provision to people with intellectual disabilities.

Palliative care and intellectual disabilities

The word *palliative* is derived from the Latin verb 'palliere' meaning to 'cloak' or 'shield' (Regnard and Kindlen, 2002). The most commonly used definition is provided by the World Health Organization, which describes palliative care as:

> 'the active total care of patients whose disease is not responsive to curative treatment.' (World Health Organization, 1990)

This incorporates an approach that improves the quality of life of patients and their families by the prevention and relief of suffering by means of early identification and thorough assessment and treatment of pain and other physical, psychological and spiritual problems. Increasingly palliative care is seen to include conditions other than cancer (see Box 9.1), although cancer remains the most common condition.

In addition to pain and symptom assessment and management, the key concepts inherent in palliative care (identified in Box 9.2) involve caring (by informal or professional carers), dignity (as perceived from the patient and carer perspectives), comfort (including physical, emotional and spiritual), knowing the patient (often perceived as an essential aspect of the 'art' of medicine), empathy (accessing the emotions of others) and supportive care (which encompasses palliative care) (Seymour, 2004). Whilst palliative care may continue over many months, or even years, terminal care is often associated with the last few days of life. Such a philosophy of holistic care incorporates the physical, psychological, emotional and spiritual aspects of the individual.

Box 9.1   Palliative care conditions

- Cancer
- Alzheimer's disease
- Dementia
- HIV and AIDS
- Multiple sclerosis
- Chronic conditions (e.g. heart disease, chronic obstructive pulmonary disease)

Box 9.2   Key concepts in palliative care nursing (Seymour, 2004)

- 'Knowing the patient'
- Teamwork
- Dignity
- Comfort
- Empathy
- Support and 'supportive care'
- Hope
- Suffering
- Quality of life

People with intellectual disabilities are described as having a reduced ability to understand new or complex information, or to learn new skills (impaired intelligence), with a reduced ability to cope independently (impaired social functioning) which started before adulthood and with a lasting effect on development (Department of Health, 2001a). Such individuals may have a whole range of different presenting competencies in communication, social skills, social functioning and/or behaviour. In recent years, community care initiatives and developments have meant a huge increase in residential and nursing care homes, yet people with intellectual disabilities remain 'amongst the most socially excluded and vulnerable groups in Britain today' (Department of Health, 2001a, p. 14). A recent report by Mencap identifies that people with intellectual disabilities:

> 'have poor health, more health needs and die younger.' (Mencap, 2004, p. 11)

This report aims to engage with health providers to improve the healthcare of people with intellectual disabilities, by raising its profile and proposing recommendations for future service developments. From a palliative care perspective, members of this population are frequently diagnosed with palliative conditions but may have difficulties accessing the appropriate assessment, treatment and subsequent care they require, often resulting in poor prognosis (Tuffrey-Wijne, 1997). The challenges inherent in providing appropriate palliative care to people with intellectual disabilities are multifactorial.

Challenges to palliative care

The initial recognition of ill health in people with an intellectual disability may be difficult since some individuals may not be able to articulate discomfort or perceive physical changes indicative of illness (e.g. weight loss, loss of appetite). Some initial signs may be observable, such as a breast lump, rectal bleeding, vomiting and anaemia (Evenhuis, 1997; Tuffrey-Wijne, 2003), which are reliant on carer perception. Should the person feel unwell, some individuals may lack the verbal skill repertoire to articulate their distress in meaningful and socially acceptable ways. Tuffrey-Wijne (2003) has identified that communication is the biggest barrier to effective medical assessment.

Changes in behaviour may be the first indicator of distress (e.g. irritability, inactivity, self-injurious behaviour or a combination of these symptoms) (Bosch et al., 1997; Evenhuis, 1997; Tuffrey-Wijne, 2003), but personal or professional carers may not recognise such changes as ill health indicators, particularly amongst people with profound and complex needs. Such diagnostic overshadowing (Brown et al., 2003) may initially mask the diagnosis of serious ill health. The illness can be identified through regular, routine screening programmes (e.g. breast and cervical) although accessing routine screening is often inconsistent and problematical for this population (Hogg et al., 2001). Once a serious illness is suspected, accessing appropriate services may be difficult, compounded by the ambivalent attitudes and communication difficulties experienced by the variety of professionals potentially involved.

Investigative procedures, important in terms of diagnosis and devising treatment plans, are often intrusive and invasive, and some individuals may not appreciate their relevance and withdraw their active co-operation. For some individuals with an intellectual impairment, consent may be a straightforward procedure, for example if they live independently, receive no specific care input, are able to articulate their preferences, and can read and write. For others, informed consent may be more difficult to establish. However,

> 'It should *never* be assumed that people are not able to make their own decisions, simply because they have a learning disability.' (Department of Health, 2001b, p. 1)

For a person's consent to be valid, the person must be capable of taking that particular decision ('competent'), be acting voluntarily and be provided with enough information to enable them to make the decision (Department of Health, 2001b). Involving the individual with an intellectual disability in issues involving treatment options may be a complex, lengthy and arduous process.

Once a firm diagnosis has been ascertained, accessing appropriate treatment may also be problematic. Professional carers working in intellectual disability services may not be fully conversant with the concept of palliative care: what this entails; what services are available; and who can offer specialist care and support. Many such services 'are built upon the concept of supported living' and focus upon the future and living well, not upon death and dying (Todd, 2004). Similarly, palliative care professionals may not be familiar with people with intellectual disabilities, and may harbour a host of negative attitudes centring on fear and the stigma associated with marginalised populations. Such challenges may delay an important diagnosis, reducing treatment options and often resulting in a poor prognosis and outcome for this population (Tuffrey-Wijne, 1997).

> **Box 9.3 Features of person-centred planning**
>
> - The person is at the centre
> - Family members and friends are partners in planning
> - The (care) plan highlights what is important to the person, capacities and what support they require
> - The (care) plan results in actions that are about life, not just services, and reflects what is possible, not just what is available
> - The (care) plan results in a process of ongoing listening, learning and further action
>
> (Department of Health, 2002b; Kilbane and Thompson, 2004)

Person-centred planning and palliative care

The government's White Paper, *Valuing People* (Department of Health 2001a), has advocated a person-centred approach to planning care for people with intellectual disabilities. It stated that planning should start with the individual (not with services), and take into account their wishes and aspirations. One of the central themes for person-centred planning is listening to the person and those who know them best, and 'honouring' their voices (Iles, 2003). This is particularly pertinent when a person with intellectual disabilities is identified as having palliative care needs. The main features of person-centred planning are identified in Box 9.3, and the reader is advised to refer to Chapters 3 and 4 for a fuller account.

One way of effectively meeting palliative care needs is to adopt a person-centred planning style or approach. O'Brien and O'Brien (2000) have identified 11 person-centred planning approaches, four of which are currently favoured in England. These four approaches are identified in Box 9.4, and their application to palliative care is delineated. One of these approaches, essential life planning, particularly lends itself to supporting the person with palliative care needs. A framework for the essential life planning approach includes recognising the salient points illustrated in Fig. 9.1.

Although Thompson and Cobb (2004) have suggested 'that for many people the use of one tool is not the complete answer', it may be, however, a starting point for professional development and service delivery. Within the person-centred plannning framework, a health action plan needs to be devised in order to meet palliative care needs.

'A health action plan details the actions needed to maintain and improve the health of an individual and any help needed to accomplish these. It is a mechanism that links the individual with a range of services and supports they will need if they are to have better health.' (Department of Health, 2002b)

A health action plan thus can be crucial from a palliative care perspective.

Box 9.4 Overview of four person-centred approaches and styles in relation to palliative care (based on Smull and Harrison, 1992; Mount, 1995; Sanderson, 2003; O'Brien and Pierpoint, 2003)

Approach	What is it?	Implementation	Application to palliative care
Planning Alternative Tomorrows with Hope (PATH)	A way of planning direct and immediate action	Focuses first on dreams and works back from a positive and a negative perspective. Future mapping out with action plans along the way	An action-orientated approach that focuses on the future and this may be limited in palliative care
Making action plans (MAPs)	Helps people to make connections with community, by focusing on a person and their gifts	Gives people opportunity to express both hopes for future (in dreaming section) and fears about future (in nightmare section). Action planning development is about working towards the dream and away from the nightmare	A creative approach that has a future orientation. The 'nightmares' may indeed have a frightening reality in the palliative care context
Personal futures planning (PFP)	Provides a way of helping to describe a person's life now, and looks at what they would like in the future. Builds upon what is working well now and a more desirable future	Develops personal profiles and ideas about what the person would like in the future, and takes action to move towards this. Involves exploring possibilities with community and what needs to change with services	A thoughtful, humanistic approach that focuses upon future perspectives
Essential lifestyle planning (ELP)	Provides details about what a person carries on doing on a day-to-day basis. Develops a life style which works for the person now. What is important for this person to stay healthy and safe.	Develops lifestyle plan based upon person's history, with life achievements important. Prioritises what is important to the person. Attempts to achieve this using an action plan, based on unresolved issues and questions to ask (reflection). Anything that is working, that requires action to make it work and if not working also requires attention	A passionate and sensitive approach that focuses upon the 'here and now', with health and safety a priority. The combined focus upon immediacy, continuity and detailed, non-negotiable priorities, makes this a useful tool within the palliative care context

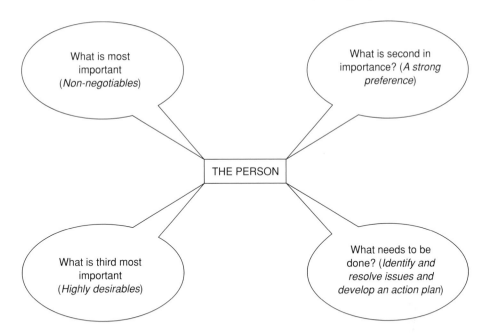

Fig. 9.1 Framework for an essential lifestyle plan approach (after Sanderson et al., 1997; Smull and Harrison, 1992; Sanderson, 2003).

Palliative care and essential lifestyle planning

Essential lifestyle planning was originally developed by Smull and Harrison (1992) to enable people with 'severe reputations' (people with extreme and complex challenges) to move from long-stay institutions to community-based facilities (Kilbane and Sanderson, 2004). It is an approach that is being increasingly used to support people who live in community-based settings. The following features of essential lifestyle planning make it useful when planning care for people with intellectual disabilities who have palliative care needs (Smull and Harrison, 1992; Sanderson, 2003):

- Identification of what is important to that person and what they require to stay healthy and safe
- Focus upon the person's life here and now (in the light of historical knowledge of the person), and ways to improve it. It also identifies what is not working properly
- Detail of support which is required on a day-to-day basis, resulting in consistent high-quality care (which is of fundamental importance to the person with intellectual disability and palliative care needs)

An essential lifestyle plan can be used throughout the care process of a person who has an intellectual disability and requires palliative care.

Person-centred approaches and palliative care

The care journey of a person with intellectual disabilities should be underpinned by a combined palliative care approach and a person-centred approach, dependent on individual need. These needs can be broken down into the following phases: recognising ill health, diagnosis, treatment and prognosis. In addition, the particular care needs identified during each phase can be mapped out and effectively met by adopting this combined approach. Case illustrations are useful in highlighting the integration of person-centred approaches within the phases of a palliative care journey. The following three case studies, in part, sensitively illustrate these phases, and highlight both general and specific points in relation to the inherent difficulties that people with intellectual disabilities may encounter when experiencing a palliative illness.

Case illustration 9.1

Joe had lived in a small nursing home for people with intellectual disabilities for 2 years; prior to that he had lived in a long-stay hospital for many years. He had a moderate intellectual disability. He appeared very happy following his move to his new home, and found the care staff very caring and helpful. He enjoyed accessing local community facilities and visiting local places of interest. He also appeared to enjoy his new lifestyle and the increased opportunities to make choices in his life. An elderly relative (who he was very fond of) visited approximately once every fortnight. Joe had been diagnosed as having a heart condition many years ago. He also had angina, and was prescribed medication to treat both medical conditions. Recently care staff had noticed that Joe had become more breathless and had difficulties in relation to his mobility. In addition he appeared to be losing weight, and generally looked unwell. Joe's GP examined him, and after consulting Joe it was decided that he would be admitted to the local hospital, where he was placed in a side room. Care staff from his care home visited him regularly. They were informed he had suffered a stroke (CVA) and he died during the night, 2 weeks after he had been admitted to hospital.

On reflection

Joe's story illustrates the importance of his carers' recognising his ill health (weight loss and increasing mobility difficulties). They also needed to identify care priorities on his behalf, in order to ensure a timely diagnosis (by his GP), treatment and subsequent care plan, based on his changing health needs. A challenge, identified in the case study, related to Joe's continuity of care as a result of his having to be admitted to hospital. Hospital care staff had differing care priorities, skills and work practices to those who worked in the nursing residential home. Joe lost the familiarity of his surroundings, friends and of those caring for him.

Case illustration 9.2

Mark had lived in a social services hostel for many years. He was a very popular and well liked man, who had Down's syndrome. He had regular contact with his elderly mother and sister, who visited him at least once a fortnight. Over the past year his care staff had noted that he was becoming increasingly forgetful, and engaging in behaviour which they were increasingly finding difficult to cope with. They also noted he was experiencing complex and multiple mood changes over a short time span. He would become very tearful for no apparent reason, and become very distressed and angry. Mark's behaviour was also impacting negatively on fellow residents in the care home where he lived. A local community learning disabilities team had provided Mark and his carers with ongoing support. Mark was initially prescribed anti-depressants, but he was eventually diagnosed as having Alzheimer's disease. He was encouraged to participate in regular meetings, which reviewed his care needs and helped plan for his future. A speech and language therapist and clinical psychologist also provided Mark with support, in order that he could actively participate in the meetings. Eventually, after consulting with Mark, a decision was made (using Holman's (1997) 'best interest' guidelines) that it would be in his best interest to have continuous nursing care. Mark moved to a nursing home within a month of the decision being made. Care staff from the hostel visited occasionally, but found it upsetting, due to a marked decline in his health status.

On reflection

Mark's story highlights palliative care issues in relation to Down's syndrome and Alzheimer's disease. Research has indicated that most people with Down's syndrome over the age of 35 years have neuropathological evidence of Alzheimer's disease (Ball and Nuttall, 1980; Wisniewski et al., 1985; McCarron, 1999). Issues connected to ill health, diagnosis and prognosis were pertinent to this study. Mark's medical diagnosis had a profound impact upon him personally and also upon those who cared for, and about, him. The main challenge for his carers was to involve him actively in the decision-making process in relation to his changing health and future care needs. The care team used 'best interest' guidelines (Holman, 1997) to influence their decision making. 'Best interest' guidelines use the Law Commission's checklist to ascertain appropriate support for those people unable to make decisions for themselves.

Case illustration 9.3

Jean had lived in supported accommodation for many years. She had a history of mental health difficulties and was regarded as a heavy smoker. Jean received ongoing support from the community learning disabilities team. She was noticed to become short of breath on exertion, and to have a 'smokers cough'. In addition she was noted to be hoarse when speaking and also to be losing weight. She was eventually diagnosed with incurable lung cancer. A 'circle of support' was identified which would offer Jean the care and support she required. The circle included a community learning disabilities nurse, a specialist Macmillan nurse, a district nurse, general practitioner, social worker, a manager and key-worker from the care home where Jean lived. The vicar from a local church, which Jean regularly attended, also formed part of the 'circle of support'.

Jean's GP informed her of the extent of her illness, in the presence of her social worker and manager from the care home. Jean stated that she wanted to die at home. Jean met regularly with people from her circle of support, and together they identified the ongoing support and care she required. The level of support and care required understandably increased, as her health deteriorated. Jean's wishes were respected, and she died a month later at home, surrounded by people from her circle of support.

On reflection

Jean's story illustrates issues surrounding diagnosis and prognosis. Jean was diagnosed with lung cancer, late in the trajectory of her illness, perhaps because of diagnostic overshadowing (Brown et al., 2003). Sadly, the prognosis for Jean was poor, but her wishes and needs were met by her 'circle of support'. A 'circle of support' involves a group of committed people who aim to break down the barriers to appropriate care; in this instance this involved palliative care.

Assessment and management of Jean's pain was of crucial importance. Pain might have been assessed using Anne's Vulvar Cancer Centre pain chart (http://annescancer.tripod.com), or the DisDat Distress Assessment tool (Regnard et al., 2003). The analgesic ladder (World Health Organization, 1996; Katz et al., 2004) is also a useful model to conceptualise pain relief for a person with Jean's specific needs. These tools are useful in assessing pain generally, but only the DisDat tool (Regnard et al., 2003) has been developed specifically for people with intellectual disabilities, and focuses upon observable behaviours as indicators of distress for people with limited communication.

Discussion of the three case illustrations

The three case studies have highlighted the various difficulties in recognising, responding to, and managing palliative care needs among people with intellectual disabilities. Recognising ill health may be difficult (as illustrated in Case illustration 9.1) and all carers need to remain vigilant in recognising any changes in a person's health and behavioural status. Involving individuals who develop complex health needs in their care may be fraught with difficulties (as identified in Case illustration 9.2).

'Knowing the patient' is a key feature of palliative care (Seymour, 2004) particularly when it involves a person with intellectual disabilities. Life story work has been used to promote the uniqueness of individuals with intellectual disabilities, and to create history and develop a heritage for individuals who may have difficulty in recollecting and describing previous life experiences. Life story books have been described as tools to help people to get to know the individual, define the person and help them to express and identify the unique personality of an individual (Hewitt, 1998). In addition to the many positive benefits of life story work generally, within a palliative care context, life story books become an invaluable resource in reminding professional carers of who the person was before the illness. They offer a rich source of information about what the person used to enjoy doing; what their hobbies were; what food they preferred; and who their family and friends are. Accompanying photographs are simple, inexpensive and concrete reminders of people, places and experiences that offer opportunities for reminiscence work with individuals, in addition to helping carers to remember the unique individual within the illness. They are relatively simple and inexpensive resources that can be used throughout the individual's life and may ultimately make a huge contribution to the quality of care delivered as the person moves towards death. Subsequently, life story approaches may play an important role within the palliative care context.

The case illustrations all highlight the necessity of adopting a person-centred approach within the holistic nature of palliative care. As previously indicated, a person-centred approach that may be well suited to addressing these needs is an essential lifestyle plan. Ideally it should be implemented while the person with intellectual disabilities is physically well, and can then be reviewed and adapted if the person develops a life-threatening illness. This will ensure they receive care of a consistently high standard, particularly when their needs are palliative in nature. If an essential lifestyle plan approach were used early in (for example) Jean's care (Case illustration 9.3), it may have incorporated the issues identified in Fig. 9.2. Here, diagnosis and treatment options were the initial essential features, together with involving and empowering Jean in the illness trajectory, and establishing a circle of support was a strong preference. However, as the illness progressed, the focus would inevitably change, and choosing and arranging the place of choice for death would perhaps have become a 'non-negotiable' factor. Fig. 9.2 is offered for illustrative purposes only, and it only recognises one space in time along the palliative care pathway; the reader needs to recognise that these four key areas could change almost on a daily basis in keeping with the person-centred approach to care within the palliative care context. As Jean approaches death, the place of death will become a non-negotiable option together with management of pain and other symptoms.

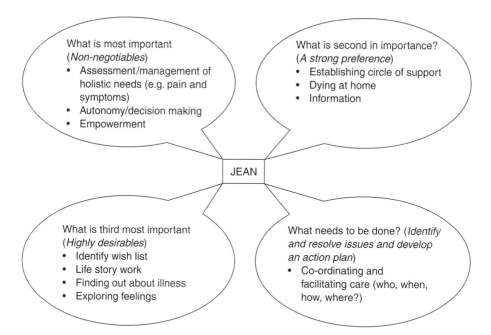

Fig. 9.2 Jean's essential lifestyle plan (after Sanderson et al., 1997; Smull and Harrison, 1992; Sanderson, 2003).

Holistic palliative care

Holistic palliative care incorporates attention to the physical, psychosocial, emotional and spiritual needs of any individual. Social needs could be met by providing practical help and support within the family, residential or nursing context (Jeffrey, 2003). The specialist social worker (intellectual disabilities) will be instrumental in addressing these needs. Psychological support might focus on helping the individual to express feelings and/or manage anxiety, anger and depression resulting from the person's illness. Support offered might range from a cognitive behavioural intervention to counselling, depending on the person's needs. The aim of these interventions is to improve the psychological and emotional well-being of the person with intellectual disabilities and palliative care needs (Jeffrey, 2003).

The difficulties that individuals have in communicating within the palliative care illustrations described, stress that people with intellectual impairment often have difficulties in recognising ill health and articulating their needs, often resulting in them becoming passive recipients of care (Keenan and McIntosh, 2000). People with intellectual disabilities are reliant on so many for so much, and often rely on personal and professional carers to recognise indicators of ill health on their behalf. Therefore, professional carers need to be reminded of the importance of maintaining an observational vigilance and remain alert to such obvious or subtle changes. Education may play an important role within this context.

Addressing the spiritual needs of an individual is also part of the holistic nature of palliative care, and is an area that may be fraught with difficulties for people with intellectual disabilities. Dimensions of spirituality include meaning and purpose, love and commitment, finding hope and strength, forgiveness, expression of personal beliefs and values, and sensing God or a deity amongst us (McSherry, 2001; Narayanasamy et al., 2002). Carers may feel uncertain regarding the spiritual dimensions of care; they may be confused about their role and lack the appropriate personal insight, precluding effective support (Swinton and Powrie, 2004). Person-centred planning and the National Institute of Clinical Excellence guidance (National Institute of Clinical Excellence, 2004) may encourage services to develop strategies that respond to the spiritual needs of individuals in a constructive and proactive way. Hatton et al. (2004) have provided an excellent training resource and guide that explores the meaning of faith and may encourage carers to work alongside people with intellectual disabilities in this difficult area of support.

Bereavement support

Death never occurs in a vacuum, but always within a social context (Costello, 2004), and the social context may be varied and affect access to appropriate palliative care (Oliviere and Munroe, 2004). Despite all the positive changes in care for people with intellectual disabilities, many are still not receiving the support they require following bereavement (Oswin, 2000) and their emotional needs in particular are often neglected (Arthur, 2003). Bereavement issues were never mentioned in any of the aforementioned case studies.

When a person dies in a residential or care setting, the impact on friends who also have an intellectual disability may be profound. A continuum of support is required, that recognises the individual needs of bereaved people and responds to these needs in proactive and reactive ways. This continuum involves the following (Read, 2005a):

- Education – opportunities to explore loss, change, death and grief as part of an educational curriculum
- Participation – nurturing a healthy response to grief by encouraging naturalistic opportunities to explore death and grief and developing resources
- Facilitation – reactive support that provides a constructive invitation to talk and explore the facts surrounding the death
- Communication in a meaningful and creative way
- Knowing when to refer on
- Therapeutic interventions – involving assessment and (for example) counselling, psychotherapy, guided morning interventions

Such a continuum of support before, during and after a death is an adult-orientated approach that helps the person to appreciate the emotional and psychological complexities of death; establishes effective coping strategies; and may ultimately reduce the need for specific therapeutic interventions (Read, 2005a). It does, however, mean that professional carers need to be proactive and have a consistent and planned approach to death and dying. Following death, some of the resources contained within a life story book can be used by family and friends as source of comfort and may help to preserve the memory of the deceased in a very concrete way.

Conclusion

Palliative care is an inherently sensitive topic, and many factors may influence how, what and, indeed, where such services are accessed. Having an intellectual disability may compound the difficulties in accessing appropriate care, and the challenges involved with this marginalised population (for example, involving practical, cognitive, philosophical and sometimes erroneous issues) have been presented for consideration in this chapter. People with intellectual disabilities who have palliative care needs have more similarities to the rest of the population than differences, and therefore the general principles of good palliative care should apply equally to them. However, as a result of the combination of the palliative care component of the condition and the learning disability itself, some people are identified as being potentially vulnerable from a death and dying perspective (Read and Elliott, 2003).

Person-centred planning has been recognised as a way of ensuring equity and parity of care for people with intellectual disabilities who develop palliative care needs, and these approaches have been explored in this chapter using case study illustrations. Essential life planning is a model that promotes good practice and has been integrated within one of the case illustrations to demonstrate its potential within the palliative care context.

The amount of research around palliative care generally is huge, but in relation to people with intellectual disabilities as a diverse population, it is sadly lacking (Tuffrey-Wijne, 2003). More empirical work is urgently required to identify the extent of the healthcare needs of this population; to disseminate examples of good practice such as the DisDat tool (Regnard et al., 2003) and evaluate their effectiveness; and to nurture the development and subsequent provision of effective education and training in this area. Collaborative working may be the key to minimising the professional challenges involved, and this means encouraging palliative care professionals and professionals in disability services to work together; they will then learn together to overcome the identified challenges to effective, holistic palliative care to this marginalised group. Such collaborative approaches also incorporate educational opportunities, as professionals have to learn together in order to minimise interdisciplinary barriers.

Acknowledgement

David Elliott would like to express his thanks to South Staffordshire Health Care Trust in supporting him in the writing of this chapter. In particular he would like to thank Mrs Judy Morris (Clinical Director – Learning Disabilities), Mrs Penny Pritchard (Clinical Co-ordinator – Learning Disabilities) and Mrs Sandra Brickley (Community Nurse Manager – Learning Disabilities), whose support he found invaluable.

References

Ahmed, N., Bestrall, J.C., Ahmedzai, S.H., Clark, D., and Noble, B. (2004) Systematic review of the problems and issues of accessing palliative care by patients, carers and health and social care professionals. *Palliative Medicine* **18** (6), 525–42.

Anne's Vulvar Cancer Centre. *Pain Chart.* http://annescancer.tripod.com/pain_chart2.html

Arthur, A.R. (2003) The emotional lives of people with learning disability. *British Journal of Learning Disabilities* **31** (1), 25–30.

Ball, M.J. and Nuttall, K. (1980) Neurofibrillary tangles, grannovacuolar degeneration, and neuron loss in Down's syndrome. Quantitative comparison with Alzheimer dementia. *Annals of Neurology* **7**, 462–5.

Bosch, J., Van Dyke, D.C., Milligan Smith, S. and Poulton, S. (1997) Role of medical conditions in the exacerbation of self-injurious behaviour: an exploratory story. *Mental Retardation* **35** (2), 124–30.

Brown, H., Burns, S. and Flynn, M. (2003) 'Please don't let it happen on my shift!' Supporting staff who are caring for people with learning disabilities who are dying. *Tizard Learning Disability Review* **8** (2), 185–6.

Costello, J. (2004) *Nursing the Dying Patient: Caring in Different Care Contexts.* Hampshire: Palgrave Macmillan.

Department of Health (2001a) *Valuing People: A New Strategy for Learning Disability for the 21st Century.* London: Department of Health.

Department of Health (2001b) *Seeking Consent: Working with People with Learning Disabilities.* London: Department of Health.

Department of Health (2002a) *Planning with People – Towards Person-Centred Approaches: Guidance for Partnership Boards.* London: Department of Health.

Department of Health (2002b) *Health Action Plans and Health Facilitation.* London: Department of Health.

Evenhuis, E. (1997) Medical aspects of ageing in a population with intellectual disability: 111. Mobility, internal conditions, and cancer. *Journal Intellectual Disability Research* **41** (1), 8–18.

Forest, M., Pearpoint. J and Rosenburg, R.L. (1997) *All my Life's a Circle. Using the Tools: Circles, MAP, and PATHS,* 2nd edn. Toronto: Inclusion Press.

Hatton, C., Turner, S. and Shah, R. (2004) *What About Faith? A Good Practice Guide for Services on Meeting the Religious Needs of People with Learning Disabilities.* London: The Foundation for People with Learning Disabilities.

Hewitt, H. (1998) Life story books for people with learning disabilities. *Nursing Times* **94** (33), 61–3.

Hogg, J., Northfield, J. and Turnbull, J. (eds.) (2001) *Cancer and People with Learning Disabilities: The Evidence from Published Studies and Experiences from Cancer Services.* Kidderminster: BILD Publications.

Holman, A. (1997) In the absence of legislation, follow the 'Best Interests' guidelines. *Community Living* **10** (3), 2.

Iles, I. (2003) Becoming a learning organization: a precondition for person centred services to people with learning difficulties. *Journal of Learning Disabilities* **7** (1), 65–77.

Jeffrey, D. (2003) What do we mean by psychosocial care in palliative care? In: *Psychosocial Issues in Palliative Care* (Lloyd-Williams, M., ed.). Oxford: Oxford University Press.

Katz, J., Komaromy, C. and Siddell, M. (2004) *Foundations in Palliative Care: A Programme for Facilitated Learning for Care Home Staff.* London: Macmillan Cancer Relief.

Keenan, P. and McIntosh, P. (2000) Learning disabilities and palliative care. *Palliative Care Today* **9**, 11–13.

Kilbane, J. and Sanderson, H. (2004) 'What' and 'how': understanding professional involvement in person centred planning styles and approaches. *Learning Disability Practice* **7** (4), 16–20.

Kilbane, J. and Thompson, J. (2004) Never ceasing our exploration: understanding person centred planning. *Learning Disability Practice* **7** (3), 28–31.

McCarron, M. (1999) Some issues in caring for people with dual disability of Down's syndrome and Alzheimer's dementia. *Journal of Learning Disabilities for Nursing, Health and Social Care* **3** (3), 123–9.

McSherry, W. (2001) Spirituality and learning disability: Are they compatible? *Learning Disability Practice* **3** (5) 35–9.

Mencap (2004) *Treat me Right! Better Healthcare for People with a Learning Disability (accessible format).* London: Mencap.

Mount, B. (1995) *Capacity Works: Finding Windows for Change using Personal Futures Planning.* New York: Graphic Futures.

Narayanasamy, A., Gates, B. and Swinton, J. (2002) Spirituality and learning disability: A qualitative study. *British Journal of Nursing* **11** (14), 948–57.

National Institute for Clinical Evidence (2004) *Improving Supportive and Palliative Care for Adults with Cancer. The Manual. Key Recommendations and Workforce Implications.* London: North East London Workforce Development Directorate Lead for Cancer Services.

O'Brien, C.L. and O'Brien, J. (2000) *The Origins of Person-centred Planning: A Community of Practice Perspective.* Responsive Systems Associates Inc. Available online at http://soeweb.syr.edu/thechp/rsapub.htm.

O'Brien, J. and Pierpoint, J. (2003) *Person-centred Planning with MAPs and PATH: A Workbook for Facilitators.* Toronto: Inclusion Press.

Oliviere, D. and Monroe, B. (eds.) (2004) *Death and Dying and Social Differences.* Oxford: Oxford University Press.

Oswin, M. (2000) *Am I Allowed to Cry?* 2nd edn. London: Souvenir Press.

Read, S. (2005a) Loss, bereavement and learning disability: Providing a continuum of support. *Learning Disability Practice* **8** (1), 31–7.

Read, S. (2005b) Learning disability and palliative care: Recognising pitfalls and exploring potential. *International Journal of Palliative Nursing* **11** (1), 15–20.

Read, S. and Elliot, D. (2003) Death and learning disability: a vulnerability perspective. *The Journal of Adult Protection* **5** (1), 5–14.

Regnard, C. and Kindlen, M. (2002) *Supportive and Palliative Care in Cancer: An Introduction*. Abingdon: Radcliffe Medical Press.

Regnard, C., Matthews, D., Gibson, L., Clarke, C. and Watson, B. (2003) Difficulties in identifying distress and its causes in people with severe communication problems. *International Journal of Palliative Nursing* **9** (3), 173–6.

Sanderson, H. (2003) Person-centred planning. In: *Learning Disabilities: Toward Inclusion*, 4th edn, (Gates, B., ed.). Edinburgh: Churchill Livingstone.

Sanderson, H., Kennedy, J., Ritchie, P. and Goodwin, G. (1997) *People, Plans and Possibilities – Exploring Person Centred Planning*. Edinburgh: Scottish Human Services Publications.

Seymour, J. (2004) A concept analysis of key terms. In: *Palliative Care Nursing: Principles and Evidence for Practice* (Payne, S., Seymour J. and Ingleton C., eds.). Berkshire: Open University Press.

Smull, M. and Harrison, S. (1992) *Supporting People with Severe Reputations in the Community*. Virginia: National Association of State Directors of Developmental Disabilities Services.

Swinton, J. and Powrie, E. (2004) *Why are we Here? Meeting the Spiritual Needs of People with Learning Disabilities*. London: The Foundation for People with Learning Disabilities.

Thompson, J. and Cobb, J. (2004) Person-centred health action planning. *Learning Disability Practice* **7** (5), 12–15.

Todd, S. (2004) Death counts: the challenge of death and dying in learning disability services. *Learning Disability Practice* **7** (10), 12–15.

Tuffrey-Wijne, I. (1997) Palliative care and learning disabilities. *Nursing Times* **93** (31), 50–1.

Tuffrey-Wijne, I. (2003) The palliative care needs of people with learning disabilities: A literature review. *Palliative Medicine* **17** (1), 55–62.

Wisniewski, K.E., Wisniewski, H.M. and Wen, G.Y. (1985) Occurrence of neuropathological changes and dementia of Alzheimer's disease in Down Syndrome. *Annals of Neurology* **17**, 278–82.

World Health Organization (1990) *Cancer Pain Relief and Palliative Care*. Technical report, Series B04. Geneva: World Health Organization.

World Health Organization (1996) *Cancer Pain Relief*. Geneva: World Health Organization.

Chapter 10

The planning and delivery of nursing care in community nursing services

Owen Barr and Maurice Devine

Introduction

The majority of people with intellectual disabilities live in community settings and many more live with family carers than live in hospitals or community-based residential accommodation (Scottish Executive, 2000; Department of Health, 2001a; McConkey et al., 2003; Barron and Mulvany, 2004). Therefore, effective collaboration between parents, family carers and community nurses is at the core of providing specialist nursing care for many people with intellectual disabilities in the community (Hubert and Hollins, 2000). The range of community settings in which the people with intellectual disabilities may live in has diversified over recent years. More opportunities now exist for people with intellectual disabilities to live in their own home, a range of supported housing options, small group homes and, for some people, larger residential or nursing home accommodation (Simons and Watson, 1999). Current national and international policy in services for people with intellectual disability continues to emphasise the importance of developing a wider range of smaller accommodation options that will enable people to live in community settings, rather than larger congregated settings (Scottish Executive, 2000; Department of Health, 2001b; DHSSPS, 2005). Integral to the growth in the availability and range of community-based residential facilities for people with intellectual disabilities have been the partnerships between statutory and independent sector providers, including private providers, housing associations and charities.

People with intellectual disabilities also use other community-based services, including day services, further education, leisure services, employment training services, and may have meaningful work in supported or open employment. Some people with intellectual disabilities may have a package of day activities that brings together time in day centres with further education, training and work in open or supported employment. These services are provided both by statutory and independent sector providers, across a number of agencies including health, social services, education and employment. Therefore community nurses need to have effective collaborative relationships with staff in community-based residential accommodation, and across a number of other agencies in order to provide effective nursing care to people living in the community. However, despite the developments in community-based services, there continues to be a reliance on parents and other family carers, and they remain the largest group of carers in the community (Department of Health, 2001a).

The changing demography of people with intellectual disabilities

The numbers of people with intellectual disabilities in the total population have been estimated on the basis of prevalence and with varying rates identified in each constituent country of the United Kingdom and the Republic of Ireland. These have been reported either as rates for people with differing levels of disability or an overall prevalence rate for all people with intellectual disability. For example, prevalence rates in Scotland and England have been reported as three to four people with profound and severe intellectual disabilities among 1000 people in the general population (Scottish Executive, 2000; Department of Health, 2001b) and between 20 and 25 people with mild/moderate intellectual disabilities per 1000 of the population (Scottish Executive, 2000; Department of Health, 2001b). Within Northern Ireland, a combined administrative prevalence of all people with intellectual disabilities has been reported as 9.7 people per 1000 people in the population (McConkey et al., 2003). Finally, the Republic of Ireland the figures for 2004 reported an administrative prevalence of 6.49 per 1000 of the population. This was comprised of prevalence rates of 2.30, 2.45, 1.01 and 0.27 for people with mild, moderate, severe and profound intellectual disabilities respectively, and included a prevalence rate of with 0.46 for people for whom a level of intellectual disability had not been verified at the time of reporting (Barron and Mulvany, 2004).

On the basis of these prevalence rates, it has been estimated there are around 210 000 people with profound and severe intellectual disabilities in England, of which approximately 65 000 are children and young people, with 120 000 adults of working age and 25 000 older people (Department of Health, 2001b). Within Scotland, the estimated number of people with intellectual disabilities has been given as 120 000 (Scottish Executive, 2000). In Northern Ireland, a population of 16 366 people with intellectual disabilities has been reported, almost evenly split between people under the age of 19 years (8150: 49.8%) and those older than 19 years of age (8216: 50.2%) (McConkey et al., 2003). In comparison, the Republic of Ireland has reported a total of 25 416 people with intellectual disabilities, of which 8680 (34.2%) are 19 years old or younger and 16 736 (65.8%) are over 19 years of age (Barron and Mulvany, 2004).

Services within Northern Ireland and the Republic of Ireland have used a measure of 'administrative prevalence'; that is, people known to services. Administrative prevalence has the strength of providing accurate figures and more detailed statistical analysis than prevalence rates based on the projection of rates from smaller studies to the overall population, which may result in over-estimation of actual numbers. However, it is recognised that administrative prevalence may provide an underestimation of actual numbers of people with mild intellectual disabilities who may only be included when they are using intellectual disability services, and of older people with intellectual disabilities, who may not have availed of services when younger and only become known to services in their later years (Barron and Mulvany, 2004).

Due largely to improvements in health and social care, people with intellectual disabilities are now living longer and there will continue to be an increasing number of older people with intellectual disabilities (Hubert and Hollins, 2000). There has also been a growth in the number of children with complex health needs living into young adulthood. Both these groups of people will present challenges to adult services as staff in these services have limited experience to date in supporting younger adults and older people with such complex needs (Jenkins, 2000).

The numbers of people with intellectual disabilities are expected to continue rising by 1% every year over the next 10–15 years (Scottish Executive, 2000; Department of Health, 2001b). This will result in a greater proportion of younger people and older people with intellectual disabilities who will have complex health needs. The increasing life expectancy of people with intellectual disabilities will also lead to a greater proportion of people with intellectual disabilities living with older parents and family carers, or outliving their parents and carers, than is the situation at present (Hubert and Hollins, 2000). This trend has already been reported in Scotland with a quarter of people with intellectual disabilities living with a family carer over 65 years of age, 20% with two carers aged 70 or over, and 11% with one carer over 70 years of age (Scottish Executive, 2000).

Reader activity 10.1

Read your local trust policy document in relation to supporting people with intellectual disabilities. Ask your local service manager for information on the ages of people and their carers within the trust in which you work.

Think of one child, one young adult and one person with intellectual disabilities over 50 years of age you have had contact with. List the professionals and services that may be involved in providing support to them. Prepare a list of the key contact points for these organisations within your local trust.

Context of community nursing services

The role and functions of community nurses for people with intellectual disabilities (referred to as community nurses within this chapter) are influenced by a number of factors. These can be grouped under three broad headings:

community healthcare nursing, principles underpinning wider intellectual disability services and service developments and restructuring.

Community healthcare nursing: role of community nurses for people with intellectual disabilities

Community nurses for people with intellectual disabilities have existed in some parts of the United Kingdom for almost 30 years, and commenced in the Republic of Ireland in 2000. From a few small services in the mid 1970s, the number of community nurses for people with intellectual disabilities has grown steadily to the current situation in which community nurses are employed in the vast majority of community intellectual disability services across the United Kingdom. Community nurses within these services are Registered Nurses (Intellectual Disabilities) and have often undertaken an additional nursing course in community nursing (Boarder, 2002; Mobbs et al., 2002; Slevin, 2004).

Initially, during the 1970s and 1980s the role of these nurses was not clearly defined and varied considerably across different areas of the country. However, during the 1990s, a clearer picture of the role of community nurses emerged and research studies reported a largely consistent range of reasons for involvement. A number of differing approaches have been used in research studies that sought to provide an understanding of the current role of community nurses. These have included research studies based on the analysis of caseloads of community nurses working with people with intellectual disabilities (Jenkins and Johnson, 1991; Parahoo and Barr, 1996; Slevin, 2004), the views of service managers (Boarder, 2002; Mobbs et al., 2002) and other professionals working in community services (Mansell and Harris, 1998; Powell et al., 2004). Overall, the results of these studies showed that community nurses reported a reasonably consistent range of reasons for visiting people with intellectual disabilities. These included support in responding to the presence of challenging behaviour, mental health problems, physical disability, epilepsy, physical care needs, issues associated with people with intellectual disabilities growing older, sexuality and sensory disability.

Principles underpinning wider intellectual disability services

A series of policy reviews in each of the four countries of the United Kingdom have taken place since 2000. This has resulted in new policy documents to guide developments in intellectual disability services within the United Kingdom. The documents for the individual countries are as follows:

- Scotland   *Same as You?* (Scottish Executive, 2000)
- England   *Valuing People* (Department of Health, 2001b)
- Northern Ireland   *Equal Lives* (DHSSPS, 2005)
- Wales   *Fulfilling the Promises* (Welsh Office, 2001) (although this was issued as 'guidance' rather than a new policy document)

Each document contains specific service principles for each jurisdiction, but there is a convergence of principles across countries within the United Kingdom and internationally. Overall the underpinning service philosophy is one of inclusion in society, including equity of access to mainstream health services (Sowney and Barr, 2004). In achieving this overall aim, revised service principles emphasise citizenship (rights, equality), person-centred approach (choice, participation) and development of skills to increase independence. Community nurses need to consider these principles in the process of planning and delivering nursing care.

Unfortunately, potentially divisive debates in relation to the use of so-called social or medical models of services continue unnecessarily to distract the energies of people in community services. These two models are often presented as irreconcilable, and have been incorrectly linked to different professional approaches, with nursing being associated with the medical model and less acceptable in developing services for people with intellectual disabilities. The social model has been linked to social services and more appropriate to under-standing the nature of, and providing services to, people with intellectual disabilities. However, the social model of disability has also underpinned nurse education in intellectual disabilities across the United Kingdom from the 1980s. Policy documents are unanimous that the social model, which highlights the need for action to be taken to alter societal attitudes and value people with intellectual disabilities, should underpin services (Scottish Executive, 2000; Department of Health, 2001b; Welsh Office, 2001; DHSSPS, 2005).

As Thomas and Woods (2003) have highlighted, however, both models have their strengths and limitations and it is important that a medical model is not mistaken for the provision of healthcare. Indeed, health must also be under-stood within a wider social context. It could be argued that the views against the perceived limitations of the so-called medical model may have contributed to the reluctance to acknowledge the additional health needs of people with intellectual disabilities and their high level of unmet health need. Future service models will be required to become more holistic and accommodate a broader 'health' perspective that incorporates physical, mental and social health (Aldridge, 2004).

Reader activity 10.2

Obtain information from nurses in a local community team on the current role of community nurses for people with intellectual disabilities on the basis of the people on their caseloads within the trust area.

Compare and contrast the current role of community nurses with the service principles as stated in the revision of policy/service principles related to the jurisdiction in which you work. In view of the current policies and role, what do you see as the future priorities in further developing care planning and care delivery by community nurses in intellectual disability services?

Principles of effective planning and delivery of nursing care in the community

Community nurses in intellectual disability, as well as other areas of community healthcare nursing, have a role in working with individuals, families and groups. Across community health nursing there is a growing recognition of the need for community nurses to have a greater role in areas of public health (Watkins et al., 2003; Sines et al., 2005). While acknowledging that, this chapter focuses on the process of planning and delivering nursing care with individuals, as this is presently the core work for the majority of community nurses.

A structured nursing assessment should provide comprehensive information on the abilities and needs of clients. On the basis of the nursing assessment, 'nursing care plans' document the prioritised needs of clients and identify the prescribed nursing actions that are considered necessary to achieve agreed objectives (Mason, 1999). In planning and delivering effective nursing care for people with intellectual disabilities in the community, nurses need to consider four broad principles that apply across all stages of care planning and care delivery, namely:

- Person-centred approach
- The requirement for valid consent
- The need to be based within a nursing framework
- A collaborative endeavour

Person-centred approach

Person-centred planning is now a key principle within services (see Chapters 3 and 4). This requires support for individuals with intellectual disabilities to facilitate them to take steps that actively involve them in developing their thoughts and feelings about their future and involve them in decisions that will impact on their life. Common to all person-centred planning approaches is the need to focus on the questions 'Who are you?', 'Who are we in your life?' and 'What can we do together to achieve a better life for you now, and in the future?' (Sanderson, 2003). Person-centred planning focuses on the person as a citizen and requires nurses involved to use an approach that leads to action and is tailored to the individual, rather than being restricted to fitting people into a limited range of options available. The emphasis should be on providing the support necessary for people to be actively involved in the process of decision making, building on their strengths and resulting in the development of further skills and independence. In seeking to achieve this level of information, community nurses must be alert to the risk of discrimination that people with intellectual disabilities may encounter and take action to promote anti-discriminatory nursing practice, for instance, in facilitating equity of access to healthcare (Thompson, 2003; Sowney and Barr, 2004).

For some people who have complex health needs, community nurses will have a role in contributing to the development of a person-centred plan. The development of an overall person-centred plan does not replace the need for a nursing care plan. Rather the assessment and planning of nursing care should incorporate the principles of person-centred planning. Once the areas of nursing support required have been identified within the overall person-centred plan, community nurses should develop more specific nursing care plans in collaboration with the person with intellectual disabilities and their family or other carers. In seeking to provide person-centred support, nurses must give due consideration to the requirements of the policies relating to consent to examination, treatment and care during this process (Department of Health, 2001c; DHSSPS, 2003).

The requirement for valid consent

Within current policies, consent is no longer limited to medical or surgical treatment (it never really was), but rather relates to examination, treatment and care. Furthermore, it is the responsibility of the health or social care professional that will be delivering interventions to obtain valid consent. Valid consent requires that provision of information about the benefits and possible limitations of any intervention is provided and that the process by which consent has been obtained is accurately documented. Valid consent is more than informed consent, because, although appropriate information must be provided, it also requires that consent is not given under duress. Therefore a signed consent form is not adequate in itself, and the process by which consent was obtained should be accurately documented.

Finally, no one can give consent for another adult; if a person with intellectual disabilities is unable to give consent, therefore, a decision must be made on the basis of their 'best interests'. However, before a 'best interests' decision can be taken it is necessary to establish that, despite providing a person who has intellectual disabilities with information in an appropriate format and giving assistance for the person to be able to make a decision, they do not have the capacity at that time to provide a valid consent. Traditionally, it has often been presumed that people with intellectual disabilities did not have the capacity to make decisions, and this has resulted in paternalistic practice. However, this assumption is no longer acceptable.

A 'best interests' decision must be made on the best interests of the person with intellectual disabilities rather than the best interests of professionals, the service or family carers. Furthermore it is essential that community nurses are familiar with the current legislation and guidance on determining a person's capacity for decision making in place within the country in which they work. The process by which a 'best interests' decision is made should follow the process laid out in current guidance in relation to consent and capacity, and is underpinned by the principle that capacity is present unless formally demonstrated otherwise (HMSO, 2000; Department of Health, 2001c; DHSSPS, 2003; Wheeler, 2003; Hutchinson, 2005; HMSO, 2005).

The reader may also like to refer to Chapter 5 at this point for further discussion on this topic. When contributing to discussions about the best interests of a person with intellectual disabilities, nurses should base their contributions on structured nursing assessments of individuals at that time and their professional interpretation of the results obtained from any nursing assessment undertaken.

Based within a nursing framework

Current services are increasingly provided within an overall person-centred approach and there is growing emphasis on the need for a single assessment and one comprehensive plan of care for the person with intellectual disabilities. This comprehensive plan is interdisciplinary in nature and brings together the assessments of a number of professionals and details the objectives, planned interventions and the responsibilities of professionals involved in relation to the components within the plan of care. This can pose a major challenge for the professional practice of community nurses who work as members of wider interdisciplinary intellectual disability teams within community services. Their role within such teams is to provide a nursing service to the person with intellectual disabilities and their families. Nurses can make a valuable contribution to the development and delivery of this overall plan of care through their involvement in the stages of assessment, planning, implementation and evaluation. As registered nurses, their contribution should be built upon the foundation of a structured nursing assessment that forms the basis of the subsequent nursing care plans. The actions to be taken by the nurses should be detailed in nursing care plans, which are in essence the prescription of nursing care for which nurses are professionally accountable. It is not enough for nurses to be involved in overall discussions about the planning and delivery of care without having completed a nursing assessment.

This nursing assessment requires nurses to select and use a structured approach to assessing an individual's abilities and nursing needs. Nursing models provide a range of such frameworks that could be used when undertaking a nursing assessment (McKenna, 1997). Intellectual disability nursing appears to have been reluctant in the past to use these frameworks (Duff, 1997; Horan et al., 2004a, b), possibly because of an erroneous belief that these represented a more medically orientated approach to service provision and were overly prescriptive, or were not consistent with a person-centred approach. Such views are a misunderstanding of the purpose of nursing models, which were developed to provide broad frameworks to guide nursing assessment and nursing practice. It was never intended that a single nursing framework would suit all people from any client group, be that intellectual disability, mental health or adult branches of nursing. At times community nurses have adapted existing nursing models to reflect more closely the aims and objectives of intellectual disability nursing practice, usually by adding some further detail. However, it is important that in doing so the model does not become so 'adapted' that the coherence of the original model is lost (Lister, 1987).

Each nursing framework is underpinned by a view of the nature of people, health environment and nursing. Nurses need to have knowledge of a range of frameworks for nursing and select the appropriate one for the person they are working with at that time (McKenna, 1997). Each model has its strengths and limitations and the role of the registered nurse is to make a professional decision which framework to use with each individual (Fraser, 1996; Aggleton and Chalmers, 2000). The past few years have seen a growing willingness to use nursing models within intellectual disability nursing practice and published articles have demonstrated the usefulness of models of nursing, such as Peplau and Orem, to nursing practice (Navrady, 1998; Horan et al., 2004a, b). Furthermore, some attempts have been made to develop models of nursing that may be more suitable to the values underpinning intellectual disability nursing practice (Lee, 1990; Aldridge, 2004).

Community nursing services should have the capacity to use a number of nursing frameworks in order to respond to the diversity of individuals they may be working with. They could foreseeably use a range of nursing models, depending on the main aim of the nursing intervention as agreed with the person with intellectual disabilities and their family carers (where appropriate). To restrict community nursing practice to the use of one nursing framework and a 'one size fits all approach' is at best professionally questionable. Such a limited approach to professional practice is nonsense and totally undermines the emphasis on working with people as individuals and the need for person-centred approaches to planning and delivery of nursing care.

Finally, it is important that community nurses use a selected nursing model across all the stages of assessment, planning, implementation and evaluation of nursing care. These nursing frameworks provide much more than checklists for assessment. They contain guidance on the nature of nursing care plans and implementation of nursing care, of which community nurses should be aware. Other professionals involved in supporting people with intellectual disabilities will also undertake assessments and bring their professional education and knowledge into the discussions about aspects of care. In working collaboratively with other professionals, people with intellectual disabilities and their families, a more co-ordinated package of care should be possible.

Reader activity 10.3

Find out what nursing framework(s) is/are used to guide the assessment, planning, implementation and evaluation of community nursing care and how the information obtained contributes to an overall person-centred plan.

Consider two other organised nursing frameworks that could be used. Compare and contrast these to the models currently being used and consider the implications of using these models for care planning and care delivery.

Collaborative endeavour

If the process of care planning and delivery is to be effective, community nurses must develop collaborative relationships with a number of people. They will need to develop relationships with the person with intellectual disabilities with whom the care plan is being developed. This relationship should encompass the principles of person-centred planning and provide opportunities to be as involved as possible in decisions about the nursing care plan being developed. The ability of community nurses to communicate effectively with a wider range of people, some of whom may be reluctant to communicate or negotiate with them, will require careful attention to the use of skills in listening, explaining and negotiation (Long, 1999).

Given that the majority of people with intellectual disabilities live with family carers, community nurses will need to take time to establish relationships with key family carers in order that they can contribute to the process of care planning and delivery. Family carers include parents of young children, a growing number of older parents of adults, adult siblings and, at times, members of the extended family (Carpenter, 1997; Vagg, 1998; Burke, 2004). Effective working relationships with family members are particularly important, as often it is they who undertake the majority of 'implementation' of the actions detailed in nursing care plans, with community nurses providing ongoing support to family members. Even when they do regularly visit the home, community nurses are not able to maintain the level of supervision possible in residential or hospital settings and are often reliant on family carers to provide information about the person with intellectual disabilities.

Therefore, community nurses need to support carers effectively in order that the agreed care plans are implemented appropriately. In working with family carers, community nurses should be sensitive to the considerable role they have had in supporting their relative. They should seek to understand the relationship carers have with the person with intellectual disabilities and how this may influence their involvement in care planning and delivery (BILD, 1998; Department of Health, 2001a). Community nurses should provide information to family members about the role of community nurses and, from the outset of their involvement, take steps to ensure family members understand what the contribution and duration of contact from community nursing, as a specialist nursing service, is likely to be. There has been some debate as to what influence care plans actually have on nursing practice. Within a general nursing context, Mason (1999) questioned the reality of nursing care plans guiding practice if these were not locally 'owned' by the people involved in developing them and they were not considered relevant to that setting. A key message was, when developing nursing care plans, that particular attention should be given to the involvement of people who will deliver and receive nursing care.

In the absence of collaborative relationships with people with intellectual disabilities and family carers, community nurses will not be effective in their work. Community nurses have no right of entry to the home of people with intellectual disabilities or their family carers. So, without investing some time in establishing working relationships with family carers and people with intellectual disabilities, they may not even get inside the home.

Community nurses are part of a wider community team within intellectual disability services, which usually includes social workers, psychologists, allied health professionals and psychiatrists. Although these professionals may not all be within a single formally structured team, they need to work collaboratively in order to provide a co-ordinated service to people with intellectual disabilities and their families (West, 2004). In addition, community nurses need to have established relationships with professionals in primary care, as well as mainstream acute general and mental health services for both children and adults, in order to achieve the aim of health facilitation (Department of Health, 2001b).

To work collaboratively, community nurses need to have a clear understanding of their own role and how this interfaces with that of other professionals involved in services. Community nurses need to take active steps to ensure the professionals with whom they are working, in intellectual disability and mainstream services, are clear about the role of community nurses for people with intellectual disabilities. Although, community nurses are valued team members and viewed as having important roles, there continues to be confusion about their role and how this interfaces with other services (Mansell and Harris, 1998; Stewart and Todd, 2001; Boarder, 2002).

In recent years some community nurses have demonstrated the benefit of working collaboratively with professionals in mainstream services (Hunt et al., 2001; Cassidy et al., 2002; Martin, 2003; McConkey et al., 2003). This has been assisted, in part, by communicating their role in practical terms, which provides examples of actions that community nurses undertake, rather than a description around broad themes, such as advocate, educator and health promoter. Informing professionals of the role of community nurses is an ongoing process and there needs to be an ongoing strategy for keeping professionals aware of the developments in the role of community nurses. This is necessary to ensure that, as professionals in local services move on, new professionals are given relevant information about the role and function of community nurses for people with intellectual disabilities.

Alongside this, community nurses need to take steps to remain up-to-date about the role of other professionals they may be working with across intellectual disability and mainstream services. They should know how their role interfaces with these professionals and identify areas in which they can work collaboratively. Community nurses need to develop collaborative links beyond intellectual disability services, and maintain contact with other professionals and community nurses outside of intellectual disability services. The development of such networks will be of assistance in promoting equity of access to mainstream services for people with intellectual disability. It should also act to increase the understanding and clarify misperceptions of other professionals about the actual and potential contributions of community nurses from intellectual disability services to supporting people with intellectual disabilities, and how they could be of assistance to other professionals. A useful approach to achieving this is to ensure community nurses for people with intellectual disabilities are invited to (or invite themselves to) wider community nurse meetings and are appropriately represented on nursing groups across the local trust. In this way community nurses in intellectual disability services should be less isolated within those services, and, through remaining up-to-date with developments across community healthcare nursing in their locality, they will be in a more informed position to contribute to debates about such developments and also to access education and opportunities open to other community nurses.

Reader activity 10.4

Obtain any printed information on the role of the community nurses for people with intellectual disabilities within your trust. In discussion with people with intellectual disabilities, family carers and staff in intellectual disability and other services, consider how useful this information is in relation to care planning and care delivery by community nurses. List suggestions for how this information may be further developed.

The process of care planning and care delivery in community nursing for people with intellectual disabilities

Action on receipt of a referral for community nursing intervention

The process of community nurses planning and delivering specialist nursing care for people with intellectual disabilities commences with a referral to the community nursing service (Fig. 10.1). Depending on local arrangements, this referral may be made directly to community nurses or through wider community intellectual disability team and then allocated to the community nurse as a team member. Some services may use a generic screening assessment at this stage, which may be undertaken by any team member, to determine who the referral would be most appropriately responded to, by a community nurse or other team member.

Upon receipt of the referral the community nurse will prepare to undertake a structured nursing assessment. This assessment commences with reviewing the information contained in the referral letter/form as this gives the background information. A specialist community nursing service should have a baseline level of information required in a referral, as this is necessary to assist nurses in preparing to undertake the nursing assessment. The level of information required and the format expected in a referral should be published in the local leaflets and other media explaining the role of community nurses for

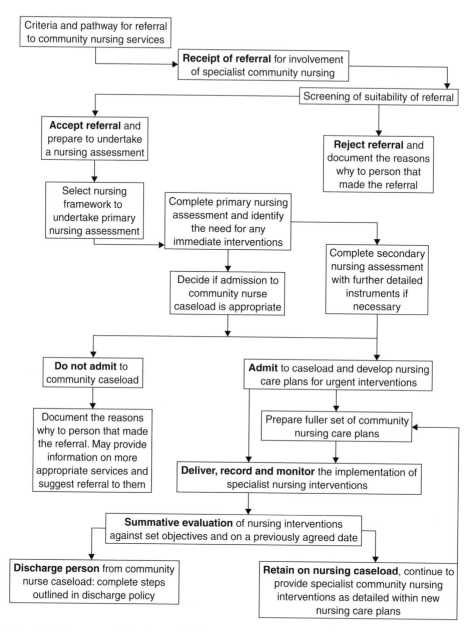

Fig. 10.1 Process of planning and delivery of nursing care by community nurses in intellectual disability services.

people with intellectual disabilities. This should also clearly state that the acceptance of referral does not mean an automatic admission to the caseload of the community nursing service. The decision about admission is made on the outcome of the nursing assessment.

Community nursing services should monitor the sources of their referrals and the profile of people referred to the service. This information is useful in determining the level of knowledge about community nursing services and the demographics of people referred to the service. By keeping this information over time, it is possible to identify trends in referrals that may indicate opportunities for co-working with local professionals. In addition, this information can provide an indication of the appropriateness and timeliness of referrals to specialist community nursing services. Recent reviews of the caseload of community nurses has indicated the reduction in referrals of children to community nursing services and concern that such referrals are not being made early enough to the gain the full benefit of early intervention (Mobbs et al., 2002; Northway, 2004; Barr, 2006).

Undertaking a nursing assessment

In preparing to undertake a nursing assessment, community nurses will be guided in part by the information contained within the referral. This should provide a clear indication for the main reason(s) for referral and the degree of urgency attached to this. Community nurses should decide which nursing framework is most appropriate to provide a structure for this initial (primary) nursing assessment in order to gain an overview of the main abilities and needs of the individual at that time. This primary assessment may indicate the need for further detailed assessment of specific aspects (secondary assessment) such as physical health, mental health or challenging behaviour (see Chapters 8 and 12). Information should be provided to the person with intellectual disabilities and, where appropriate, their family carers about the purpose and nature of the assessment process, in order for them to decide if they wish the assessment to proceed. In undertaking these additional assessments community nurses often work in collaboration with other professionals to access information already known to other services, if it is appropriate for this to be shared.

Assessments are more complete once community nurses, people with intellectual disabilities and family carers have the opportunity to build a working relationship, and community nurses do not feel like strangers to the person. However, when a referral requests an urgent assessment, it may be necessary to undertake an assessment focused on the area of particular concern within the referral in the first instance. This may involve the use of more detailed assessment schedules depending on the area of concern. The results of this aspect of the assessment may provide an indication of the initial nursing care that could be provided in the first instance. However, this does not remove the need for a more comprehensive nursing assessment, as this may reveal additional information relevant to the area of concern. Therefore, community nurses should then broaden the assessment to provide a complete nursing assessment (Aldridge, 2004). If there is a need to complete an urgent assessment, the community nurse involved should also seek to establish why the referral was not made to their service earlier and take action to prevent this happening with future referrals.

In undertaking a nursing assessment, community nurses will gather information about the family environment and family carers, to the extent that it relates to the assessment of the person with intellectual disabilities. However, seeking information about family carers within an assessment of the person with intellectual disability should not be confused with a carer's assessment. Family carers should be made aware of their right to a separate carer's assessment and arrangements promptly made for this to be undertaken if they wish to have this completed. Community nurses must also be mindful of any cultural considerations that need to be planned for or responded to in undertaking a nursing assessment in families from various cultural backgrounds. For instance, who is it acceptable to ask for information, how may questions be asked, the need for interpreters or having other people present (Nursing and Midwifery Council, 2004).

The results of the nursing assessment should be summarised to identify the current abilities and needs of the person with intellectual disabilities. It is important that both abilities and needs are considered, as an understanding of a person's abilities will assist the nurse develop nursing interventions that will be more appropriate and provide opportunities for the person to be involved in their own care. On the basis of this information, community nurses must reach a decision about those nursing needs that require specialist nursing care and whether it is appropriate for them to become involved in responding to these needs. If they consider this appropriate, the person should be admitted to a community nurse's caseload, or waiting list, depending on the availability of community nurses. Where community nurses work as part of wider interdisciplinary teams, the decision to admit or not admit someone to a nursing caseload is a decision that can only be made by the community nurse, and one that they are accountable for.

An alternative possibility is that following assessment, although it is established that the person has needs requiring a response, these are not at the level of requiring specialist nursing support. The needs identified in the assessment should be responded to by another service, either within intellectual disability services or the wider health and social services. When this is outcome of the assessment, the rationale for this decision should be documented and promptly explained to the person with intellectual disabilities, family carers and person making the referral (without breaching confidentiality of detail obtained during assessment) and documented. Following this, information should be provided about another agency that is considered more appropriate, together with information on how to make a referral to that service. However, the person should not be admitted to a community nurse's caseload. This can be a challenge for community nurses, who may know how they could help and may be tempted to intervene. The difficulty with this is that community nurses can end up filling gaps in services, rather than focusing their interventions on areas where their specialist knowledge and skills can achieve the greatest impact.

Preparing community nursing care plans and planning of interventions

When developing nursing care plans, community nurses will work from the priorities identified within the nursing assessment. They should also consider how these priorities relate to any overall interdisciplinary care plan that may have been developed as part of a person-centred planning process. Nurses should consider the interface between the nursing care plan, nursing interventions and overall person-centred plan; they must remain cognisant that, as autonomous nurses, they are accountable for the quality of the nursing care plan developed and how this is documented (Nursing and Midwifery Council, 2004 and 2005).

Within a nursing care plan, the areas of nursing need identified within the assessment are restated as nursing problems and objectives to be achieved are set. Community nurses should take care to state clearly the area of nursing needs, providing the wider context and the impact on the person with intellectual disabilities; for example, 'John is currently overweight (providing his weight and body mass index), and becomes breathless on walking more than 40–50 metres, which restricts in opportunities to attend leisure activities outside his home'. John may have associated objectives relating to cardiovascular health. Such broader statements place the difficulties the person experiences within the wider context of their life and can indicate further areas for nursing intervention. Community nurses should avoid the temptation to use short phrases or single words in outlining the nursing needs, such as 'obesity' or 'restricted mobility', 'lack of leisure opportunities', without providing the wider context and contributing factors.

The areas identified for attention will in part be influenced by the nursing framework or model being used to structure the nursing intervention, for example, Orem (1991), Peplau (1991), Roper et al. (2001) or Aldridge (2004) (also see Chapters 1, 8 and 13). Similarly, the objectives within the nursing care plans should reflect the type of care plan being written as outlined within the nursing frameworks, for example, 'supporting or comforting' are key to care planning with Roper et al. (2001), and care plans within Orem (1991) may be described as 'wholly compensatory, partially compensatory or educative' in nature.

Objectives should be client centred and provide a clear statement of the skill/ knowledge the person with intellectual disabilities is seeking to achieve, the support they will need to do this and the criteria that will be used to establish when the objectives have been achieved. This could incorporate some aspect of measurement of success, either by using a recognised instrument or self-reports from the person with intellectual disabilities and family carers. Objectives also need to be realistic and achievable within a few weeks. Therefore, community nurses may need to break down longer-term objectives, which may take several months to achieve, into manageable periods of intervention that will be completed and evaluated every few weeks. Each objective should have a specific date for evaluation, rather than 'in 4 weeks' or the date for evaluation being described as 'ongoing'. This level of specificity helps to keep a focus on the interventions and provides regular feedback of progress.

There are two key limitations to the way objectives are at times written in some nursing care plans. Firstly, the objectives are stated as something to be achieved by the community nurse rather than the person with intellectual disabilities, for example 'to maintain safety, or to maintain independence'. Such objectives are not person centred and, although the nurse may feel they have achieved the objective, little may have changed for the person with intellectual disabilities. Secondly, objectives do not include clear descriptions of the knowledge or skills to be achieved, and often do not have statements about the conditions or criteria for the achievement of the objectives. Broad objectives such as 'maximise independence' are given, as opposed to 'John will be able to go to the toilet independently', or 'Mary will self administer her prescribed medication without error for 5 consecutive days'. The absence of clear statements in relation to knowledge, skills and criteria makes it almost impossible to establish when nursing interventions have been successful, as there are no set criteria or conditions to measure them against, therefore care plans may be considered to remain ongoing. This, in turn, can result in difficulties in deciding when to discharge people from the community nursing caseload.

The use of pre-written 'core nursing care plans' is not inconsistent with a person-centred approach, as long as the 'core' plan is appropriately individualised for each person, with additional interventions added as necessary and those listed in the core plan which are not relevant deleted. However, nurses need to be aware professional accountability issues associated within using core plans which are not individualised before use. This may result in the nursing care plan not accurately reflecting the nursing interventions, in which situation nurses are not providing care as prescribed in the nursing care plan and may be undertaking interventions that are not listed in the nursing care plan.

Having agreed the statements of nursing need and objectives of the nursing care plan, community nurses should outline the nursing interventions that they will complete in order to achieve the objectives of the care plan. The statement of nursing interventions should be clear and easily understood by everyone who will need to read the care plan. Community nurses should be able to provide a rationale for their proposed actions and are increasingly expected to be able to demonstrate an evidence base for their proposed nursing interventions (Freshwater and Rolfe, 2004). Nursing interventions should be written as statements of what nurses will do, giving an indication of the time commitment to specific aspects of work to be undertaken, for example, a skills development intervention a may involve a 1-hour session each week for 6 weeks.

Care plans should also indicate what other carers will be expected to do. Agreed nursing interventions should be practical given the living environment of the person with intellectual disabilities and other people who live there. Therefore, in agreeing interventions to be undertaken, community nurses should consider how practical these are given the accommodation people live in and the resources available to them. Community nurses should remain alert to the fact that what may work in one family setting might not be suitable in another, or what worked in a larger residential or hospital setting, may not be appropriate for a family home, due to the resources required or the potential disruption to other people living there.

Once nursing interventions and actions of other people are agreed, community nurses should identify any resources that will be necessary for these interventions to take place, such as the provision of equipment and training for family carers or other staff. If community nurses are involved in providing training to other staff and family members, in particular to undertake invasive procedures, clear protocols should exist outlining how this training will be delivered and how competence should be assessed. It is advisable that such protocols should clarify the professional accountability of community nurses in undertaking this work. If answers to particular questions about the limits of accountability are unclear, these should be discussed with the appropriate representatives of the Nursing and Midwifery Council. The care plan cannot be implemented until these resources are in place. In the absence of the necessary resources nurses should consider if the nursing care plan needs amending or that it cannot be implemented. If required resources are not available, this should be identified as an unmet need and the appropriate person within the trust notified (Nursing and Midwifery Council, 2004). When notifying people of unmet needs, community nurses should document and keep copies of correspondence relating to this in client records.

To complete the nursing care plan, a date for implementation and review should be added to the care plan document. As already stated, these should be actual dates, rather than 'in 2 weeks' or 'review monthly'. When admitting someone to their caseload, community nurses should clearly signal that their intervention is focused on the objectives set and when these are achieved the person will be considered for discharge. By sensitively identifying their role in such a focused and potentially time-limited context during the process of care planning, people with intellectual disabilities, family carers and other professionals should have a more realistic understanding of the likely involvement of community nurses.

Implementation: the delivery of specialist nursing care

During the implementation phase nursing care plans provide the blueprint of the actions to be taken and how this will be co-ordinated. In supporting people with intellectual disabilities, community nurses will carry out the agreed interventions as detailed within the care plan to achieve the set objectives. This will involve working directly with the person with intellectual disabilities, their family carers and liaising with other professionals involved. Each time a community nurse makes a visit in relation to a person on their caseload they should have specific objectives for that visit. The focus of the interventions by community nurses should relate directly to the actions identified within the nursing care plan. If new issues are introduced during a visit, these may take precedence depending on the urgency attached to the issues, and the planned objectives for the visit may be deferred to another time. On completion of the visit the community nurse should evaluate if these objectives have been achieved (formative evaluation) and what the next steps should be. The outcome of this evaluation may indicate the need for nursing interventions to be amended and, if this is the situation, the nursing care plans should be amended accordingly and new care plans agreed following that visit.

Integral to the effective implementation of nursing care is the need to ensure all people involved regularly share information and no gaps in communication arise. This requires community nurses to keep in touch with all people involved in the delivery of the nursing care plan, and other key people who may be involved in providing other related support, as part of an overall person-centred plan or care management package of support. A clear record should be kept of the communication that occurs with other people during the implementation phase.

Recording and reporting by community nurses must receive a high priority. The importance of this has been recently highlighted by the Nursing and Midwifery Council, who stated that:

> 'record keeping is an integral part of nursing, midwifery and specialist community public health nursing practice. It is a tool of professional practice and one that should help the care process. It is not separate from this process and it is not an optional extra to be fitted in if circumstances allow.' (Nursing and Midwifery Council, 2005, p. 6)

The Nursing and Midwifery Council guidance (Nursing and Midwifery Council, 2005) goes on to state that records should be:

- Factual, consistent and accurate
- Written as soon as possible after an event has occurred, providing current information on the care and condition of the patient or client
- Written clearly and in such a manner that the text cannot be erased
- Written in such a manner that any alterations or additions are dated, timed and signed in such a way that the original entry can still be read clearly
- Accurately dated, timed and signed, with the signature printed alongside the first entry
- Not include abbreviations, jargon, meaningless phrases, irrelevant speculation and offensive subjective statements
- Readable on any photocopies
- Be written, wherever possible, with the involvement of the patient, client or their carer

- Written in terms that the patient or client can understand
- Consecutive
- Identify problems that have arisen and the action taken to rectify them
- Provide clear evidence of the care planned, the decisions made, the care delivered and the information shared

Records are required to be completed as soon as possible after a visit and accurately dated and timed for when the record was written. Within a working day, therefore, community nurses should have time scheduled in their diary to maintain adequate records. If it is often a few hours before nurses are able to make a record in a client's nursing notes, they should make some notes in their diary after each visit and these will form the basis of the entry into the nursing file. Some community nurses may choose to use a dictaphone that they carry with them, as this allows them quickly to record more detailed information shortly after a visit. They should be aware that it is now an offence in many countries to use a hand-held dictaphone or mobile phone when driving. In using either approach, community nurses must treat their diaries and any dictaphone recordings as confidential documents and store these securely.

In keeping a record of each visit in the nursing notes, community nurses should use a structured approach in which they document the objectives for that visit, the interaction that occurred during the visit, their conclusion on whether the visit objectives were achieved and the outline plan for the next visit. If new information arose during the visit indicating a need to amend the nursing care plan this should be promptly amended and communicated to people who have copy of the original care plan. The initial implementation phase of care delivery is completed on the first date set for review of the nursing care plan.

Summative evaluation of nursing interventions

In evaluating the effectiveness of nursing interventions community nurses should review the progress that has been made towards achieving the objectives that were set during the care planning stage. It is here that the time spent focusing the objectives and setting criteria for evaluation is reinforced. When objectives have been clearly stated it should possible to establish the extent to which the person has achieved the objective. In reaching this decision community nurses should speak to the person with intellectual disabilities, their family carers and other professionals who are able to provide feedback on the achievement of the objective. Community nurses should also review the information within their nursing records from the period of implementation.

Once the progress towards achieving the objectives outlined within the nursing care plan has been established, the evidence for reaching this decision should be documented in the nursing records. Community nurses then need to make a decision about their further involvement with the person. If it is established that objectives have been achieved and no future objectives were planned, then the community nurse should actively consider discharging the person from their caseload (Caffery and Todd, 2002; Walker et al., 2003). This does not mean that the person with intellectual disabilities does not have ongoing needs, indeed they often have. Rather, it means that those needs do not require the support of a specialist community nursing service at that time. As with the decision to admit someone to a community nursing caseload, the decision to discharge is a nursing decision. This does not mean that the person will not receive support from other members of the community team, but is a decision to conclude the nurse's interventions.

Community nurses should be cautious about keeping someone on a caseload that they will visit infrequently and 'monitor' just in case some further nursing needs arise or because of a reluctance to discharge, as a re-admission would necessitate further paperwork. It is questionable what impact a 'specialist' community nurse can have if they are only visiting someone every few months. This limited involvement also raises questions about the level of nursing objectives that have been set and how nurses are managing their continuing professional accountability for nursing interventions for people they are visiting infrequently.

Community nursing services should have robust clinical supervision and discharge policies in place, to facilitate the discharge of people from the nursing caseload. These polices should state the steps to be followed in discharging people including how the decision to discharge someone from a nursing caseload is made and how this information is communicated to people with intellectual disabilities, family carers and other professionals (including the person who wrote the original referral). It should also state how the discharge should be recorded in nursing notes, and what information is provided to the person with intellectual disabilities and family carers about any further referral to community nursing services. Finally, it should provide clear guidance on the storage of nursing notes from people discharged from the community nurse caseloads.

It may be the situation that the objectives within the nursing care plan were the first set of objectives, but were part of a longer-term plan of nursing care, and that it was expected that further objectives will need to be set. In this situation, new nursing care plans, with revised objectives, nursing interventions and specific review dates, should be set. It may also become apparent during the process of evaluation that further needs have arisen and, as above, if these are within the remit of community nurses then new care plans should be developed and, following nursing interventions, these should be evaluated.

If the conclusion of evaluation is that no or little progress has been made towards the achievement of the objectives, this needs to be further explored. Community nurses need to review the original care plans and their record of interventions to establish why limited progress has been made. Following this a decision should be taken about the need for continuing support from community nursing services. If these continue to be required then new care plans should be developed, implemented and further evaluated.

Conclusion

Community nursing services for people with intellectual disabilities have their origins in the need to support people living with family carers. Research evidence demonstrates the changing role of community nurses across the United Kingdom, with an increasing focus on supporting people with more complex physical and mental health needs living in a growing range of community settings. It is also envisaged that the future role of specialist community nursing services for people with intellectual disabilities will have to be underpinned by a more health-orientated model than previously (Boarder, 2002; Mobbs et al., 2002; Aldridge, 2004).

Community nurses need to become more proactive in identifying areas of specialist nursing interventions that can assist people with intellectual disabilities, and less reactive to filling gaps in services. These should be identified as unmet needs and not 'mopped up' by the community nurses in intellectual disability services. Nurses need to take steps to communicate their role to a wider group of professionals, within and outside intellectual disability services, in order to increase the appropriateness and timeliness of referrals to their service. Perhaps the biggest challenge for community nurses is to be more focused on developing approaches to nurse care planning and care delivery that are more time limited, providing intensive aspects of work which focus on agreed objectives within nursing care plans, and then discharge people for whom these objectives have been achieved.

References

Aggleton, P. and Chalmers, H. (2000) *Nursing Models and Nursing Practice*, 2nd edn. Basingstoke: Palgrave.

Aldridge, J. (2004) Learning disability nursing: a model for practice. In: *Learning Disability Nursing* (Turnbull, J., ed.). Oxford: Blackwell Publishing, pp. 169–87.

Barr, O. (2006) The evolving role of community nurses for people with learning disabilities: changes over an 11-year period. *Journal of Clinical Nursing* **15** (1), 72–82.

Barron, S. and Mulvany, F. (2004) *National Intellectual Disability Database Committee: Annual Report for 2004*. Dublin: Health Research Board.

Boarder, J. (2002) The perceptions of experienced community learning disability nurses of their roles and ways of working: an exploratory study. *Journal of Learning Disabilities* **6** (3), 281–96.

British Institute of Learning Disabilities (1998) *Working with Older Carers: Guidance for Service Providers in Learning Disability*. Kidderminster: British Institute of Learning Disabilities.

Burke, P. (2004) *Brothers and Sisters of Disabled Children*. London: Jessica Kingsley Publishers.

Caffery, A. and Todd, M. (2002) Community learning disability teams: the need for objective methods of prioritisation and discharge planning. *Health Services Management Research* **15** (4), 223–31.

Carpenter, B. (1997) *Families in Context: Emerging Trends in Family Support and Early Intervention.* London: David Fulton Publishers.

Cassidy, G., Martin, D.M., Martin, G.H.B. and Roy, A. (2002) Health checks for people with learning disabilities: community learning disability teams working with general practitioners and primary care teams. *Journal of Learning Disabilities* **6** (2), 123–36.

Department of Health (2001a) *Family Matters.* London: The Stationery Office.

Department of Health (2001b) *Valuing People. A New Strategy for Learning Disability for the 21st Century.* London: The Stationery Office.

Department of Health (2001c) *Good Practice in the Consent Implementation Guide: Consent to Examination or Treatment.* London: The Stationery Office.

Department of Health, Social Services and Public Safety (2003) *Good Practice in Consent: Consent for Examination, Treatment or Care: Handbook for HPSS.* Belfast: Department of Health, Social Services and Public Safety.

Department of Health, Social Services and Public Safety (2005) *Equal Lives: Draft Report of the Learning Disability Committee.* Belfast: Department of Health, Social Services and Public Safety.

Duff, G. (1997) Using models in learning disability nursing. *Professional Nurse* **12** (10), 702–4.

Fraser, M. (1996) *Conceptual Nursing in Practice: A Research Based Approach,* 2nd edn. London: Chapman & Hall.

Freshwater, D. and Rolfe, G. (2004) *Deconstructing Evidence-based Practice.* London: Routledge.

Her Majesty's Stationery Office (2000) *Adults with Incapacity (Scotland) Act 2000.* London: Her Majesty's Stationery Office.

Her Majesty's Stationery Office (2005) *Mental Capacity Act 2005.* London: Her Majesty's Stationery Office.

Horan, P., Doran, A. and Timmins, F. (2004a) Exploring Orem's self-care deficit nursing theory in learning disability nursing: Philosophical parity paper: Part 1. *Learning Disability Practice* **7** (4), 28–33.

Horan, P., Doran, A. and Timmins, F. (2004b) Exploring Orem's self-care deficit nursing theory in learning disability nursing: Practical application paper: Part 2. *Learning Disability Practice* **7** (4), 33–7.

Hubert, J. and Hollins S. (2000) Working with elderly carers of people with learning disabilities and planning for the future. *Advances in Psychiatric Treatment* **6**, 41–4.

Hunt, C., Wakefield, S. and Hunt, G. (2001) Community nurse learning disabilities – a case study of the use of an evidence-based health screening tool to identify and meet health needs of people with learning disabilities. *Journal of Learning Disabilities* **5** (1), 9–18.

Hutchinson, C. (2005) Addressing issues related to adult patients who lack capacity to give consent. *Nursing Standard* **19** (23), 47–53.

Jenkins, R. (2000) Learning disability nursing. The needs of older people with learning disabilities. *British Journal of Nursing* **9** (19), 2080, 2082–5, 2088–9.

Jenkins, J. and Johnson, B. (1991) Community nursing learning disability survey. In: *The Community Mental Handicap Nurse-specialist Practitioner in the 1990s* (Kelly, P., ed.). Penarth: Mental Handicap Nurses Association.

Lee, T. (1990) A framework to cater for all abilities. SEPP: a model for mental handicap nursing. *The Professional Nurse* December, 142–4.

Lister, P. (1987) The misunderstood model. *Nursing Times* **83** (41), 40–2.

Long, A. ed. (1999) *Interaction for Practice in Community Nursing*. London: Macmillan.

McConkey, R., Moore, G. and Marshall, D. (2002) Changes in the attitudes of GPs to health screening of patients with learning disabilities. *Journal of Learning Disabilities* **6** (4), 373–84.

McConkey, R., Spollen, M. and Jamison, J. (2003) *Administrative Prevalence of Learning Disability in Northern Ireland. A Report to the Department of Health, Social Services and Public Safety*. Belfast: Department of Health, Social Services and Public Safety.

McKenna, H. (1997) *Nursing Theories and Models*. London: Routledge.

Martin, G. (2003) Annual health reviews for patients with severe learning disabilities: five years of a combined GP/CLDN Clinic. *Journal of Learning Disabilities* **7** (1), 9–22.

Mansell, I. and Harris, P. (1998) Role of the registered nurse learning disability within community support teams for people with learning disabilities. *Journal of Learning Disabilities for Nursing, Health and Social Care* **2** (4), 190–5.

Mason, C. (1999) Guide to practice, or 'load of rubbish'? The influence of care plans on nursing practice in five clinical areas in Northern Ireland. *Journal of Advanced Nursing* **29** (2), 380–7.

Mobbs, C., Hadley, S., Wittering, R. and Bailey, N.M. (2002) An exploration of the role of the community nurse, learning disability, in England. *British Journal of Learning Disabilities* **30**, 13–8.

Navrady, E. (1998) Challenging behaviour; Palau's model of nursing. *Learning Disability Practice* **1** (2), 18–21.

Northway, R. (2004) Right from the start. *Learning Disability Practice* **7** (7), 3.

Nursing and Midwifery Council (2004) *Code of Professional Conduct: Standards for Conduct, Performance and Ethics*. London: Nursing and Midwifery Council.

Nursing and Midwifery Council (2005) *Guidelines for Records and Record Keeping*. London: Nursing and Midwifery Council.

Orem, D.E. (1991) *Nursing: Concepts of Practice*. St Louis: Mosby-Year Book.

Parahoo, K. and Barr, O. (1996) Community mental handicap nursing services in Northern Ireland: a profile of clients and selected working practices. *Journal of Clinical Nursing* **5**, 211–28.

Peplau, H. (1991) *Interpersonal Relationships in Nursing: A Conceptual Frame of Reference*. New York: Springer.

Powell, H., Murray, G. and McKenize, K. (2004) Staff perceptions of community learning disability nurses' role. *Nursing Times* **100** (19), 40–2.

Roper, N., Logan, W. and Tierney, A. (2001) *The Elements of Nursing a Model for Nursing. Based on a Model for Living*. London: Churchill Livingstone.

Royal College of Nursing (2003) *Defining Nursing*. London: Royal College of Nursing.

Sanderson, H. (2003) Person centred planning. In: *Learning Disabilities: Toward Inclusion*, 4th edn, (Gates, B., ed.). Edinburgh: Churchill Livingstone.

Scottish Executive (2000) *The Same as You? A Review of the Services for People with Learning Disabilities*. Edinburgh: Scottish Executive.

Simons, K. and Watson, D. (1999) *The View from Arthur's Seat: Review of Services for People with Learning Disabilities – A Literature Review of Housing and Support Options beyond Scotland*. Edinburgh: Scottish Executive Central Research Unit.

Sines, D., Appleby, F. and Frost, M. (eds.) (2005) *Community Health Care Nursing*, 3rd edn. Oxford: Blackwell Science.

Slevin, E. (2004) Learning disabilities: a survey of community nurse for people with prevalence of challenging behaviour and contact demands. *Journal of Clinical Nursing* **13**, 571–9.

Sowney, M. and Barr, O. (2004) Equity of access to healthcare for people with learning disabilities: a concept analysis. *Journal of Learning Disabilities* **8** (3), 247–66.

Stewart, D. and Todd, M. (2001) Role and contribution of nurses for people with learning disabilities: a local study in a county of the Oxford-Anglia region. *British Journal of Learning Disabilities* **29**, 145–50.

Thomas, D. and Woods, H. (2003) *Working with People with Learning Disabilities: Theory and Practice*. London: Jessica Kingsley Publishers.

Thompson, N. (2003) *Promoting Equality: Challenging Discrimination and Oppression*, 2nd edn. London: Palgrave Macmillan.

Vagg, J. (1998) A lifetime of caring. In: *Standards and Learning Disabilities*, 2nd edn (Thompson, T. and Mathias, P., eds.). London: Baillière Tindall, in association with the RCN.

Walker, T., Stead, J. and Read, S.G. (2003) Caseload management in community learning disability teams; influences on decision-making. *Journal of Learning Disabilities* **7** (4), 297–321.

Watkins, D., Edwards, J. and Gastrell, P. eds. (2003) *Community Health Nursing: Frameworks for Practice*, 2nd edn. London: Baillière Tindall.

Welsh Office (2001) *Fulfilling the Promises*. Cardiff: Welsh Assembly.

West, M. (2004) *Effective Teamwork: Practical Lessons from Organisational Research*. Oxford: Blackwell Publishing.

Wheeler, P. (2003) Patients' rights: consent to treatment for men and women with a learning disability or who are otherwise mentally incapacitated. *Learning Disability Practice* **6** (5), 29–37.

Further reading and resources

Overall policy reviews and guidance

Despite the fact that the following reviews and guidance have been around for a number of years, many community nurses have not read the original documents and, instead, their understanding is based on secondary references or brief summaries. As the documents cover a number of areas relevant to community nursing it is important that nurses have a copy and at least read the document for their country, although reading other reviews would also be helpful. Several of these documents are available on their respective websites.

Department of Health (2001) *Valuing People. A New Strategy for Learning Disability for 21st Century*. London: The Stationery Office. (www.valuingpeople.gov.uk)

Department of Health, Social Services and Public Safety (2004) *Equal Lives: Draft Report of Learning Disability Committee*. Belfast: Department of Health, Social Services and Public Safety. (www.rmhldni.gov.uk)

Scottish Executive (2000) *The Same as You? A Review of the Services for People with Learning Disabilities*. Edinburgh: Scottish Executive. (www.scotland.gov.uk)

Welsh Office (2001) *Fulfilling the Promises*. Cardiff: Welsh Assembly.

Consent and capacity

Throughout the UK there have been considerable changes to policy in relation to consent and it has been highlighted that the requirements for consent extends well beyond medical intervention. Community nurses regularly undertake interventions that require consent or a decision based on 'best interests'. Nurses should read and have a reference copy of the latest guidance on consent for examination, treatment and care. In addition they will need to keep up to date with new guidance becoming available on establishing capacity/incapacity which are currently being written.

Department of Health (2001) *Good Practice in the Consent Implementation Guide: Consent to Examination or Treatment*. London: The Stationery Office.

Department of Health, Social Services and Public Safety (2003) *Good Practice in Consent: Consent for Examination, Treatment or Care: Handbook for HPSS*. Belfast: Department of Health, Social Services and Public Safety.

Her Majesty's Stationery Office (2005) *Mental Capacity Act (2005)*. London: Her Majesty's Stationery Office. www.hmso.gov.uk/acts/acts2005/20050009.htm

Adults with Incapacity (Scotland) Act 2000: www.scotland-legislation.hmso.gov.uk/acts/acts2000/20000004.htm

Northern Ireland legislation under preparation at the time of writing this chapter: www.dhsspsni.gov.uk.

The wider role of community nurses

This chapter has focused on the role of community nurses in intellectual disability services when planning and delivering care on an individual basis, whilst noting the role of community nurse also involves an increasing public health role. Community nurses in intellectual disability services should also read texts on wider community nursing issues, as they are first and foremost community nurses.

Long, A. (ed.) (1999) *Interaction for Practice in Community Nursing*. London: Macmillan.

Sines, D., Appleby, F. and Frost, M. (eds.) (2005) *Community Health Care Nursing*, 3rd edn. London: Blackwell Publishing.

Watkins, D., Edwards, J. and Gastrell, P. (eds.) (2003) *Community Health Nursing: Frameworks for Practice*, 2nd edn. London: Baillière Tindall.

Websites

The website addresses listed below are examples of websites that are updated on an ongoing basis and provide largely current information in relation to service policy, research and views of people with learning disabilities. It is useful to browse these regularly in order to be aware of key issues and research that should be considered when planning and delivering nursing care.

Policy development and implementation
Valuing People Support Team website with updates on the progress of the implementation of *Valuing People*: www.valuingpeople.gov.uk

Scottish Executive site, which contains information on the implementation of *Same as You?*: www.scotland.gov.uk/Topics/Health/care/17548/9026

Review of Mental Health and Learning Disability (Northern Ireland), with learning disability link for updates on progress relating to *Equal Lives*: www.rmhldni.gov.uk

National Electronic Library for Health, specialist library for learning disabilities: http://libraries.nelh.nhs.uk/learningdisabilities

Nursing networks
National Network for Learning Disability Nurses. Also contains link to Access to Acute (A2A) network: www.nnldn.org.uk

Professional guidance
Nursing and Midwifery Council in the United Kingdom, responsible for the professional regulation of nursing and midwifery in the UK: www.nmc-uk.org

An Bord Altranais is the body responsible for the professional regulation of nursing and midwifery in the Republic of Ireland: www.nursingboard.ie

Some research centres with a particular interest in learning disabilities

Developmental Disabilities and Child Health Research Group at the University of Ulster: www.science.ulster.ac.uk/inr/developmental
Institute of Health Research, Lancaster University: www.lancs.ac.uk/fss/ihr
Unit for the Development of Intellectual Disabilities, University of Glamorgan: www.glam.ac.uk/socs/research/UDID
White Top Research Unit, University of Dundee: www.dundee.ac.uk/wtru

Chapter 11

Care planning in residential settings

Robert Jenkins, Paul Wheeler and Neil James

Introduction

Central to the role of the intellectual disability nurse within residential settings is an imperative that a framework is established that will direct the way in which services and therapeutic approaches are provided. This chapter will explore issues concerning the provision of accommodation for people with intellectual disabilities. It considers the purpose of nursing, the historical development of services and the role of the intellectual disability nurse. The central focus of this chapter will consider how a concept of quality of life may be used as a framework for care planning. Three case illustrations are provided in order to demonstrate an application of a quality of life framework to practice situations.

Residential alternatives

People may predominantly associate nursing with residential healthcare settings (Mitchell, 2004) but nurses frequently play a role in the management of a wide variety of residential settings, including local authority, voluntary and private agencies. Although Perry and Felce (2003) state that people with intellectual disabilities are increasingly finding themselves housed in small-scale residential settings, some individuals with intellectual disabilities may be housed in medium-sized secure units. Such varied provision may be seen to be increasing as a result of the changes in strategies and policies that have and are being developed in an attempt to recognise and address the needs of people with intellectual disabilities. Gates (2003) highlighted that residential care in the UK has historically been influenced by political, ideological and economic factors. Despite the fact that there is such a wide range of places in which intellectual disability nurses may work, there is a range of factors that will apply in whatever setting that they find themselves. Additionally there is a continuing need for the development of the services provided.

In the United Kingdom, the Royal College of Nursing definition of nursing suggests that the purpose of nursing is to promote and maintain health; to care for people when their health is compromised; to assist recovery; to facilitate independence; to meet needs and to improve/maintain well-being/quality of life (Royal College of Nursing, 2003). Nursing in the field of intellectual disabilities has continually been striving to define itself and the role that it fulfils in meeting the needs of this specific group of people (Alaszewski et al., 2001). In their practice intellectual disability nurses draw upon knowledge from a diverse range of academic and professional disciplines. We would, therefore, argue that it is the application of the amalgam of this knowledge that places the intellectual disability nurse in a unique position from which the basis of holistic care planning can be undertaken. Within residential settings there is a need for a framework for care planning that will provide the intellectual disability nurses with the scope to ensure that the people they support are achieving optimal autonomy and quality of life outcomes (Northway and Jenkins, 2003).

Since the 1959 Mental Health Act, the introduction of the principles of normalisation and the 1971 White Paper, *Better Services for the Mentally Handicapped* (Department of Health, 1971), there has been a developing policy aimed at integrating people with intellectual disabilities into the wider community and providing access to appropriate occupational and recreational activities. This movement towards integration has culminated in legislation, such as the 1990 National Health Service and Community Care Act, and the publication of more recent policy documents, such as *Valuing People* (Department of Health, 2001), *Fulfilling the Promises* (National Assembly for Wales, 2001), *Same As You* (Scottish Executive, 2000) and *Equal Lives* (DHSSPS, 2004). Whilst we have seen a move away from large-scale residential care, there remains, and always will, a need for residential care and this will be for a variety of reasons. For example, Jenkins (2005) has highlighted that as a result of advances in medical technology, children with profound and multiple disabilities who previously might have died in childhood are surviving to adulthood. Likewise, the life expectancy of adults with intellectual disability is increasing. This undoubtedly has implications for the care-planning process to meet the particular needs of these and other individuals who may experience epilepsy, cerebral palsy, challenging behaviour, autism, profound and multiple intellectual disability and poor mental health.

The process of planning will need to encompass the possible needs that such individuals may experience and be vulnerable to. For example, Jenkins and Davies (2004) have argued that individuals with profound and multiple intellectual disabilities and people who exhibit challenging behaviour may be more vulnerable to abuse due to additional risk factors. Vulnerability to abuse can also be heightened by living in residential care environments due to poor management practices and clients being made to feel powerless (Wardhaugh and Wilding, 1998). Vulnerability may also be greater during the transition from child to adult services, a key area in which the intellectual disability nurse can be involved in the planning process. Finally, older people with intellectual disabilities may be susceptible to degenerative conditions, such as dementia and other cognitive and physical declines that can accompany the ageing process (Jenkins, 2005).

An awareness of the diversity of cultural and spiritual needs is also important so that these can be incorporated within the planning process. It is recognised that cultural and spiritual needs may be complex issues for care staff to respond to. For example, there is difficulty in defining what constitutes spirituality. However, it is important that learning disability nurses recognise and acknowledge such needs (McSherry et al., 2004). These issues will have an impact when planning and delivering care that recognises peoples' individuality, based on such things as their origins, background and history. The intellectual disability nurse will be required to be able to plan care in conjunction with others, thereby enabling individuals to gain access to services or facilities that will promote their social and spiritual well-being. This is undoubtedly compatible with the person-centred planning approach that is promoted by current policy (Department of Health, 2001).

The role of the intellectual disability nurse in care planning

Whilst nurses have a multi-faceted role in residential care settings, some of the activities most widely valued by other carers and professionals include direct care, management and administration, liaison work and educational activity (Alaszewski et al., 2001). Alaszewski et al. (2001) have also stated that people with intellectual disabilities themselves saw the role of the intellectual disability nurse in a similar light, but also as a helper and enabler, as a friend and as possessing specialist knowledge in relationship to intellectual disabilities.

In order to provide holistic and person-centred assessment, planning and implementation of care, appropriate knowledge, skills and attitudes are important in ensuring quality of life. Whilst professionals, such as psychologists and social workers, may undertake post-registration training in working with people with intellectual disability, intellectual disability nurses are the only professionals who gain a specialist qualification that is exclusively concerned with addressing the needs of people with an intellectual disability. Throughout their training students will have been exposed to a wide variety of disciplines that include sociological, psychological, educational and philosophical theory. In addition students are placed in a variety of care settings where they can, under supervision, apply the theory learned to practical situations, thereby addressing the needs of individuals with intellectual disabilities and their carers.

In respect of skills, the intellectual disability nurse should be adaptable and possess the ability to work as part of multi-professional team. They should be able to co-ordinate and manage systems of working whilst being pro-active within political fora. They should also take a role in the education of a variety of persons, including people with intellectual disabilities, families and carers, primary health care workers, other professionals and social care workers. This requires that the intellectual disability nurse possesses and uses research skills to ensure the promotion and adoption of evidenced-based practice. When nurses are employed as home managers or care managers their role maybe less 'hands on' and more advisory than in a 'continual healthcare setting'. For example, they may provide advice about access to services, on transition from child to adult services and in relation to primary healthcare needs.

There may be a reduction in 'hands on' care as a result of the promotion of the use of and access to social and generic services, but intellectual disability nurses are likely to have to undertake assessments and produce clear individual plans for others to implement. Additionally, as a result of the move to social care, many people with an intellectual disability have unmet health needs (Kerr et al., 2003). The intellectual disability nurse should play a major role in detecting ill health and promoting positive health in a wide range of areas, including nutrition (Mughal, 2002), management of epilepsy (Kerr, 2003), promotion of positive sleep patterns, promotion of continence, promotion of personal safety and prevention of injury (Sherrard et al., 2004), monitoring the effects of medication (Jenkins, 2000) and promoting positive mental health (Priest and Gibbs, 2004).

Reader activity 11.1

In your area of practice identify how many clients may need the services of an advocate and why. If you were going to advocate on behalf of a client in the care-planning process what considerations would you need to take? For example would you act on the client's wishes or 'best interests' or both?

Encompassing and inherent in all these roles, the intellectual disability nurse will have a role to play in advocacy. Intellectual disability nurses may not be ideally situated to act as an advocate for individuals, but they are in a position where they can teach self-advocacy skills and provide links between clients and independent advocacy services (Wheeler, 2000). The attitudes of intellectual disability nurses are shaped by their underlying value base that helps them recognise the ability of individuals to achieve their potential in all areas of life. Attitudes may give rise to the application of tools or frameworks such as 'person-centred planning' or 'quality of life' that promote autonomy, empowerment, respect, inclusion, working in partnership, and enable people with intellectual disabilities to participate actively in decision making relevant to their lives. On completion of education, intellectual disability nurses are required to be fit for award, purpose and practice. This level of fitness is a prerequisite to being able holistically to plan care in the multifarious residential settings in which people with intellectual disabilities may live.

Enhancing quality of life

Northway and Jenkins (2003) have highlighted that many nursing models use domains or dimensions in planning care. For example, the popular 'activities of daily living' model (Roper et al., 1996) is made up 12 activities of daily living (see Chapter 13 for example). The influence of nursing models on intellectual disability nursing has been variable with some nurses rejecting them because they feel they reflect a medical model, which is not compatible with current philosophies of care. This lack of influence may in part be due to the fact that there have been very few models developed specifically for intellectual disability nurses. Interestingly some of the models which have been developed have focused on types of factors, which could be likened to domains, which impact on the lives of people with intellectual disabilities. For example, Lee (1990) developed a model with the acronym SEPP which focused on four areas – social, educational, psychological and physical. Biley and Donlan (1990) have used a number of dimensions to create a model for community intellectual disability nurses. Domains and dimensions have again been used in a recent model developed by Aldridge (2003), although this primarily focuses only on the healthcare needs of people with intellectual disabilities. However, there are still attempts at applying a traditional nursing model (Orem's) to meeting the needs of people with intellectual disabilities (Horan et al., 2004). Implicit in many of these models is the attempt to improve matters for people with intellectual disabilities. If the ultimate aim of care planning is to enhance the quality of life of the individual then why not use the concept of quality of life as a framework to assess, plan, implement and evaluate care?

The concept of quality of life has emerged in recent years as a prominent focus for research, education and practice in the field of intellectual disabilities (Schalock, 2004). However, there are still difficulties in providing a suitable definition which can be used as a measurable outcome. Keith (2001) believed that the complex process of doing so would present too many technical and philosophical difficulties. In spite of this, there now seems to be some consensus in the belief that it is a multi-dimensional concept (Felce, 1997; Keith, 2001; Schalock, 2004). Edgerton (1990) felt that it is unlikely that one single measure would be able to encapsulate quality of life as experienced by each individual. Therefore, Felce (1997) has argued for the use of core domains as a way of capturing different aspects of a person's quality of life. Keith (2001) believed that international consensus favours the eight core dimensional model developed by Schalock (1996) (Box 11.1).

Quality of life as a basis for developing collaborative care planning

Jenkins (2002) has highlighted a number of advantages in using quality of life as an organising concept for delivering collaborative care planning:

Box 11.1   Quality of life core domains and indicators (adapted from Schalock, 2004)

Core domains	Indicators
Emotional well-being	• Contentment • Self image • Stress
Interpersonal relations	• Interactions • Relationships/friendships • Personal supports and networks
Material well-being	• Financial status • Employment • Housing/environment
Personal development	• Education • Personal competence • Performance
Physical well-being	• Health • Self-help skills • Leisure/hobbies
Self-determination	• Autonomy/personal control • Goals and personal values • Choices
Social inclusion	• Community integration and participation • Community roles • Social supports
Rights	• Human • Legal

- The core domains cover most aspects of people's lives and as such a holistic approach can be taken
- A number of objective assessment measures which focus on particular aspects of an individual's quality of life are available
- It can also be used to assess the quality of service provided to the client
- By focusing on what really matters in the client's life, it has the potential to improve happiness and satisfaction

Northway and Jenkins (2003) have further emphasised that quality of life can be used as a sensitizing concept, a basis for collaborative care planning and as an evaluation tool. They offer a framework in which a person-centred quality of life approach can be adopted when planning and delivering care in partnership with people with intellectual disabilities in any setting. This is in keeping with Schalock (2004) who advocated that:

'any proposed quality of life model must recognize the need for a multi-element framework, the realization that people know what is important to them, and that the essential characteristic of any set of domains is that they represent in aggregate the complete quality of life construct.'

Assessing the quality of an individual's life can be a problematic area; assessment needs to include both subjective and objective measures (Keith, 2001). In the past more reliance was placed on objective rather than subjective measures of quality of life (Cummins, 1997). This was due in part to the belief that people with intellectual disabilities were unable to express their opinions because of cognitive and communication problems. However, there is a growing realisation that people with intellectual disabilities are capable of expressing their opinions if they are given the appropriate support (Felce, 1996; Cummins, 1997; McVilly and Rawlinson, 1998; Prosser and Bromley, 1998). Northway and Jenkins (2003) have highlighted that even when people with intellectual disabilities are able to express their opinions, others are needed to listen and respect their viewpoints.

Inevitably, there will be some clients in residential care that will be unable to express their views and preferences. Examples include individuals with profound and multiple intellectual disabilities or older people who may be in the later stages of dementia. The use of an advocate would be helpful in such circumstances. However, Jenkins and Northway (2002) have suggested that intellectual disability nurses are not always best placed to act as advocates for people with intellectual disabilities. Instead they feel that nurses have an indirect role in promoting the use of independent advocates who can speak up on behalf of clients. Indeed, Wheeler (2000) has stated that any nurse who thinks of acting as an advocate should consider this option very carefully. A key advantage of having an independent advocate is that they are independent of the organisation providing the service to the client. Therefore they should not have a conflict of interest when representing the individual in the care-planning process. The use of such advocates in residential care may also help in preventing abuse (Davies and Jenkins, 2004).

Reader activity 11.2

Discuss some of the factors in residential settings which may have a negative impact on an individual's quality of life, for example, lack of personal space, sharing with others and drab furniture.

Guidance for using a person-centred quality of life framework

The eight key domains and indicators should cover all aspects of the individual's life. However, there may be a great deal of overlap between domains and indicators. For example, health is given as an indicator under the physical well-being domain. Health can impact on any one of the other domains, but the important issue here is that it is highlighted and acts as a source of reference in the care-planning process. In reality clients may be more bothered about a particular aspect of their health rather than which heading health is put under. Renwick et al. (2000) have argued that quality of life has the potential to be a powerful force for change if it is directed in a person-centred fashion. They stated that this can only be done if people who apply the person-centred quality of life concept:

- 'Understand clearly and value each person's ways of expressing needs and goals related to core life domains
- Understand that the expressions of needs and goals are unique to the person and should not be the same as those of others
- Understand how a person's unique expressions of needs and goals add to, or detract from, quality within his or her life.' (Renwick et al., 2000, p. 9)

The following stages are guidance on how the person-centred quality of life framework described by Northway and Jenkins (2003) could be used to organise and plan care.

Stage one: assessment

This involves gathering information to identify a particular need. The quality of life framework acts as a source of reference (see Box 11.1). The client is the first person to indicate their needs followed by family/direct care staff and finally professional assessment (see Box 11.2). In instances where the client has difficulty in communication or has opted for the services of an advocate then they will represent the clients' viewpoint. If clients are unable to communicate verbally, strong emphasis needs to be placed on observation and the interpretation of what the client is trying to tell us. A number of objective indicators/

Box 11.2   General assessment and evaluation record

Domain	Client	Carer/family	Professional	Objective measure
Emotional well-being				
Interpersonal relations				
Material well-being				
Personal development				
Physical well-being				
Self-determination				
Social inclusion				
Rights				

measures may be available which can be used to supplement the assessment; for example, quality of life issues related to community involvement and daily activities may be assessed using the index of community involvement (Raynes et al., 1989a) and the index of participation in domestic tasks (Raynes et al., 1989b). Schalock and Verdugo (2002) provide a useful overview of measurement techniques and tools currently used in quality of life research.

Stage two: areas for intervention

This stage involves agreeing areas for intervention by ensuring that a person-centred approach is adhered to. It is essential that client's views are taken seriously when developing areas for intervention. However, because the quality of life domains and indicators cover a wide range of areas, there may be instances where a large number of areas for intervention will be identified. Therefore a priority list will need to be agreed upon in which needs can be met.

Stage three: goals and strategies

Once areas for intervention have been identified, it will be necessary to agree on goals and strategies for their achievement (see Box 11.3). Goals set must be achievable, measurable and realistic. Strategies which are developed to achieve the set goals must have the consent of the client and the support and commitment of all those concerned.

Box 11.3 Specific domain area for intervention (adapted from Schalock, 2004)

Domain: Emotional well-being	Identified need	Specified aim/goal	Action required to meet need	Resources required
Contentment (personal satisfaction and enjoyment)				
Self-concept (personal identity, self worth, self esteem)				
Stress (predictability and control)				

Stage four: evaluation

It is important that interventions achieve what they set out to do and where this does not happen that we know why. Therefore an evaluation of the progress and final outcome takes place. The client is often the best person to evaluate the success or failure of each of the goals set. However, it is equally important for services and professionals to be accountable for the actions taken. Therefore, the use of valid and reliable objective measures highlighted in the assessment process can be useful tools in evaluating whether clients' quality of lives are being enhanced or not.

Case illustrations

Case illustration 11.1

David is a 42-year-old individual who has an intellectual disability and additional mental health needs (schizophrenia). He communicates well when he is lucid, although recently he has become withdrawn and complaining that people are 'picking' on him. He is currently an inpatient on a local NHS trust's assessment and treatment unit after having been sectioned under the Mental Health Act. He has spent most of his life at home with his parents and does not like restrictions on his freedom to go where he wants.

Case illustration 11.2

Alison is an 18-year-old lady who is blind, has profound and multiple intellectual disabilities and has been in residential care for most of her life. Her parents visit on a regular basis. She is unable to communicate effectively and is totally dependent on others for her needs. Her epilepsy is not well controlled and she has reduced lung capacity due to repeated chest infections.

Case illustration 11.3

Nora is a 63-year-old lady with intellectual disabilities. She has spent most of her life in a large intellectual disability hospital but it is planned for her to move into a group home with three other ladies as part of a resettlement programme. She has some communication skills but tends to be understood only by people who know her well. She is set in her ways and does not like changes in staff or her routines.

The following discussions around the three case illustrations identify different perspectives within the format of Box 11.2 in order to give a general overview of some of the factors to consider in using the quality of life framework.

Reader activity 11.3

In each of the three case illustrations consider the other quality of life domains which are not used. For example, in Case illustration 11.1 the domains of rights, self-determination and social inclusion are discussed. Apply the domains of emotional well-being, interpersonal relations, material well-being, personal development and physical well-being to David's case.

Discussion of case illustrations

Case illustration 11.1

There are several issues resulting from being in an assessment and treatment unit that will impact on David's quality of life. Clearly one of the major impacts will be the fact that he has been admitted under the Mental Health Act into a more restrictive environment. Many of the domains contained in the quality of life framework will therefore have significance for David. For example, David will have restrictions placed on his ability to exert control and choice as a result of legal requirements that will impact on his autonomy. However, for the purpose of this discussion we will concentrate on three specific domains: rights, self-determination and social inclusion.

Client's perspective
Under the domain of rights and social inclusion David feels that he should be allowed to come and go as he pleases and not under staff escort. He believes that his right to freedom has been denied by the doctors placing him on a 'section'. He is unwilling to accept medication as he says that it is poisonous and he is being made to take it by staff.

Family perspective
His family are in agreement with professionals as to the need for medication but they feel he should have more freedom, especially home visits to provide some 'normality' in his life.

Professional perspective
The professionals feel that it is important to ensure David's security and reduce his access to the local community until the medication can be seen to have had

a positive effect on his psychotic symptoms and hence reduce the perceived risks to him and others.

Objective measures
Possible objective measures would include the use of mini PAS-ADD (Prosser et al., 1996) or the Reiss screen for maladaptive behaviour (1994) (see Chapter 8). Achievement of goals might also be independently audited by the Mental Health Act Commissioners Mental Health Review Tribunal. Given his unwillingness to consent to medical treatment, a second opinion doctor would need to be consulted in order to comply with mental health legislation.

Possible interventions
In relation to the three identified domains the following interventions might be considered. Firstly, under the domain of rights, care staff would ensure that he is made aware of his rights under the Mental Health Act. They would also seek to ensure that he was able to benefit from his human rights to as great a level as possible given the restrictions of the environment. Under the domain of self-determination, staff at the unit would seek to enhance his choices in relation to other aspects of his life, for example, when he goes to bed and when he gets up. They would also ensure he was offered access to an independent advocate and/or solicitor. In relation to the domain of social inclusion, staff would seek to maintain David's relationships within the community by providing him with support to attend family and social occasions which he would normally access; they will also encourage his family and friends to visit.

Case illustration 11.2

As with the previous case illustration there are a number of issues that may impact on the domains of quality of life for Alison. However, the domains we have selected as being important in relation to provision of care for Alison include material well-being, personal development and physical well-being.

Clients' perspective
Although Alison has no speech or sign language she is able to communicate likes and dislikes using facial expressions and by vocalising. For example, her whining, facial grimacing and recoiling body movements indicate discomfort, sadness and pain following a seizure. Staff who know her feel, via her identified communicative strategies, that she enjoys getting 'dressed up', having make-up applied and being taken to the swimming pool and to pop concerts.

Parent's perspective
Alison's parents find it upsetting when they visit her, particularly if she is having a seizure. They want Alison to live her life without any pain whilst also having access to a variety of different activities. When they arrive to visit Alison they expect to find her bathed, dressed and ready to go out. They also

want to have more control over her finances so that they can decide what her money is spent on.

Professionals' perspective

Of particular concern to the professionals involved in her care is her physical well-being. Due to her profound and multiple disabilities she is at greater risk of infection, skin disorders and various others disorders. They are also concerned that Alison's epilepsy does not appear to be well controlled at present.

Objective measures

Possible objective measures would include continual monitoring and recording of her seizures in relation to frequency, severity and duration. Other monitoring would include the impact that epilepsy is having on her social inclusion and the effects of anti-convulsant medication. A further objective measure might be the use of regular health screening and monitoring of such things as chest infections and skin conditions.

Possible interventions

There could be development of an epilepsy profile with an appropriate care plan and risk assessment. Referral to a specialist in epilepsy may result in alternative and a more efficacious medication regime. The use of pain tools would be researched and developed to fit the needs of Alison and support staff in the assessment and appropriate relief of pain. Referral to speech and language therapy service for assessment of communication needs and competence may benefit all parties in ensuring that her desires are being met rather than those of others being imposed upon her; for example, although Alison appears to enjoy getting dressed up and going to pop concerts, she may prefer to develop in other ways. In respect of finances, her parents could be given greater involvement in what her limited resources are spent on by consultation and discussion with the appointed person.

Case illustration 11.3

In this final case illustration we are going to focus on the domains of emotional well-being and interpersonal relations, although the other domains clearly have significance for Nora.

Client's perspective

Nora is concerned that she will have to get to know new staff who may not understand her as well as those currently supporting her. Nora also has anxieties over having to identify with her new staff the things that she likes and how she is cared for with regard to her hygiene needs. Although she likes the idea of having her own room and living in a small community environment, she is not welcoming of the idea that she will have to participate in the preparation of food and other household activities.

Parent/carers perspective
Nora's parents are deceased and she has had no contact with other family members since her admission to an intellectual disability hospital some 40 years previously.

Professional perspective
Having spent over 40 years of her life in an intellectual disability hospital, staff feel that they have developed a good understanding of Nora and her needs. Based on their knowledge of Nora their major concern is the possible impact that the transition to a group home may have on her emotional well-being and interpersonal relations; for example, the group home is a considerable way from the location of her current network of friends. Additionally, they are concerned that she may have difficulty in coping with the stress of moving and this may present itself in exhibition of challenging behaviours and reduction of interaction with fellow residents and staff.

Objective measures
A monitoring and recording chart may be used to monitor the maintenance of interpersonal relationships.

Possible interventions
The development of a person-centred plan will seek to involve Nora in the planning process and take into account her wants and desires. Communication, anxiety management and assertiveness training will equip her with skills to communicate her desires in an appropriate manner. Staff working closely with her will also need to be involved in any training in communication techniques. The introduction of 'active support' (Mansell et al., 2004) should be considered to maintain and improve her current skill levels, especially with domestic tasks.

Conclusion

Using a quality of life framework this chapter has explored how intellectual disability nurses can plan and deliver good quality care for people with intellectual disabilities in a variety of residential settings. The quality of life framework outlined in this chapter organises planning within eight key domains. This makes it a valuable planning tool as it covers all aspects of a person's life and is arguably preferable, when compared to the majority of nursing models commonly used in the UK. This model also lends itself to the concept of person-centred planning, as it seeks to ascertain the view of the person with intellectual disability. In the situation where a person with intellectual disability is unable to express their views and preferences then the use of an advocate has been recommended, and this must be seen as good practice. Finally, the use of a quality of life framework should ensure that the focus always remains on the enhancement of an individual's quality of life.

References

Alaszewski, A., Gates, B., Motherby, E., Manthorpe, J. and Ayer, S. (2001) *Educational Preparation for Learning Disability Nursing: Outcomes Evaluation of Learning Disability Nurses within the Multi-professional, Multi-agency Team.* London: English National Board for Nursing, Midwifery and Health Visiting.

Aldridge, J. (2003) The ecology of health model. In: *Contemporary Learning Disability Practice* (Jukes, M. and Bollard, M., eds.). Salisbury: Quay Books.

Biley, F. and Donlan, M. (1990) A model for mental handicap nursing. *Nursing Standard* **4** (29), 36–9.

Brown, I. (1999) Embracing quality of life in times of spending restraint. *Journal of Intellectual and Developmental Disability* **24** (4) 299–308.

Cummins, R.A. (1997) Self-rated quality of life scales for people with an intellectual disability: a review. *Journal of Applied Research in Intellectual Disabilities* **10** (3) 199–216.

Davies, R. and Jenkins, R. (2004) Protecting people with learning disabilities from abuse: a key role for learning disability nurses. *The Journal of Adult Protection* **6** (2) 31–41.

Department of Health (2001) *Valuing People: A New Strategy for Learning Disability for the 21st Century.* London: Department of Health.

Department of Health, Social Services and Public Safety (2004) *Equal Lives: Draft Report of Learning Disability Committee.* Belfast: Department of Health, Social Services and Public Safety.

Department of Health and Social Services and the Welsh Office (1971) *Better Services for the Mentally Handicapped.* London: Department of Health.

Dickens, P. (1994) *Quality and Excellence in Human Service.* Chichester: Wiley.

Edgerton, R.B. (1990) Quality of life from a longitudinal research perspective. In: *Quality of Life: Perspectives and Issues* (Schalock, R.L., ed.). Washington: American Association on Mental Retardation.

Felce, D. (1996) Ways to measure quality of outcome: an essential ingredient in quality assurance. *Tizard Learning Disability Review* **1** (2), 38–44.

Felce, D. (1997) Defining and applying the concept of quality of life. *Journal of Intellectual Disability Research* **41** (2), 126–35.

Gates, B. (2003) Residential alternatives for people with learning disabilities In: *Learning Disabilities: Toward Inclusion,* 4th edn, (Gates, B., ed.). Edinburgh: Churchill Livingstone.

Horan, P., Doran, A. and Timmins, F. (2004) Exploring Orem's self-care deficit nursing theory in learning disability nursing: Philosophical parity paper: Part 1. *Learning Disability Practice* **7** (4), 28–33.

Jenkins, R. (2000) Use of psychotropic medication in people with a learning disability. *British Journal of Nursing* **9** (13), 844–50.

Jenkins, R. (2002) Enhancing quality of life for people with learning disabilities. *Learning Disability Practice* **5** (9), 29–35.

Jenkins, R. (2005) Older people with learning disabilities. Part 1: individuals, ageing and health. *Nursing Older People* **16** (10), 30–3.

Jenkins, R. and Davies, R. (2004) The abuse of adults with learning disabilities and the role of the learning disability nurse *Learning Disability Practice* **7** (2), 30–8.

Jenkins, R. and Northway, R. (2002) Advocacy and the learning disability nurse. *British Journal of Learning Disabilities* **30** (1) 8–12.

Keith, K.D. (2001) International quality of life: current conceptual, measurement, and implementation issues. *International Review of Research in Mental Retardation* **24**, 49–74.

Kerr, M. (2003) Epilepsy. In: *Seminars in the Psychiatry of Learning Disabilities* (Fraser, W., ed.). Glasgow: Gaskell.

Kerr A.M., McCullough, D., Oliver, K., McLean, B., Coleman, E., Law, T., Beaton, P., Wallace, S., Newell, E., Eccles, T. and Prescott, R.J. (2003) Medical needs of people with an intellectual disability require regular assessment, and the provision of client- and carer-held reports. *Journal of Intellectual Disability Research* **47** (2), 134–45.

Lee, T. (1990) A framework to cater for all abilities. SEPP: A model for mental handicap nursing. *Professional Nurse* **6** (3), 142–4.

Mansell, J., Beadle Brown, J., Ashman, B. and Ockenden, J. (2004) *Person-Centred Active Support.* Brighton: Pavilion Publishing.

McSherry, W., Cash, K. and Ross, L. (2004) Meaning of spirituality: implications for nursing practice. *Journal of Clinical Nursing* **13** (8), 934–41.

McVilly, K. and Rawlinson, R.B. (1998) Quality of life issues in the development and evaluation of services for people with intellectual disability. *Journal of Intellectual and Developmental Disability* **23** (3), 199–218.

Mitchell, D. (2004) Keynote review: learning disability nursing. *British Journal of Learning Disabilities* **32** (3), 115–18.

Mughal, T.M. (2002) Nutrition and physical health. In: *Physical Health of Adults with Intellectual Disabilities* (Prasher, V.P. and Janicki, M.P., eds.). Oxford: Blackwell Publishing.

National Assembly for Wales (2001) *Fulfilling the Promises: Proposals for a Framework for Services for People with Learning Disabilities.* Cardiff: Learning Disability Advisory Group, National Assembly for Wales.

Northway, R. and Jenkins, R. (2003) Quality of life as a concept for developing learning disability nursing practice? *Journal of Clinical Nursing* **12** (1), 57–66.

O'Brien, J. (1987) A guide to life-style planning: Using the Activities Catolog to integrate services and natural support systems. In: *A Comprehensive Guide to The Activities Catolog: An Alternative Curriculum for Youth and Adults with Severe Disabilities* (Wilcox, B. and Bellamy, G.T., eds.). Baltimore: Paul H Brookes Publishing.

Perry, J. and Felce, D. (2003) Quality of life outcomes for people with intellectual disabilities living in staffed community housing services: a stratified random sample of statutory, voluntary and private agency provision. *Journal of Applied Research in Intellectual Disabilities* **16** (1), 11–28.

Priest, H. and Gibbs, M. (2004) *Mental Health Care for People with Learning Disabilities.* London: Churchill Livingstone.

Prosser, H. and Bromley, J. (1998) Interviewing people with learning disabilities. In: *Clinical Psychology and People with Intellectual Disabilities* (Emerson, E., Hatton, C., Bromley, J. and Caine, A., eds.). Chichester: John Wiley.

Prosser, H., Moss, S., Costello, H., Simpson, N. and Patel, P. (1996) *The Mini PAS-ADD: an Assessment Schedule for the Detection of Mental Health Problems in Adults with Developmental Disabilities.* University of Manchester: Hester Adrian Research Centre.

Raynes, N.V., Sumpton, R.C. and Pettipher, C. (1989a) *The Index of Community Involvement.* Manchester University: Department of Social Policy and Social Work.

Raynes, N.V., Sumpton, R.C. and Pettipher, C. (1989b) *The Index of Participation in Domestic Tasks.* Manchester University: Department of Social Policy and Social Work.

Reiss, S. (1994) *The Reiss Screen for Maladaptive Behaviour Test Manual,* 2nd edn. Worthington OH: IDS Publishing.

Renwick, R., Brown, I. and Raphael, D. (2000) Person-centred quality of life: contributions from Canada to an international understanding. In: *Cross-Cultural Perspectives on Quality of Life* (Keith, K.D. and Schalock, R.L., eds.). Washington: American Association on Mental Retardation.

Roper, N., Logan, W. and Tierney, A. (1996) *The Elements of Nursing*, 4th edn. Edinburgh: Churchill Livingstone.

Royal College of Nursing (2003) *Defining Nursing: def. Nursing is . . .* London: Royal College of Nursing.

Schalock, R.L. (1996) Reconsidering the conceptualisation and measurement of quality of life. In: Quality of Life: Vol. 1. *Conceptualization and Measurement* (Schalock, R.L., ed.). Washington DC: American Association on Mental Retardation.

Schalock, R.L. (2000) Three decades of quality of life. *Focus on Autism and Other Developmental Disabilities* **15** (2), 116–27.

Schalock, R. (2004) The concept of quality of life: what we know and do not know. *Journal of Intellectual Disability Research* **48** (3), 203–16.

Schalock, R.L. and Verdugo, M. (2002) *Handbook on Quality of life for Human Service Practitioners*. Washington DC: American Association on Mental Retardation.

Scottish Executive (2000) *The Same as You? A Review of Services for People with Learning Disabilities*. Edinburgh: Scottish Executive.

Sherrard, J.J., Ozanne-Smith, J. and Staines, C. (2004) Prevention of unintentional injury to people with intellectual disability: a review of the evidence. *Journal of Intellectual Disability Research* **48** (7), 639–45.

Wardhaugh, J. and Wilding, P. (1998) Towards and explanation of the corruption of care In: *Understanding Health and Social Care: An Introductory Reader* (Allott, M. and Robb, M., eds.). London: Sage/Open University Press.

Wheeler, P. (2000) Is advocacy at the heart of professional practice? *Nursing Standard* **14** (3), 39–41.

Further reading and resources

Cattermole, M. and Blunden, R. (2002) *My Life. A Person-centred Approach to Checking Outcomes for People with Learning Difficulties*. Kidderminster: BILD.

Cattermole, M., McGowan, C., Brunning, K. and Blunden, R. (2002) *Using My life. A Guide to Conducting a Quality Network Review*. Kidderminster: BILD.

Jack, R. (ed.) (1999) *Residential Versus Community Care: the Role of Institutions in Welfare Provision*. London: Macmillan.

Keith, K.D. and Schalock, R.L. (eds.) (2000) *Cross-cultural Perspectives on Quality of Life*. Washington: American Association on Mental Retardation.

Sanderson, H., Kennedy, J., Richie, P. and Goodwin, G. (1997) *People, Plans and Possibilities – Exploring Person Centred Planning*. Edinburgh: SHS.

Websites

Person-centred planning
www.valuingpeople.gov.uk/pcp.htm
www.learningdisabilities.org.uk/index.cfm
www.bild.org.uk/factsheets/person_centred_planning.htm

General
www.learningdisabilities.org.uk/index.cfm
www.bild.org.uk/

Quality of life
ww2.audit-commission.gov.uk/pis/quality-of-life-indicators.shtml

Intellectual disability nursing
www.nnldn.org.uk/
www.nhsinherts.nhs.uk/hp/health_topics/learning_disabilities/
learning_disabilities_links.htm

Chapter 12

Care planning for good health in intellectual disabilities

Helen Atherton

Introduction

Over the past two decades, healthcare provision for people with intellectual disabilities has undergone a significant change and this is particularly so in the UK. Historically, services for this group were predominantly provided by specialist intellectual disability professionals within segregated settings, such as long-stay hospitals. However, in the early 1970s, the inception of the principles of normalisation into service design for people with intellectual disabilities served to challenge the appropriateness of the institutional model of care, advocating instead the integration of this group within society (Wolfensberger, 1972). A central facet of this integration was community presence and participation that included the use of mainstream healthcare provision (O'Brien and Tyne, 1981). The necessity of providing healthcare in this manner was to be further consolidated in a range of policy documents throughout the 1970s and 1980s, culminating in the NHS and Community Care Act (1990), which advocated a 'mixed economy of care'. In line with such policy and legislation healthcare provision for this group has increasingly become the responsibility of mainstream healthcare providers, although there remains a distinct and essential set of specialist intellectual disability services catering for those whose healthcare needs fall outside the remit of ordinary services, such as people with profound intellectual disabilities and complex needs, mental health problems and/or behavioural difficulties (Department of Health, 2001a).

The move from the use of specialist to mainstream health services in the UK has not been unproblematic. Whilst it is recognised that people with intellectual disabilities have more profound and numerous healthcare needs than those of the general population (Van Schrojenstein Lantman-De Valk et al., 2000), access to appropriate healthcare is beset with difficulties (Singh, 1997; Band, 1998; Mencap, 2004). Coupled with this is evidence that suggests that the process of care planning and implementation for this group is often disempowering rather than empowering, in which important facets, such as choice, partnership and ownership, remain unrecognised (Hart, 1999; Williams and Robinson, 2000). Limitations in current healthcare provision for people with intellectual disabilities have been recognised in a number of health-related policy and advisory documents (Department of Health, 1995; NHS Executive, 1998 and 1999) culminating in the most recent White Paper for England in intellectual disabilities, *Valuing People: A New Strategy for Learning Disability for the 21st Century* (Department of Health, 2001a). Within this document, the system of healthcare facilitation that includes the development of individualised health action plans has been outlined as a way in which access to healthcare for people with intellectual disabilities may be improved.

This chapter discusses the principles of care planning in meeting the health needs of people with intellectual disabilities within the context of health facilitation and health action planning. Whilst it has been suggested that the role of health facilitator may be adopted by a range of different people, including both professionals and lay carers (Department of Health, 2002a), it has been recognised that the already present knowledge and skills of intellectual disability nurses ensures that they are in a key position to lead on this role (Hunt et al., 2001). A central feature of health facilitation is the necessity of working in a way that promotes rights, independence, choice and inclusion for people with intellectual disabilities (Department of Health, 2001a). This involves adopting the key principles of person-centred planning (Department of Health, 2002b) and this will be discussed in this chapter with specific reference to addressing healthcare needs through health action planning. Throughout the chapter, best practice examples will be amassed and used to consolidate recommended approaches to improving access to healthcare for people with intellectual disabilities. To contextualise the necessity of adopting these new ways of delivering care, the following section of this chapter explores the current healthcare status of people with intellectual disabilities.

Current healthcare status of people with intellectual disabilities

People with intellectual disabilities, especially those with severe to profound intellectual disabilities, are known to have more complex healthcare needs than those of the general population (Van Schrojenstein Lantman-De Valk et al., 2000). Health conditions known to be significantly more prevalent amongst this group include mental health problems, epilepsy, visual and hearing impairments, thyroid dysfunction and skeletal malformations caused by conditions such as osteoporosis (Hatton et al., 2003). The most prevalent causes of death, however, have been identified as respiratory disease, followed by cancer (Durvasula et al., 2002). Whilst unusually high incidence rates of some of these health problems could be attributed to the clinical features of certain genetic conditions within intellectual disabilities, such as Prader–Willi syndrome (Smith et al., 2003) or tuberous sclerosis (Lewis et al., 2004), others could be related to the social, economic and employment circumstances of individuals (Turner, 2001). Other factors known to predispose this group to poor health include a lack of information, lack of exercise, poor mobility and eating habits and the side effects of some medication, including the stimulation of appetite and obesity (Van Schrojenstein Lantman-De Valk et al., 2000). Additionally, there is evidence to suggest that the rate of smoking amongst this group may also be increasing (Emerson and Turnbull, 2005).

The aetiology and demography of intellectual disabilities is changing, the most prominent change being increased life expectancy. In the case of people with mild intellectual disabilities, life expectancy is now said to be equivalent to that of the general population (Patja et al., 2000). The advancement of antibiotics and the introduction of new forms of anticonvulsant therapy, improved quality of care and new surgical techniques have all been listed as important factors in increasing life expectancy for all people with intellectual disabilities, but particularly those with Down's syndrome (Hollins et al., 1998). Recent estimates have suggested that around 80% of people with Down's syndrome are now living over the age of 50 years, compared to an average life expectancy of 12 years in 1949 (Kerr, 1997). This increased life expectancy, however, is matched by an increased prevalence of previously unrecognised conditions amongst this group, such as presenile dementia which is currently presenting a significant challenge to services (Waterman, 2003).

Despite increasing longevity of life, mortality rates amongst people with intellectual disabilities remain higher than those of the general population (Durvasula at al., 2002), with preventable deaths recorded as being as much as four times higher (Dupont and Mortenson, 1990). In one study undertaken in two London boroughs, it was estimated that the risk of dying amongst people with intellectual disabilities was 58 times higher than that found in the population of England and Wales (Hollins et al., 1998). Significantly it has been argued that many recordable deaths amongst people with intellectual disabilities would have been preventable with regular health surveillance (Durvasula et al., 2002). It has been shown, however, that provision of preventative health interventions and level of uptake of health surveillance is mismatched with the level of actual need (Kerr et al., 1996; Turner, 1996). This is situation is supported by research evidence detailing the scale of unmet health needs amongst people with intellectual disabilities (Meehan et al., 1995; Barr et al., 1999; Webb and Rogers, 1999; Cassidy et al., 2002; Lennox et al., 2003), culminating in a more recent piece of evidence that has prompted the first formal inquiry into health equalities experienced by this group (Disability Rights Commission, 2004).

It has been argued that existing health inequalities for people with intellectual disabilities may be largely attributed to the range of barriers that currently exist for this group at an individual, carer and organisational level (Alborz et al., 2003), barriers which are often cited in the personal recollections of both people with intellectual disabilities and their carers (Band, 1998; Fox and Wilson, 1999; Rutter and Seyman, 1999; Mencap, 2004). A number of the barriers from the work of Alborz et al. (2003) are shown in Box 12.1.

Box 12.1   Barriers to healthcare for people with intellectual disabilities

Individual
- Limitations in ability to identify and communicate healthcare needs
- Fear of accessing services
- Fear of encountering negative attitudes amongst healthcare providers

Carer
- Failure to recognise a gradual deterioration in health loss
- Fear of upsetting the individual with intellectual disabilities

Organisational
- Physical inaccessibility
- Communication difficulties
- Time constraints
- Lack of knowledge
- 'Unhelpful attitudes'

Coupled with the barriers to healthcare experienced by people with intellectual disabilities is a failure on the part of some professionals actively to involve them in the planning of their own care (Redworth and Philips, 1997). Recommendations in policy documents relate to the necessity of working in partnership with people with intellectual disabilities and their carers to instigate packages of care that meet self-defined needs (NHS Executive, 1998). Research evidence, however, would suggest that this group are commonly on the periphery of decisions made about their care (Hart, 1999; Fovargue et al., 2000) and that the tools and processes used to determine their needs are often inaccessible, thereby leaving them with no measurable level of control (Williams and Robinson, 2000).

One particular area of difficulty is in the provision of informed consent to healthcare interventions. It has been suggested that there remains a presumption on the part of some healthcare professionals that people with intellectual disabilities lack the capacity to give informed consent, and therefore little is done to help facilitate the decision-making process (Joseph Rowntree Foundation, 2001; Cea and Fisher, 2003). This is particularly noticeable in the case of people with profound intellectual disabilities who may have no formal communication skills and where it has been argued that a lack of commitment on the part of the professional to elicit their views may lead to care being based solely on 'inferences' (Ware, 2004).

Whilst the health of people with intellectual disabilities has been the subject of much policy guidance over the last few years (Department of Health, 1995; NHS Executive, 1998 and 1999), difficulties in providing a high-quality service to this group remain. Recent policy guidance would suggest that what is essentially needed is a proactive rather than reactive approach to healthcare delivery, achievable through the processes of health facilitation and health action planning (Department of Health, 2001a).

Reader activity 12.1

Imagine that you have been feeling ill and need to visit the doctor. Make a list of the personal skills that you would be required to draw upon in order to achieve your goal. Consider the difficulties that a person with intellectual disabilities may have when attempting the same activity.

Responding to a new agenda for health

The term 'health facilitation' was first introduced in the recent White Paper, *Valuing People* (Department of Health, 2001a), although it is acknowledged that its intrinsic processes have evolved out of the roles traditionally held by both professionals and family members involved in the care of people with intellectual disabilities (Department of Health, 2002a). Broadly speaking, health facilitation aims to promote access to mainstream services for people with intellectual disabilities, whilst aiding those very same services to develop the necessary skills to accommodate the individual needs of this group (Department of Health, 2002a). Health facilitation is therefore seen to be operating on two distinct levels: level 1, which is described as *self-development work*, and involves developing, auditing and monitoring health initiatives at local and national levels, and level 2 which is described as *person to person work with people with learning disabilities*, of which health action planning is a central facet (Department of Health, 2002a). A health action plan has been described as one which:

> 'details the actions needed to maintain and improve the health of an individual and any help needed to accomplish these. It is a mechanism to link the individual and the range of services and supports they need, if they are to have better health.' (Department of Health, 2002a)

It has been concluded that whilst health action plans have the potential for improving healthcare delivery to all people with intellectual disabilities, their main focus should be upon those groups who are most vulnerable to the risk of exclusion, particularly those undergoing some form of life transition, such as moving from child to adult services, leaving home or retiring (Department of Health, 2002a). This same guidance also recommends that a health action plan be offered to those who are experiencing a significant change in health status, where a health problem is suspected or for those whose health status may be compromised because they are unable to advocate on their own behalf. Research detailing the effectiveness of health action plans in improving access to relevant care to people with intellectual disabilities is currently scarce, although results from the evaluation of similar mediums of communication, for example 'health logs' and 'personal health records', reveal that they may prompt the identification and monitoring of health needs, referral to appropriate services and greater consideration of an individual's health history (Curtice and Long, 2002; Turk and Burchell, 2003).

The processes of both health facilitation and health action planning are underpinned by the principles of person-centred planning that are more fully discussed in Chapter 4 of this book. The central facets of this type of planning are the active and central involvement of the person with intellectual disabilities in decision making, a process that has previously been observed as a way in which the balance of power between users and service providers can be equalised (Redworth and Philips, 1997). Good practice guidance argues that the two methods of planning must complement each other rather than be regarded as separate entities (Department of Health, 2002a) and ways in which this can be achieved across different stages of the health planning process will be discussed in the following section.

Initiation of a health action plan

Whilst it is the intention to offer all people with intellectual disabilities the opportunity to develop their own health action plan, it has been recognised that, wherever possible, such a decision must be based upon informed choice, which involves helping a person understand the nature of the planning process and the range of potential outcomes (Department of Health, 2002a). In some cases this may be achieved through discussion with an individual and supported by easy-to-read information on health action planning (Department of Health, 2002c). Access to health information material remains somewhat problematic for people with intellectual disabilities, as it is often pitched at inappropriate levels (Taylor and Smithurst, 2001). It has been concluded, therefore, that, in order for people with intellectual disabilities to benefit from such material, it must be in a format that takes into account both sensory impairments and languages in use (NHS Executive, 1998). This may include the use of large bold font, pictures, photographs and symbols (Townsley, 1999). Promoting access to such material in this way optimises the chance of healthcare decisions, including the initiation of health action plans, being based upon informed consent.

Obtaining informed consent is crucial to ensuring that all people with intellectual disabilities have a clear choice when meeting their healthcare needs and should be obtained at each stage of the health action planning process. This reflects the necessity of viewing the mechanisms of achieving informed consent as a 'process' and not a one-off event, thereby recognising the right of an individual to withdraw it at any one time (Department of Health, 2001b). Central to this process is an assessment of 'capacity', that is the degree to which a person is able to make an informed decision, and this measurement of capacity will form part of the role of the health facilitator (Department of Health, 2001b). In many cases, people with learning disabilities will be able to make healthcare decisions based upon careful scrutiny of available information

(Fovargue et al., 2000). In other cases, people's 'capacity' may be drawn into question, such as those who have non-conventional forms of communication, although it has been argued that this should not deter people from attempting to elicit such consent, as there is evidence to suggest that this group can make decisions if appropriately supported and sufficient time is taken (Ware, 2004; Cannella et al., 2005). In such instances, augmentative forms of communication may be usefully employed; one recent example of this is 'talking mats', where picture symbols are used to help a person explore their own thoughts and ideas (Brewster, 2004).

Realistically, however, despite best efforts, some people with intellectual disabilities will be unable to provide informed consent for the instigation of healthcare interventions. In such circumstances, the health facilitator may find themselves having to act in the 'best interests' of that person (Department of Health, 2001c). The decision to resort to best interests is one that should not be taken lightly, and should reflect an adherence to current policy recommendations in this area which includes a multi-disciplinary approach to decision making and the necessity of attaining consensual agreement (Department of Health, 2001b, c). Part of this process should involve obtaining the views of those who have intimate knowledge of the person, and it is suggested that the processes used to make decisions about an individual's healthcare may reflect those used in person-centred planning (Sanderson et al., 1997). It is envisaged that such an approach will also minimise the risk of care being based on 'inferences' made about a person's needs (Ware, 2004). A further strategy discussed by Ware is the use of advocates or 'proxies', although it has been acknowledged that the best people to assume this role are not necessarily the people closest to the individual as there may be competing agendas and conflicts (Redworth and Philips, 1997; Fovargue et al., 2000). In such circumstances, citizen advocates may be usefully employed to ensure objectivity and promote the rights of an individual (Gates, 1994).

In addition to exploring the process and potential outcomes of health action planning, the health facilitator must establish an understanding as to the way in which an individual with learning disabilities perceives the nature of 'health issues' (Department of Health, 2002a). Such information is considered necessary as it may provide a basis for prioritising health needs and informing decisions made about care later in the planning process. In general, the concept of health means different things to different people (Saunders, 2001). Such a concept may be influenced by a range of variables, including genetic factors, ethnicity, family, physical/social environment, age and level of intellectual functioning (Alborz et al., 2003). It has been argued that a failure to acknowledge the views of a client or patient on what constitutes good and/or bad health may lead to both ineffectual healthcare practices and a lack of commitment on the part of the individual (Kerns et al., 2003). The necessity of exploring the concept of health with an individual with intellectual disabilities is even more pertinent in light of evidence that suggests that this group may still be viewed as 'suffering' from their disability (Alderson, 2001). Emerging research would suggest that, even in the presence of a chronic health condition or long-term disability, a person may report being in good health (Lindsey, 1996; Moch, 1998).

Strategies discussed in the attainment of informed consent may also be usefully employed in establishing an individual's conceptualisation of health. This may include facilitated discussion supported by health-related literature that meets an individual's communication needs, such as the recent Department of Health publication *Choosing Health* (Department of Health, 2004), which is available as an easy-to read document and on CD-ROM. In the case of people with profound learning disabilities, where their understanding of health may be difficult to gauge, information about the person's likes and dislikes may be gleaned through the process of person-centred planning (Sanderson et al., 1997). Such likes and dislikes may form the basis of 'preference assessments' that could be used to increase the health facilitator's understanding of what an individual is likely to perceive as representing good or bad health (Cannella et al., 2005).

Assessing healthcare needs in learning disabilities

Once an agreement has been reached either directly or indirectly that supports the necessity of health action plan, an assessment of an individual's health needs forms the next step (Department of Health, 2002a). It has been argued that structured and systematic assessment processes may lead to the identification of health needs and potential health problems amongst people with intellectual disabilities (Matthews and Hegarty, 1997). Research studies that have adopted such an approach during the health screening of this group have shown that this results in the detection of a large number of unmet healthcare needs and the instigation of appropriate remedial actions (Barr et al., 1999; Hunt et al., 2001; Lennox et al., 2001). Department of Health guidance on health action planning advises that the tools used in the assessment of healthcare needs amongst people with intellectual disabilities should demonstrate a number of important properties, including being evidence based, being able to identify healthcare needs particular to both an individual and to those of people with intellectual disabilities in general, reflect current health policy and have the capacity to be administered in a person-centred way (Department of Health, 2002a). Attention is drawn to a number of tools designed specifically for the measurement of healthcare needs amongst people with intellectual disabilities, and these include the Cardiff health check and the St Georges Hospital Medical School health check, although there is currently a lack of data to support their validity and reliability. The OK health check (Matthews and Hegarty, 1997), on the other hand, has demonstrated clear psychometric properties and has been found systematically to identify a range of unmet healthcare needs amongst people with intellectual disabilities (Hunt et al., 2001). Another tool is the comprehensive health assessment tool, which again has demonstrated comprehensibility when assessing both type and level of healthcare need amongst this group (Lennox et al., 2001). Other assessment tools identified by the Department of Health target only one area of health, such as PAS-ADD (psychiatric assessment schedule for adults with a developmental disability) (Moss et al., 1993), but it is acknowledged that they could be used as part of a general assessment of health need (Department of Health, 2002a). Such an approach supports the necessity of employing an eclectic mix of models when assessing an individual with a number of complex healthcare needs.

Previous research has drawn attention to the inaccessibility of assessment processes for people with intellectual disabilities, and this includes the documentation used (Williams and Robinson, 2000). It has been recognised that the active involvement of an individual in the assessment of their own healthcare needs could optimised by using clear words and language, illustrations, photographs and augmentative communication systems, such as Makation or Rebus symbols (Townsley, 1999). In others with more severe forms of learning disability this may be more problematic due to restrictions in their ability to communicate signs of ill health (Mencap, 2004). In such circumstances, a consensus about the current health status of the individual may be ascertained from information generated from those individuals significant to the person, again using the process of person-centred planning (Sanderson et al., 1997). An alternative approach explored in the literature, however, is the observation and subsequent classification of an individual's behaviours as a predictor of different health statuses (Callan et al., 1995).

For all people, however, regardless of the level of intellectual disability, attention has been drawn to the necessity of a multi-disciplinary approach to the assessment of healthcare need in providing access to different types of clinical knowledge and skill, increasing the ease to which relevant information is shared and promoting collaborative decision making (Hunt et al., 2001; Cassidy et al., 2002). Identifying those people who could make a significant contribution to facilitating healthcare for an individual with intellectual disabilities forms the second part of the assessment process (Department of Health, 2002a). At this stage the level of support that an individual currently has and the level that may be required to address health needs are assessed and may be usefully explored by developing a relationship circle (Sanderson et al., 1997). In saying this, however, the right of the individual to choose who is involved in their care is one that should be adhered to throughout the planning process and again reflects the philosophy of person-centred planning (Sanderson et al., 1997).

Creating a plan of care to meet healthcare needs

Once the health needs of an individual have been identified a plan of appropriate action must be devised to reflect the outcome of the assessment process. This process of planning requires the development of 'goals' or 'health actions' (Department of Health, 2002a). In accordance with the general guidance on care planning, the action plan should reflect a mixture of both short-term goals (those that can be attained in hours or days) and long-term goals (those that need to be met over a longer period such as months or years) (Heath, 1995). Heath also draws attention to the necessity of such goals being specific, reflecting a clear time frame, being achievable and measurable, being based on patient-partnership and stating 'who' and 'how' (STAMPS). In particular, she highlights the importance of ensuring that the goals devised for people with intellectual disabilities are realistic and achievable, as she argues that verging on the side of caution is better than being unduly optimistic, thereby risking 'catastrophic failure' (Heath, 1995).

Once the goals have been identified, collaboration between the health facilitator, the person with intellectual disabilities and/or relevant others, should lead to the ranking of the goals based on priority of need. Levels of priority include high (the presence of a condition which, if left untreated, may result in harm to themselves); intermediate (the presence of a non-emergency or life-threatening condition) or low (where a need is not directly linked to current health need) (Heath, 1995). Again, in line with the philosophy of person-centred planning, such collaboration ensures that the subsequent health action plan reflects the wishes and desires of the individual and not those of the professional (Department of Health, 2002b). The result of this collaboration must be presented in the health action plan in an accessible format, that may use some of the media advocated by Townsley (1999).

The self-determination of goals is a desirable outcome of the collaborative process, but it must be acknowledged that this may also involve accepting the right of a person with intellectual disabilities to make potentially 'unhealthy' decisions (Hunt et al., 2001). Such a situation may result in a health facilitator experiencing an ethical dilemma resulting from a conflict between their 'duty to care' and the necessity of supporting the autonomy of an individual (Fovargue et al., 2000). In such circumstances, a level of risk must be accepted as part of the process, so it is crucial that the health facilitator has assessed both the capacity of the individual to make an informed decision and has provided them with all the necessary information in an accessible format (Marshall et al., 2002). Such information may encompass the respective benefits and risks of proposed treatment, the implications of having or not having the treatment and any available alternatives (Department of Health, 2001c). In cases where the health facilitator is unsure about an individual's capability, further support could be sought from a variety of sources that include peer supervision and relevant policy documentation (Holloway, 2004). In such circumstances, it is essential that the health facilitator clearly documents both the process of obtaining consent and the outcome (Department of Health, 2001c).

Implementing a health action plan

Following the identification of health needs, consideration must be given to the way in which such needs may be addressed. The key aim of any health action plan is improved health status through increased accessibility to a range of healthcare interventions (Department of Health, 2001a). The collective term for such interventions is health promotion, and this is observed to operate on three distinct levels (Nightingale, 1992):

- Primary prevention, in which ill health and disease are prevented
- Secondary prevention, which involves early detection and treatment of disease
- Tertiary prevention, which aims to inhibit the progression of an existing health condition

Health promotion activities have been categorised as having either a medical, behavioural or educational focus, in addition to those which specifically seek to promote empowerment within an individual or elicit a social change that involves improving access to healthcare for people with intellectual disabilities at an organisational level (Ewles and Simnett, 1992). A range of appropriate health promotion activities for people with intellectual disabilities can be found in some policy guidelines and include further investigations and treatment that may also involve referral to more specialised health and screening services, incentives for becoming involved in sport and leisure activities and the awarding of 'certificates of achievement of good health' (NHS Executive, 1998). Yearly screening programmes have also been recommended as a minimum level of healthcare input for people with intellectual disabilities, although it recognised that this frequency must reflect the changing health status of an individual (Cassidy et al., 2002).

Central to any health promotion activity for people with intellectual disabilities is the health facilitator, whose role may differ according to the needs of an individual. Practice examples suggest that this role may involve the following (Hunt et al., 2001):

- Giving information prior to a medical procedure, arranging pre-visits
- Providing explanations for necessary care interventions or procedures
- Attending appointments to support the individual and/or carer and facilitating communication between all parties
- Supporting and educating mainstream health professionals in order that they may provide a service that successfully meets the needs of an individual

Regardless of the type of intervention, informed consent must be sought, and fundamental to this process is the provision of health information that may be achieved through the structured process of health education.

Health education has been defined in terms of three interrelated functions that are as follows (Whitehead, 2004):

- The provision of information to influence values and beliefs, attitudes and motivations
- The encouragement of health or illness related learning through the acquirement and appraisal of knowledge
- The development of skills and modification of health-related behaviours

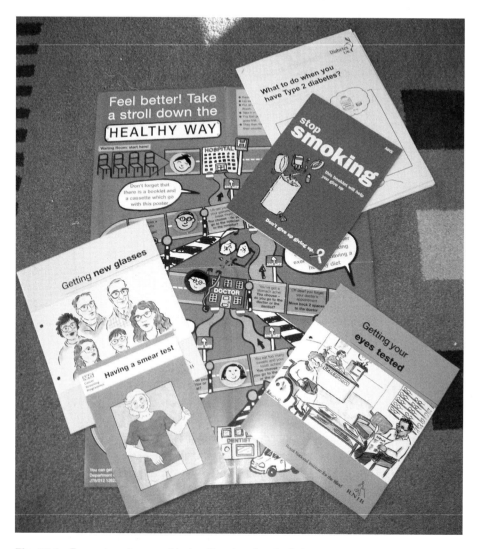

Fig. 12.1   Examples of accessible health education leaflets.

Health education may target carers as well as people with intellectual disabilities themselves, as it has been acknowledged that this group may also have limited knowledge about leading a healthier lifestyle (NHS Executive, 1999). A variety of media may be used to elicit positive changes in health behaviours amongst people with intellectual disabilities. Increasingly, health education material for this group is being developed and there are some good examples of where a combination of easy-to-read text, symbols and pictures increase the accessibility of relevant information (Figure 12.1; Royal National Institute for the Blind, 1999; Diabetes UK, 2000; Department of Health, 2000; NHS Cancer Screening Programmes, 2000). Another good example of accessible

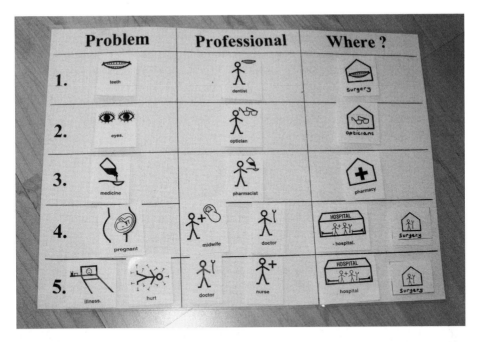

Fig. 12.2   Example of a health education game.

health education material is that which can be found in the Books Beyond Words series, that includes titles such as *Looking After My Breasts* (Hollins and Perez, 2000) and *Looking After My Balls* (Hollins and Wilson, 2004).

Despite the increasing availability of such educational material it has been concluded that they alone cannot generate a change in the health behaviours of people with intellectual disabilities, and that a multi-faceted approach needs to be adopted (Lindsay et al., 1998). Good practice examples of where a combination of different teaching methods (for example, quizzes, role play, videos and games) have been used with this group include breast awareness (Cowie and Fletcher, 1998); weight reduction (Marshall et al., 2002); alcohol awareness (Forbat, 1999); HIV/AIDS awareness (Cambridge, 1996); smoking (Kelman et al., 1997); and healthy eating (Richardson, 1993). Fig 12.2 is an example of such a health education game. Attention has also been drawn to the necessity of a multi-disciplinary approach in implementing the actions necessary to meet the identified heathcare needs (Department of Health, 2002a). Again, regardless of the type of action, all planned interventions must be clearly recorded in an accessible format in the health action plan.

Reviewing the health action plan

The final stage of the health action planning involves reviewing the effectiveness of the health action plan in improving an individual's health status. Policy guidance recommends that this should involve checking that any required actions have been implemented, that the required assistance was given, evaluating the relative effectiveness of respective actions and assessing the need for new action (Department of Health, 2002a). The necessity of undertaking this evaluation in collaboration with the person with intellectual disabilities and/or their significant others further emphasises both the philosophy of person-centred planning (Sanderson et al., 1997) and the necessity of having accessible methods of evaluation. Research literature exploring the effectiveness of different health interventions in eliciting positive health behaviours reveals a number of ways of evaluating care. These include physiological measurements, such as body mass index (BMI), which could be used to evaluate the effectiveness of a weight loss programme (Jolly and Jamieson, 1999), and health quizzes and verbal questionnaires (Cowie and Fletcher, 1998) that may be used to assess the degree to which health information has been both acquired and retained (Forbat, 1999). Other studies point to the use of accessible scales on which people with intellectual disabilities could express their satisfaction with respect to health action planning process (Money and Collins, 1999). This includes the necessity of using observation skills to evaluate changes in those individuals with non-conventional forms of communication, thereby re-emphasising the importance of using behaviours to evaluate health status (Callan et al., 1995).

Conclusion

This chapter has explored the process of care planning when addressing healthcare needs amongst people with intellectual disabilities. Recent policy guidance in this area points to the necessity of adopting a person-centred approach to the delivery of healthcare in this area which encompasses the processes of health facilitation and health action planning. Throughout, this chapter has drawn on contemporary research to provide concrete examples as to ways in which the central involvement of people with intellectual disabilities in decisions made about their own health can be achieved. It has recognised the importance of facilitating choice and informed decision making, which also takes account of the rights of this group to decide who will be involved in their care. It is acknowledged that whilst ways in which access to healthcare for people with learning disabilities can be achieved will continue to be developed and become more innovative, the basic rights of the individual to have an optimum level of control over this process must be maintained.

The following case illustration and health action plan consolidate the information that has been provided in this chapter. It is a working example of how the health issues of an individual with intellectual disabilities may be both identified and addressed. It recognises the importance of a person-centred approach to health action planning in addition to working in partnership with significant others.

Appendix 12.1
Example of a health action plan

Health action plan			
Name: Mohammed	Date of Birth: 15-01-71		Date of plan: 25-04-06
Identified healthcare need	**Health action required**	**Action by**	**Date of review**
Mohammed has difficulty understanding about foods that are good and bad for him	To teach Mohammed about healthy eating	Sally, Community Learning Disability Nurse	25-10-06

References

Alborz, A., McNally, R., Swallow, A. and Glendinning, C. (2003) *From the Cradle to the Grave: A Literature Review of Access to Health Care for People with Learning Disabilities across the Lifespan*: Report for the National Co-ordinating Centre for NHS Service Delivery and Organisation R&D. London: NCCSDO.

Alderson, P. (2001) Down's syndrome: cost, quality and value of life. *Social Science and Medicine* **53** (5), 627–38.

Band, R. (1998) *The NHS – Health for All?* London: Mencap.

Barr, O., Gilgunn, J., Kane, T. and Moore, G. (1999) Health screening for people with learning disabilities by a community learning disability nursing service in Northern Ireland. *Journal of Advanced Nursing* **29** (6), 1482–91.

Brewster, S.J. (2004) Putting words into their mouths? Interviewing people with learning disabilities and little/no speech. *British Journal of Learning Disabilities* **32** (4), 166–9.

Callan, L., Gilbert, T., Golding, K., Lockyer, T. and Rafter, K. (1995) Assessing health needs in people with severe learning disabilities: a qualitative approach. *Journal of Clinical Nursing* **4** (5), 295–302.

Cambridge, P. (1996) Assessing and meeting needs in HIV and learning disability. *British Journal of Learning Disabilities* **24** (2), 52–7.

Cannella, H.I., O'Reilly, M.F. and Lancioni, G.E. (2005) Choice and preference assessment research with people with severe and profound developmental disabilities: a review of the literature. *Research in Developmental Disabilities* **26** (1), 1–15.

Cardiff Health Check. Available at: http: www.uwcm.ac.uk/study/ (Accessed 14 January 2005).

Cassidy, G., Martin, D.M., Martin, G.H.B. and Roy, A. (2002) Health checks for people with learning disabilities. *Journal of Learning Disabilities* **6** (2), 123–36.

Cea, C.D. and Fisher, C.B. (2003) Health care decision-making by adults with mental retardation. *Mental Retardation* **41** (2), 78–87.

Cowie, M. and Fletcher, J. (1998) Breast awareness project for women with a learning disability. *British Journal of Nursing* **7** (13), 774–8.

Curtice, L. and Long, L. (2002) The health log: developing a health monitoring tool for people with learning disabilities within a community support agency. *British Journal of Learning Disabilities* **30** (2), 68–72.

Department of Health (1995) *The Health of the Nation: A Strategy for People with Learning Disabilities*. London: Her Majesty's Stationery Office.

Department of Health (2000) *Stop Smoking*. London: Department of Health.

Department of Health (2001a) *Valuing People: A New Strategy for Learning Disability for the 21st Century*. London: Department of Health.

Department of Health (2001b) *Seeking Consent: Working with People with Learning Disabilities*. London: Department of Health.

Department of Health (2001c) *Reference Guide to Consent for Examination or Treatment*. London: Department of Health.

Department of Health (2002a) *Action for Health – Health Action Plans and Health Facilitation*. London: Department of Health.

Department of Health (2002b) *Planning with People: Towards Person Centred Approaches – Guidance for Implementation Groups*. London: Department of Health.

Department of Health (2002c) *Health Action Plans: What are they? How do you get one?* London: Department of Health.

Department of Health (2004) *Choosing Health: A Booklet about Plans for Improving People's Health*. London: Department of Health.

Diabetes, U.K. (2000) *What to do when you have Type 1 Diabetes*. London: Diabetes, UK.

Disability Rights Commission (2004) *Equal Treatment: Closing the Gap*. London: Disability Rights Commission.

Dupont, A. and Mortenson, P.B. (1990) Avoidable death in a cohort of severely mentally retarded. In: *Key Issues in Mental Retardation* (Fraser, W.I., ed.). London: Routledge.

Durvasula, S., Beange, H. and Baker, W. (2002) Mortality of people with intellectual disability in Northern Sydney. *Journal of Intellectual and Developmental Disability* **27** (4), 255–64.

Emerson, E. and Turnbull, L. (2005) Self-reported smoking and alcohol use among adolescents with intellectual disabilities. *Journal of Learning Disabilities* **9** (1), 58–69.

Ewles, L. and Simnett, L. (1992) *Promoting Health: A Practical Guide to Health Education*. Chichester: Wiley.

Forbat, L. (1999) Developing an alcohol awareness course for clients with a learning disability. *British Journal of Learning Disabilities* **27** (1), 16–19.

Fovargue, S., Keywood, K. and Flynn, M. (2000) Participation in health care decision-making by adults with learning disabilities. *Mental Health and Learning Disabilities Care* **3** (10), 341–4.

Fox, D. and Wilson, D. (1999) Parents' experiences of general hospital admission for adults with learning disabilities. *Journal of Clinical Nursing* **8** (5), 610–14.

Gates, B. (1994) *Advocacy: A Nurse's Guide*. London: Scutari Press.

Hart, S. (1999) Meaningful choices: consent to treatment in general health care settings for people with learning disabilities. *Journal of Learning Disabilities Nursing, Health and Social Care* **3** (1), 20–6.

Hatton, C., Elliot, J. and Emerson, E. (2003) *Key Highlights of Research Evidence on the Health of People with Learning Disabilities in Improvement, Expansion and Reform – ensuring that all means all*. Available at: www.doh.gov.uk/vpst/documents/AllMeansAll.pdf (Accessed 2 November 2004).

Heath, H.B.M. (ed.) (1995) *Potter and Perry's Foundation in Nursing Theory and Practice*. Edinburgh: Harcourt Publishers.

Hollins, S., Attard, M.T., Von Fraunhofer, N., McGuigan, S. and Sedgwick, P. (1998) Mortality in people with learning disability: risks, causes, and death certification findings in London. *Developmental Medicine and Child Neurology* **40** (1), 50–6.

Hollins, S. and Perez, W. (2000) *Looking After My Breasts*. London: Gaskell, Royal College of Psychiatrists.

Hollins, S. and Wilson, J. (2004) *Looking After My Balls*. London: Gaskell, Royal College of Psychiatrists.

Holloway, D. (2004) Ethical dilemmas in community learning disabilities nursing. *Journal of Learning Disabilities* **8** (3), 283–98.

Hunt, C., Wakefield, S. and Hunt, G. (2001) Community nurse learning disabilities: a case study of the use of an evidence based screening tool to identify and meet the health needs of people with learning disabilities. *Journal of Learning Disabilities* **5** (1), 9–18.

Jolly, C. and Jamieson, J.M. (1999) The nutritional problems of adults with severe learning disabilities living in the community. *Journal of Human Nutrition and Dietetics* **12** (1), 29–34.

Joseph Rowntree Foundation (2001) *Demonstrating Control of Decisions by Adults with Learning Difficulties who have High Support Needs*. York: Joseph Rowntree Foundation.

Kelman, L.V., Lindsay, W.R., McPherson, F.M. and Mathewson, Z. (1997) Smoking education for people with learning disabilities. *British Journal of Learning Disabilities* **25** (3), 95–9.

Kerns, C.J., Meehan, N.K., Carr, R.L. and Park, L.I. (2003) Using cross-cultural definitions of health care. *The Nurse Practitioner* **28** (1), 61–2.

Kerr, M.P., Richards, D. and Glover, G. (1996) Primary care for people with an intellectual disability – a group practice survey. *Journal of Applied Research in Intellectual Disabilities* **9** (4), 347–52.

Kerr, D. (1997) *Down's Syndrome and Dementia: A Practitioner's Guide.* Birmingham: Venture.

Lennox, N., Green, M., Diggens, J. and Ugoni, A. (2001) Audit and comprehensive health assessment programme in the primary health care of adults with learning disability: a pilot study. *Journal of Intellectual Disability Research* **45** (3), 226–32.

Lennox, T.N., Nadkarni, J., Moffat, P. and Robertson, C. (2003) Access to services and meeting the needs of people with learning disabilities. *Journal of Learning Disabilities* **7** (1), 34–50.

Lewis, J.C., Thomas, H.V., Murphy, K.C. and Sampson, J.R. (2004) Genotype and psychological phenotype in tuberous sclerosis. *Journal of Medical Genetics* **41** (3), 203–7.

Lindsay, W.R., McPherson, F.M. and Kelman, L.V. (1998) The Chief Scientist reports . . . health promotion and people with learning disabilities: the design and evaluation of three programmes. *Health Bulletin* **56** (3), 694–8.

Lindsey, E. (1996) Health within illness: experiences of chronically ill/disabled people. *Journal of Advanced Nursing* **24** (3), 465–72.

Marshall, D., McConkey, R. and Moore, G. (2002) Obesity in people with intellectual disabilities; the impact of nurse-led health screenings and health promotion activities. *Journal of Advanced Nursing* **41** (2), 147–53.

Matthews, D. and Hegarty, J. (1997) The OK health check: a health assessment checklist for people with learning disabilities. *British Journal of Learning Disabilities* **25** (4), 138–43.

Meehan, S., Moore, G. and Barr, O. (1995) Specialist services for people with learning disabilities. *Nursing Times* **91** (13), 33–5.

Mencap (2004) *Treat me Right! Better Healthcare for People with a Learning Disability.* London: Mencap.

Moch, S.D. (1998) Health-within-illness: concept development through research and practice. *Journal of Advanced Nursing* **28** (2), 305–10.

Money, D. and Collins, G. (1999) Satisfaction for all: a framework for assessing life satisfaction for all people with learning disabilities. *British Journal of Learning Disabilities* **27** (2), 52–7.

Moss, S.C., Patel, P., Prosser, H., Goldberg, D.P., Simpson, N., Rowe, S. and Lucchino, R. (1993) Psychiatric morbidity in older people with moderate and severe learning disability (mental retardation). Part 1: Development and reliability of the patient interview (the PAS-ADD). *British Journal of Psychiatry* **163**, 471–80.

National Health Service and Community Care Act (1990) London: Her Majesty's Stationery Office.

NHS Executive (1998) *Signposts for Success in the Commissioning and Providing of Health Services for People with Learning Disabilities.* London: NHS Executive.

NHS Executive (1999) *Once a Day.* London: NHS Executive.

NHS Cancer Screening Programmes (2000) *Having a Smear Test.* Sheffield: NHS Cancer Screening Programmes.

Nightingale, C. (1992) Pointing to the way ahead in health education for people with learning disabilities. *Professional Nurse* **7** (9), 612–15.

O'Brien, J. and Tyne, A. (1981) *The Principle of Normalisation: A Foundation for Effective Services.* London: The Campaign for Mentally Handicapped People.

Patja, K., Livanainen, M., Vesala, H., Oksanen, H. and Ruoppila, I. (2000) Life expectancy of people with intellectual disability: a 35-year follow-up study. *Journal of Intellectual Disability Research* **44** (5), 591–9.

Richardson, N. (1993) Fit for the future. *Nursing Times* **89** (44), 36–8.

Redworth, M. and Philips, G. (1997) Involving people with learning disabilities in community care planning *British Journal of Learning Disabilities* **25** (1), 31–5.

Royal National Institute for the Blind (1999) *Getting your Eyes Tested.* London: Royal National Institute for the Blind.

Rutter, S. and Seyman, S. (1999) *He'll Never Join the Army.* London: DSA.

Sanderson, H., Kennedy, J., Ritchie, P. and Goodwin, G. (1997) *People, Plans and Possibilities: Exploring Person Centred Planning.* Edinburgh: SHS.

Saunders, M. (2001) Concepts of health and disability. In: *Meeting the Health Needs of People who have a Learning Disability* (Thompson, J. and Pickering, S. eds.). London: Baillière Tindall.

Singh, P. (1997) *Prescription for Change.* London: Mencap.

Smith, A., Loughnan, G. and Steinbeck, K. (2003) Death in adults with Prader-Will syndrome may be correlated with maternal uniparental disomy. *Journal of Medical Genetics* **40** (5), 63–6.

St Georges Hospital Medical School health check. Available at: www.sghms.ac.uk/depts/psychdis (accessed 14 January 2005).

Taylor, N. and Smithurst, S. (2001) Accessing health information. In: *Meeting the Health Needs of People who have a Learning Disability* (Thompson, J. and Pickering, S. eds.). London: Baillière Tindall.

Townsley, R. (1999) Putting it plainly: producing easy-to understand information for people with learning difficulties. *Frontline* **40**, 12–13.

Turk, V. and Burchell, S. (2003) Developing and evaluating personal health records for adults with learning disabilities. *Tizard Learning Disability Review* **8** (4), 33–41.

Turner, S. (1996) Promoting healthy lifestyles for people with learning disabilities: a survey of provider organisations. *British Journal of Learning Disabilities* **24** (4), 138–44.

Turner, S. (2001) Health needs of people who have a learning disability. In: *Meeting the Health Needs of People who have a Learning Disability* (Thompson, J. and Pickering, S. eds.). London: Baillière Tindall.

Van Schrojenstein Lantman-De Valk, H.M.J., Metsemakers, J.F.M., Haveman, M.J. and Crebolder, H.F.J.M. (2000) Health problems in people with intellectual disability in general practice: a comparative study. *Family Practice* **17** (5), 405–7.

Ware, J. (2004) Ascertaining the views of people with profound and multiple learning disabilities. *British Journal of Learning Disabilities* **32** (4), 175–9.

Waterman, K. (2003) Why wait for dementia. *Journal of Learning Disabilities* **7** (3), 221–30.

Webb, O.J. and Rogers, L. (1999) Health screening for people with intellectual disability: the New Zealand experience. *Journal of Intellectual Disability Research* **43** (6), 497–503.

Whitehead, D. (2004) Health promotion and health education: advancing the concepts. *Journal of Advanced Nursing* **47** (3), 311–20.

Williams, V. and Robinson, C. (2000) 'Tick this, tick that': the views of people with learning disabilities on their assessments. *Journal of Learning Disabilities* **4** (4), 293–305.

Wolfensberger, W. (1972) *The Principle of Normalisation in Human Management Services.* Toronto: National Institute of Mental Retardation.

Further reading and resources

Davison, P., Janicki, M.P. and Prasher, V. (2003) *Mental Health, Intellectual Disabilities and the Aging Process.* Oxford: Blackwell Science.

Hogenboom, M. (2001) *Living with Genetic Syndromes Associated with Intellectual Disability.* London: Jessica Kingsley Publishers.

Hogg, J., Northfield, J. and Turnbull, J. (2001) *Cancer and People with Learning Disabilities: the Evidence from Published Studies and Experiences from Cancer Services.* Kidderminster: British Institute of Learning Disabilities.

Prasher, V.P. and Janicki, M.P. (2002) *Physical Health of Adults with Intellectual Disabilities.* Oxford: Blackwell Science.

Priest, H. and Gibbs, M. (2004) *Mental Health Care for People with Learning Disabilities.* London: Jessica Kingsley Publishers.

Walsh, P.N. and Heller, T. (2002) *Health of Women with Intellectual Disabilities.* Oxford: Blackwell Publishing.

Teaching resources

British Institute of Learning Disabilities (1998) *Your Good Health.* Kidderminster: British Institute of Learning Disabilities.
A collection of 12 illustrated booklets exploring health issues that include alcohol and smoking, exercise and seeing and hearing

Dodd, K. and Brunker, J. (1998) *Feeling Poorly.* Brighton: Pavilion.
A training pack design to help people with learning disabilities communicate pain and the symptoms of illness

Health Education Authority (1999) *Health Related Resources for People with Learning Disabilities.* London: Health Education Authority.
A catalogue of health education material for people with learning disabilities

McCarthy, M. and Thompson, D. (1994) *Sex and Staff Training: Sexuality, Sexual Abuse and Safer Sex.* Brighton: Pavilion.
A training manual to introduce both staff and people with learning disabilities to issues of sex and sex education

McIntosh, P.A. and O'Neil, J.M. (1999) *Food, Fitness and Fun: A training pack in weight management for people with learning disabilities.* Brighton: Pavilion.
A training pack for educating people with learning disabilities about healthy eating

Websites

www.valuingpeople.gov.uk/documents/HealthListOfResources.pdf
Health resource material for people with learning disabilities.

www.intellectualdisability.info/home.htm
Information about the health needs of people with learning disabilities.

Chapter 13

Care planning and delivery for people with profound intellectual disabilities and complex needs

Julie Clark and Bob Gates

Introduction

Arguably people with profound intellectual disabilities and complex needs represent one of the most marginalised groups in western society. They are at risk from social exclusion and experience poorer health than the rest of the population. Therefore, care planning is particularly relevant for this group of people because of the high level of dependence they may have on others throughout their lives. Care plans should be regarded as a way of systematically planning and documenting interventions to meet their needs to support them in all aspects of their life. This chapter considers the intellectual disability nurse's role in care planning and delivery for this group of people.

Defining profound intellectual disabilities and complex needs

Lacey (1998) has defined profound and multiple intellectual disabilities as comprising the following characteristics:

- Profound intellectual impairment (which refers to people who score below twenty on an IQ test (World Health Organization, 1992); and
- Additional disabilities, which may include sensory disabilities, physical disabilities, autism or mental illness

Although definitions are arguably necessary for the planning and delivery of care (Ho, 2004), Mencap (2005) have reminded us that people with profound intellectual disabilities and complex needs are all different and should be treated as individuals. People with profound intellectual disabilities and complex needs should not be perceived as a list of ailments (Carnaby, 2001) but as people first, capable of experiencing the same range of human experiences as their fellow citizens (Davies and Evans, 2001).

A number of labels have been used to refer to this group of people and these include 'severe disabilities and complex needs', 'profound learning disabilities' and 'the most severely disabled' (PMLD Network, 2002). This can lead to confusion, not least for parents and carers and difficulties with accessing appropriate services. The term learning disabilities is associated with the medical model (Ho, 2004) which has arguably become outdated. Therefore, for the purposes of this chapter the term 'profound intellectual disabilities and complex needs' will be used and will refer to the definition that has already been provided by Lacey (1998).

How many people have profound intellectual disabilities and complex needs?

Calculating the incidence of intellectual disability is fraught with problems. This is because it is only the obvious manifestations of intellectual disability that can be detected at birth; for example in Down's syndrome the physical characteristics enable an early diagnosis and therefore the ability to calculate incidence of this disorder. Where there is no obvious physical manifestation, one must wait for significant delay in development in order to ascertain whether a child has intellectual disability. Therefore, it is more common in intellectual disability to talk of prevalence that is concerned with an estimation of the number of people with a condition, disorder or disease as a proportion of the whole population.

Given that a large number of people never come into contact with caring agencies, it is more common to refer to 'administrative prevalence'. Administrative prevalence refers to the number of people who have received some form of service and are therefore known to caring agencies.

Historically, there has been a general consensus that the overall prevalence of moderate and severe intellectual disability was approximately 3–4 persons per 1000 of the general population (see, for example, Open University, 1987; Department of Health, 1992). Based on more contemporary and extensive epidemiological data this has more recently been confirmed (Emerson et al., 2001). Further, such prevalence would appear to be universally common; for example, Craft (1985) has suggested that international studies have identified prevalence for severe and moderate intellectual disability as 3.7 per 1000 population.

In the UK it has been further calculated that of the 3–4 persons per 1000 population with intellectual disability, approximately 30% will present with severe or profound learning disabilities. Within this group it is not uncommon to find multiple disability that includes physical and/or sensory impairments or disability as well as behavioural difficulties. Based on these estimates it can be assumed that there are some 230 000–350 000 persons with severe learning disabilities in the UK.

People with profound intellectual disabilities and complex needs clearly represent a significant section of society and, according to The Foundation for People with Learning Disabilities (Emerson et al., 2001), this number is continuing to increase as a result of developments in medical technology, better control of epilepsy and an increase in the use of tube feeding (Mencap,

2001). These people generally require lifelong support to carry out activities of daily living and, like other citizens, they are entitled to access the resources that enable them to meet their health and social care needs as and when required.

It must be emphasised that intellectual disabilities are a state of being that lasts for life, so when we talk of people with profound intellectual disabilities and complex needs we are talking of children and adults as well as older people. This makes having access to good epidemiological data essential in order to assess contemporary as well as projected need and plan for the development of appropriate services accordingly (PMLD Network, 2002). The reader might care to refer back to Chapter 10 where a composite picture of prevalence rates is outlined in relation to the changing demography of people with intellectual disabilities.

Attitudes toward people with profound intellectual disabilities and complex needs

There remains considerable ignorance both in the general public, and health and social care professions about people with profound intellectual disabilities and complex needs. Consider the following statements from parents:

> 'You shouldn't have to look after someone like that. He should be in an institution.'
> 'If you will keep her at home what do you expect?'
> 'At the end of the day people thought my sons were worthless, utterly worthless, and we were too. I thought they were very special.'
>
> (Mencap, 2001)

And in relation to healthcare professionals, parents report on equally disturbing attitudes expressed:

> 'I overheard the doctor say: "That's not coming in my room. It will destroy the equipment." We had to stay with Anthony from 10am to 10pm because no one was feeding him.' (Mencap, 2004)

> 'Victoria was rushed to hospital after a series of seizures. She needed to be put on a ventilator. The doctor came up and spoke to us. He was suggesting that it wasn't worth trying to save her.' (Mencap, 2004)

It is not unheard of for people to say that they have never seen or met a person with profound intellectual disabilities and complex needs (PMLD Network, 2002). One explanation for this might be that these people have historically been 'shut away' from the communities in which they live. Even today many children with profound intellectual disabilities and complex needs attend a special school resulting in fewer opportunities to interact with the wider community (Oakes, 2003). In the past the majority of people with profound intellectual disabilities and complex needs lived as 'in-patients' in long-stay hospitals for the mentally handicapped where they were cared for predominantly by nursing and medical staff. Most of these hospitals have now closed and the 'patients' now live in community-based settings where they are regarded as 'clients' or 'service users'. Also, because of the hospital closures many children and adults now live in their family home or in a small residential home where they are often cared for by relatives or unqualified social care staff (Ward, 1999). Intellectual disability nurses must therefore be able to work in collaboration with a wide variety of people, including family members, paid carers and professionals from other disciplines, in a number of environmental settings.

Since the closure of the majority of long-stay hospitals and the beginnings of implementation of the White Paper, *Valuing People* (Department of Health, 2001), some progress has been made towards the social acceptance and inclusion of people with profound intellectual disabilities and complex needs but there is still a long way to go (McNally, 2004; Gooding, 2004). The PMLD Network (2002) has argued that this group of people still needs to be made more visible to society.

Carnaby (2001) has suggested that this group have been perceived as 'difficult to engage', 'passive' and an 'expensive' demand on resources. Such negative perceptions can be damaging and must be challenged if attitudes are to improve. Klotz (2004) has argued that people with profound intellectual disabilities and complex needs can, and do, live socially meaningful lives and The Human Rights Act 1998 has made it clear that everyone has a fundamental right to life. Additionally nurses are bound by a professional Code of Conduct which has explicitly stated that all patients and clients must be treated with respect and dignity (Nursing and Midwifery Council, 2004). These values are also central to the policies set out by the learning disabilities White Paper, *Valuing People* (Department of Health, 2001).

Respect and dignity are abstract concepts that can be interpreted in multiple ways. Some interpretations have led to the idea that in order to treat people with profound intellectual disabilities and complex needs with respect they must be treated in a way that is appropriate to their chronological age. However, the dictionary definitions of the terms 'respect' and 'dignity' arguably lend support to Carnaby's view that the most respectful and dignified approach to interaction involves consideration of an individual's specific abilities and disabilities (Carnaby, 2001). Respect has been defined as:

> 'a feeling of deep admiration for someone elicited by their qualities or achievements' or 'due regard for the feelings or rights of other' (Oxford English Dictionary, 2002)

and dignity as:

> 'the state or quality of being worthy of honour or respect.' (Oxford English Dictionary, 2002)

Treating an adult as an 'eternal child' could be equally disrespectful and could also hinder an individual's development (Wolverson, 2003). Therefore, approaches must be adopted which balance the necessity for developmental appropriateness with that for socially acceptable age-appropriateness.

Who decides on the content of care plans?

Nurses have a duty of care to patients, which means that clients are entitled to receive safe and competent care which should be informed by evidence-based practice (Nursing and Midwifery Council, 2004). In the context of this chapter evidence-based practice refers to a way of managing nursing interventions by making clinical decisions that use the best available research evidence, clinical expertise and an understanding of patient preferences (Craig and Smyth, 2002). However, little evidence has been established concerning people with profound intellectual disabilities and complex needs and therefore good practice is sometimes based on research that has been undertaken with people with mild and moderate intellectual disabilities (Carnaby, 2001; Klotz, 2004). This should necessarily cause us to question both the validity and reliability of 'evidence' gathered from one population and then applied to another (Gates and Wray, 2000; Gates and Atherton, 2001). The issue of referring to and treating people with intellectual disabilities as one homogenous group is commonplace but problematic.

Even the recent White Paper, *Valuing People* (Department of Health, 2001), made very little reference to the needs of people with profound intellectual disabilities and complex needs (Aylott, 2001). The policies set out by *Valuing People* were based on the principles of rights, independence, choice and inclusion. Putting these values into practice for people with profound intellectual disabilities and complex needs poses specific challenges. For example, some people are extremely limited in their abilities to make and communicate choices, and the ways in which these people require support will therefore be different. The Profound and Multiple Learning Disabilities Network have argued that the policies set out in *Valuing People* are of little use for this group and, in conjunction with Mencap, they have published their own report which has recommended that the government should make addressing the needs of this group a priority (Mencap, 2001).

When developing care plans for people whose contribution is potentially limited, it is extremely important to include family members, people who know and care for the person, as well as all relevant professionals. Carnaby (2001) has stressed the importance of joint working between professionals for providing comprehensive, seamless care. The appointment of a key worker is thought to be essential for joint working to be effective (Mencap, 2001; Wake, 2003).

In Case illustration 13.1 Abdul is presented as someone with profound intellectual disabilities and complex needs. Abdul is a young man who presents with potential threats and challenges to his health, which include epilepsy, nutritional problems, chest infections, constipation, pressure areas and visual impairments.

Case illustration 13.1

Abdul has profound intellectual disabilities and complex needs. He is 16 years old and lives in his family home with his parents and a younger brother and sister. Abdul has cerebral palsy and is unable to walk, sit up unaided or control the movements of his limbs and hands. Abdul spends his days in a wheelchair which he is reliant on others to manoeuvre. He also relies on others to wash, dress and feed him. Abdul is unable to speak and he communicates through eye contact, facial expressions and vocalisations. Abdul's parent's first language is Urdu and his Mum speaks very little English. The family belong to the Muslim faith.

Abdul experiences a number of health problems including:

- Epilepsy
- He is underweight
- Constipation
- Frequent chest infections
- He has developed pressure sores on his ankles in the past
- Poor eyesight

Abdul attends a local school for people with special educational needs. He has respite care for two nights a month at a unit for people with complex health needs.

Reader activity 13.1

Take some time to think about some of the people who might be involved in Abdul's care. Construct a realistic list and then compare your list to those identified in Box 13.1.

Are there any people listed in Box 13.1 that you have not thought of or have you listed people that we have not identified? Either way it might be worth spending some time to think about these lists and accounting for any differences with a colleague.

Constructing care plans for people with profound intellectual disabilities and complex needs

Firstly, as has been identified consistently throughout this text, all care plans must be constructed in a person-centred way, and this is especially important for those with profound intellectual disabilities and complex needs. This is because in many instances this group of people can be entirely dependent on their carers in all respects. This dependency can include, for example, having

Box 13.1   Some people who might be involved in Abdul's care

- Family
- Consultant
- GP
- Neurologist
- Community nurse
- Speech and language therapist
- Physiotherapist
- Occupational therapist
- Continence nurse
- Dietician
- Advocate
- Interpreter to communicate with the family in Urdu
- School teacher
- School nurse
- Transition worker
- Respite care staff

to be fed, toileted, moved, positioned, washed, bathed, dressed and even assisted with body elimination. With this in mind the PMLD Network (Mencap, 2001) has argued that person-centred planning can be used effectively with people who have limited communication abilities if a 'circle of support' is in place to support the planning process. A circle of support is a group of people who know and care about the person and are committed to spending time developing a deep understanding of them in order to plan and advocate for services that might improve the person's life. Care plans must be written in such a way that the people providing direct care can understand and follow them. In the field of intellectual disabilities it has been estimated that approximately 75% of the workforce is unqualified (Ward, 1999). Care plans must therefore be constructed in such a way that they can be readily understood by staff that come from a variety of backgrounds and bring various prior experiences and knowledge with them. Consistency of care is important in terms of effective outcomes but also for fostering a sense of security and predictability for the person with profound intellectual disabilities and complex needs. Ideally, day or education services, residential care and family carers should all be following the same care plans. In order to maintain confidentiality, care plans must contain information and be shared on a need-to-know basis.

> 'The practical use of clear and well constructed care plans or protocols which are regularly reviewed can help support staff to know what is expected of them.' (UKCC, 1998 p. 11)

People with profound intellectual disabilities and complex needs present with a wide range of needs. Focusing on one particular area of need can result in the neglect of other areas of care. For example, Male (1996) has found that at a special school for people with profound intellectual disabilities and complex needs, high levels of personal and healthcare support reduced opportunities for social and educational activities. Care plans must ensure that the full range of needs is addressed.

There is also a risk of needs being neglected when all aspects of life take place in one location (Goffman, 1961). Most people conduct, work, leisure and relaxation activities in different places. For people with profound intellectual disabilities and complex needs, it is just possible that all these activities could take place within the person's home. This inevitably is likely to lead to a risk of social exclusion, whereas access to a number and variety of environments might provide wider social, leisure and educational opportunities and, therefore, a more inclusive lifestyle.

Arguably, neither a medical nor social model of care on its own can adequately meet the care needs of this group. Current ideas about nursing emphasise the importance of holistic care. Narayanasamy et al. (2002) have argued that there is a need for a holistic approach to care that includes attention to mind, body and spirit. The challenge for nurses who are planning care for people with profound intellectual disabilities and complex needs is to balance a high level of need related to the 'body' with needs related to the 'mind' and 'spirit'. It is generally accepted that all three areas have an impact on quality of life (Narayanasamy et al., 2002; Shalock, 2004) but psychological and spiritual needs tend to be lower in the order of priorities.

Numerous nursing models have been devised to help organise the planning and provision of care. The remainder of this chapter discusses care planning through the use of the Roper, Logan and Tierney model of nursing (Box 13.2).

Box 13.2   The Model of Living (after Roper et al., 1996; see Holland et al., 2003)

Factors influencing activities of living	Activities of living	Dependence/ independence continuum
Biological	Maintaining a safe environment	⟵⟶
Psychological	Communicating	⟵⟶
Sociocultural	Breathing	⟵⟶
Environmental	Eating and drinking	⟵⟶
Politicoeconomic	Eliminating	⟵⟶
	Personal cleansing and dressing	⟵⟶
	Controlling body temperature	⟵⟶
	Mobilising	⟵⟶
	Working and playing	⟵⟶
	Expressing sexuality	⟵⟶
	Sleeping	⟵⟶
	Dying	⟵⟶

This model has been chosen because it is one of the most well known and used within the nursing profession. Nurses might find other models that are equally useful and may also find that with experience they rely less on a model for care planning, and more on their own knowledge, skills and understanding.

Tierney (1998) has argued that the strength of the Roper, Logan and Tierney model is that it focuses on holistic care and is based on the concept of health rather than illness and disease. Arguably, these factors make it an appropriate model for intellectual disability nursing. The model also has practical utility because it focuses on understanding the needs of people in terms of the activities they perform. The model embraces the idea that independence and dependence operate along a continuum relating to each activity of living separately. This is consistent with the generally accepted idea that the level of skills of people with intellectual disabilities can vary across different domains (American Association on Mental Retardation, 1997).

The model can be put into practice in a systematic way using the four stages of the nursing process: assessment, planning, implementation and evaluation (Yura and Walsh, 1978). The first stage, assessment, involves determining an individual's ability to carry out each of the twelve activities of living listed in Box 13.2. In the planning stage problems are identified and documented along with the goals that aim to address these problems. In relation to people with profound intellectual disabilities and complex needs, improvements are likely to be small and goals identified should reflect this. Care plans can include specific nursing interventions, but the emphasis is on the person and nurse working together towards the goals. The nursing process advocates that care plans should be implemented within normal daily routines as much as possible (Holland et al., 2003).

The final stage of the nursing process is 'evaluation'. This is an ongoing process in which the individual's ability to carry out these activities of daily living should be re-examined to see if the goals have been met. Due to the severity and enduring nature of profound learning disabilities and complex needs an appropriate goal might be to maintain a condition or prevent its deterioration. Care plans should be adjusted according to the outcome of evaluation and this can be done by using the nursing process in a cyclical way.

In order to use the Roper, Logan and Tierney model effectively, nurses must have an understanding of the five factors (biological, psychological, sociocultural, environmental and politico-economic) that influence the activities of living (Holland et al., 2003). Fig. 13.1 gives some examples of how the model and the factors that influence the activities of living might be used to develop a care plan for Abdul.

Having considered how these factors may influence the activities of daily living, the following sections discuss each of the activities of living in turn. The case illustration of Abdul is used throughout to consider how care planning might be carried out. Some of the more general issues that may arise when applying this model to the care of people with profound intellectual disabilities and complex needs are also considered.

Name: Abdul
Activity concerned: Maintaining a safe environment
Problem: Uncontrolled, tonic–clonic epileptic seizures
Goals:

- To ensure that Abdul does not suffer injury whilst having a seizure
- To respond appropriately when Abdul has a seizure
- To provide appropriate emotional support
- To monitor and record Abdul's seizures
- To monitor Abdul's medication
- To access appropriate health and medical care
- To liaise with epilepsy specialists

To be achieved by: Ongoing, to be reviewed at regular intervals

Nursing intervention (this should be based on a consideration of the five factors that affect the activities of living):

Physical: Physical effects of a seizure

- History of seizures
- Type of seizures
- Medication

Psychological: Behavioural signs of seizure activity

- Mood and behaviour following a seizure
- Psychological effects of epilepsy
- Emotional support needed to cope with epilepsy

Sociological: Restrictions of epilepsy on daily life

- Reactions of others who may witness a seizure
- Disruption of routines
- Concerns of others, information for carers and relatives

Environmental: Seizure triggers

- Risks of injury from the environment

Politicoeconomic: Ability of carers to manage epilepsy (training)

- Access to services
- Availability and access to an epilepsy nurse and neurologist

Fig. 13.1   An example of a care plan.

Maintaining a safe environment

A large number of people with profound intellectual disabilities and complex needs have epilepsy, and it is thought that approximately 50% of people with severe intellectual disabilities have some form of epilepsy (The National Society for Epilepsy, 2002). Carers play a vital role in monitoring and managing epilepsy and ensuring that these people receive appropriate care from specialist health services. Carers are the most likely people to witness seizures and it is vital that they are able to record a thorough description as this can help medical professionals to make an accurate diagnosis. A thorough knowledge of the person's medication is also essential in order to monitor its use and be alert to possible side effects.

Abdul has been diagnosed with generalised, tonic–clonic seizures. This type of seizure is characterised by a stiffening of the muscles, followed by rhythmical relaxing and tightening of the muscles which causes the body to jerk and shake. During a seizure Abdul's breathing becomes more difficult and his skin turns a blue–grey colour. When the jerking stops, his breathing and colour go back to normal and he usually sleeps for a few hours. Witnessing a seizure can be a frightening experience. Along with training, comprehensive care plans should enable carers to know how to respond in the event of a seizure (see Fig. 13.1).

Communicating

People with profound intellectual disabilities and complex needs are often unable to use formal methods of communication and rely on others to interpret their facial expressions and non-verbal behaviours. Hogg (1998) found that carers often believed that they were able to interpret needs and emotions through facial expressions, vocalisations, eye contact and posture but that these were not always reliable and valid interpretations. Improving communication with people who have profound intellectual disabilities and complex needs is therefore an important part of the carer's role and due attention should be given to this aspect of care within the care planning process.

A speech and language therapist can be asked to carry out a communication assessment and has the necessary skills to recommend appropriate communication strategies for that person (Bradshaw, 2001). One strategy which has been thought to improve communication with people who have profound intellectual disabilities and complex needs is the use of a 'communication profile'. A communication passport aims to help carers understand and interpret choices, preferences, likes and dislikes and gives specific information about how to communicate with an individual based on their level specific profile of abilities. If the communication passport is produced in a user-friendly, accessible format it is more likely to be used. It can also provide the individual with more opportunities to communicate effectively with a larger number of people who they come into contact with, within their home, the services they use and in the community.

Another communication strategy that is beneficial for some people who are at a very early stage of development is 'intensive interaction' (Nind and Hewett, 2001). Intensive interaction involves developing the repetitive, pre-linguistic behaviours that are used routinely by the individual into a shared 'language' which is thought to enable others to gain access to the person's world (Caldwell, 1997). In this way, it is thought that meaningful communication sequences can be experienced that are mutually enjoyable and relaxing (Hewett, 2005).

In order to perceive and understand the world, people with profound intellectual disabilities and complex needs are thought to rely more heavily on multiple sources of sensory stimulation (Ayer, 1998). However, it is common for this group to experience sensory impairments which might further disadvantage their ability to communicate and experience the world (Bradshaw, 2001). Regular hearing and sight assessments are therefore vital to pick up and respond to problems as early as possible. Appointment details should be recorded and strategies should be in place to ensure that the results of assessments are disseminated to everyone involved in the person's direct care.

It is thought that by documenting responses to a range of choices offered over time patterns may emerge which suggest that consistent, valid choices are being made. Aylott (2001) used the term 'choices inventory' to refer to this strategy. Belfiore and Toro-Zambrana (1994) have developed a protocol which aims to achieve this. They make a distinction between choice and preference: a choice is essentially a selection of one option from a number of options that are offered, whereas a preference refers to a relatively predictable behaviour. This can be applied in a systematic way by observing and recording how an individual responds to various environmental stimuli. For example, if it is observed that someone becomes distressed when there is a lot of noise and relaxed when it is quiet, then it could be inferred that the individual is demonstrating a preference for quietness. This information can help carers to support people to make choices and exercise some degree of control over their environment. This kind of approach to careful monitoring and reporting on preference has been more recently reported by the Joseph Rowntree Foundation where it identified that control of decisions could be enabled by:

> 'a rigorous approach to building evidence of the process, including careful and creative recording and monitoring.' (Values into Action, 2001)

Therefore over a period of time it would be possible to establish a range of preferences for Abdul and incorporate these into his care plan.

Breathing

Respiratory problems are common in people with profound intellectual disabilities and complex need and this group is particularly susceptible to chest infections (Wake, 2003). One study has found that respiratory disorders were a leading cause of death for people with intellectual disabilities (Hollins et al., 1998).

For people like Abdul, who experience difficulties with breathing, a care plan might need to address methods of enhancing respiratory function. This could include instructions on:

- Appropriate positioning
- Postural drainage to remove excess sputum
- Oral and nasal suction
- Minimising the risks of aspiration
- Methods of promoting awareness amongst carers of the signs to look for to identify chest infections promptly

Carers also need to be alert to signs and symptoms of asthma and hay fever which can further exacerbate breathing difficulties.

Eating and drinking

The term 'dysphagia' means difficulties with swallowing. This can be a serious condition which can cause aspiration and choking. It is common in people with cerebral palsy, who may have poor muscle tone in the mouth area, poor reflexes and immature feeding skills. Difficulties with eating and drinking can lead to malnourishment and dehydration, which can be prevented by monitoring food and fluid intake and weight, and responding promptly if problems arise.

Abdul is underweight and is continuing to lose weight. He does not eat very much and is frequently constipated. This is concerning and indicates the urgent need for a thorough multi-disciplinary assessment. A speech and language therapist, who has been specially trained in feeding difficulties and management, should be asked to assess Abdul's specific difficulties and recommend a strategy to ensure that he receives adequate nutrition safely. A dietician could also be involved to assess the nutritional content of Abdul's diet and make recommendations for how his diet might be improved. In addition to the difficulties Abdul has with eating and drinking, he also suffers from frequent chest infections. Both of these problems are signs of aspiration. Aspiration is potentially life threatening and needs to be addressed as a matter of urgency and a referral should be made to the speech and language therapist who specialises in this area.

If Abdul is able to eat orally, the care plan would need to include details about the appropriate consistency of food, how often and how much he should be fed, the appropriate utensils to use and how to ensure that he maintains a posture that maximises his ability to eat safely. A high risk of aspiration can indicate the need for non-oral feeding by gastrostomy. Wake (2003) has provided an excellent introduction to gastrostomy feeding for people with profound intellectual disabilities and complex needs. Even if Abdul is unable to eat orally, he should not miss out on the shared mealtime experience with his family. This can be an important social time when families get together not only to eat but to share one another's company and conversation.

Eliminating

Constipation is relatively common among people with profound intellectual disabilities and complex needs and, amongst other causes, it can be caused by lack of fibre in the diet and lack of mobility. Improving the condition can be achieved by increasing the amount high-fibre foods, such as vegetables, pulses and fruits, in the diet, as this is a natural way of increasing bulk and fibre. For people with difficulties in chewing or swallowing the use of 'smoothies' can be a pleasurable way to increase the fibre content of the diet. If this does not solve the problem, Abdul's GP could prescribe medication, but this should be used as a last resort. The use of all medications should be closely monitored and regularly reviewed. Swimming (hydrotherapy) can be a useful and enjoyable physical exercise and can assist in making the abdominal wall 'work' and thereby encouraging bowel movement. Alternative therapies, such as bowel massage, have also been shown to improve the condition for some people (Emly et al., 2001). However, the availability of these therapies is variable across different geographical areas.

Washing and dressing

Personal and intimate care is a significant and time-consuming part of life for many people with profound intellectual disabilities and complex needs. When developing a care plan for Abdul, safety is of paramount importance for both carers and Abdul. Moving and handling guidelines must be adhered to as well as the policies that are in place to protect vulnerable people from abuse (Cambridge and Carnaby, 2000a). The family will need support to ensure they have the correct equipment and training to enable them to carry out care tasks safely. When providing personal care, consideration should be given to individual preferences and cultural customs. Advice should be sought from an appropriate Muslim organisation and these issues should be discussed with Abdul's family.

Personal care provides a valuable opportunity for sensory experiences and one to one interaction (Cambridge and Carnaby, 2000b). It should not be rushed, but used as a time for social interaction and the development of skills.

Due to the nature of their disabilities, many people with profound intellectual disabilities and complex needs are incontinent. Continence care involves invading a person's intimacy and must be attended to with sensitivity. Privacy and respect are vital when carrying out all aspects of personal and intimate care. This means more than simply closing the door when providing care. It means being careful not to make insensitive comments in front of other people and giving undivided attention whilst carrying out care activities. Carers should try to avoid becoming blasé about continence care even though it can become a routine part of their work.

People with incontinence are particularly susceptible to perineal dermatitis (Gray et al., 2002). Protecting the skin is therefore a prime consideration when carrying out continence care. The care plan should detail routine preventative measures, the signs of skin breakdown and a treatment plan to follow if skin breakdown does occur. Preventative measures include the use of appropriate continence pads, keeping the skin clean and dry without scrubbing and using appropriate cleaning and moisturising products (Gray et al., 2002). Some people with sensitive skin have allergies to certain products and in these cases the use of detergents, biological washing agents, talcum powder and products containing lanolin or perfume should be avoided (Gibbons, 1996). Alternatives, such as emollients, non-biological washing agents and perfume-free products, are readily available. The pharmacist or GP can give advice on the choice and use of these products to suit an individual's needs.

People with profound intellectual disabilities and complex needs are reliant on others to ensure that their teeth are cleaned at least twice a day and checked by the dentist every 6 months. However, some people with intellectual disabilities do not like having their teeth cleaned and this can cause difficulties. If this is the case, it is worth checking with the dentist to find out if the person has a dental problem that makes brushing painful. Using a small, soft toothbrush and trying different flavoured toothpastes may also be preferred. In some areas specialist services give advice on dental care for people with intellectual disabilities. Dental care is necessary for maintaining good health and for preventing halitosis which is important for social acceptability.

One particularly important consideration in respect to medication in the management of epilepsy concerns the use of phenytoin. This particular medicine is responsible for causing both gingival hyperplasia and hypertrophy that makes the management of oral hygiene even more critical and the advice of a dentist and oral hygienist should be sought.

Maintaining body temperature

It may be more difficult for people with profound intellectual disabilities and complex needs to maintain their body temperature due to poor circulation caused by restricted mobility. Regular monitoring of Abdul's temperature is important to enable carers to respond promptly and appropriately if he develops a high or low temperature as this could indicate an underlying health problem. Abdul would be unable to communicate if he was too hot or cold, and carers must therefore be mindful to weather conditions and ensure that he wears appropriate clothing, which might include gloves, hats and scarves in the winter and cool cotton clothing in the summer. Clothing should also be comfortable and suitable for Abdul's age and culture.

Sunburn and heatstroke should be prevented by applying high-factor sun cream and ensuring that the sun is avoided around mid-day and at particularly hot times. Carers should remember that dark skins are susceptible to sunburn. Fluid intake should be increased when the weather is hot to avoid dehydration.

Mobilising

Issues of mobility are highly relevant for people who have physical disabilities. Abdul is completely reliant on others for his comfort and to ensure that the correct measures are taken to improve and maintain his posture. The role of a physiotherapist would be to assess Abdul's needs for orthotics, wheelchairs, seating and special footwear and to carry out a review at prescribed intervals in order to determine any changes in need. This is particularly important at Abdul's stage in life as he is going through puberty and is likely to require larger equipment on account of his growth.

Abdul's care plan should describe the correct use of equipment such as hoists, splints and body braces and give instructions about how to carry out interventions as recommended by the physiotherapist. His care plan might include a series of passive exercises and the correct use of equipment such as a standing frame to improve or maintain his posture.

When considering issues of mobility for people with very restricted movement, carers should be mindful of the effects this might have on an individual. Being located in one plane of orientation for prolonged periods of time can make sudden or extreme movements seem unpleasant and even frightening. Carers should remember that for some people with profound intellectual disabilities and complex needs they can, in a sense, be physically locked into their own body and this may result in a lack self-determination on their part and a total reliance on others for movement.

Hydrotherapy is thought to be a particularly valuable way of increasing mobility and maintaining posture and also offers the individual an opportunity to experience weightlessness for the period of time that they are in the water; this can be particularly helpful for the management of pressure areas.

Working and playing

Providing meaningful activities to people with profound intellectual disabilities and complex needs can be challenging. This group is reliant on others to initiate activities and their involvement may largely be passive. It is also difficult to assess how meaningful the activity is for someone who has limited communication abilities. Choice of activities should therefore be based on understanding the individual's abilities and preferences, which can be developed through the use of a communication profile and choices inventory, as discussed previously in this chapter.

Studies have shown that people with profound intellectual disabilities and complex needs often spend large periods of time unengaged (Bradshaw, 2001). This is likely to reduce their capacity and motivation to learn and practice communication skills. It is conceivable that the development of communication strategies could be achieved alongside the provision of meaningful activities.

Multi-sensory rooms or 'snoezelens' are often found in special schools, day centres and larger residential homes. The literature suggests that multi-sensory rooms can be used for relaxation, sensory stimulation, leisure and entertainment (Ayer, 1998). Their purpose is, therefore, not entirely clear and will probably depend on how they are used. If multi-sensory rooms are to be used effectively and meaningfully their use should therefore be based on individual assessment and observation. Hirstwood and Gray (1995) have suggested that these rooms can be used as 'dumping grounds' whilst staff carry out activities in other areas. This is unacceptable for someone with profound intellectual disabilities and complex needs that requires the support of other people to benefit from the environment and have a meaningful experience. It would also be dangerous for Abdul due to the risk of him having an epileptic seizure. Care plans should specify the precise aims of the multi-sensory room and be accompanied by risk assessments which detail how the room should be used safely.

Carers should not forget that the world is full of natural and man-made environments that could provide stimulation, enjoyment and opportunities for social interaction for this group. Including people with profound intellectual disabilities and complex needs in everyday activities, such as cooking, is important and an individual's preferences for such activities can be monitored by developing a choices inventory. Occupational therapists and local Mencap organisations are two possible sources of ideas for providing suitable activities.

Expressing sexuality

The sexuality of people with learning disabilities is poorly understood and has often been neglected by health and social services (Oakes, 2003). Over recent years a move away from the medical model of care towards a holistic model of health care has led to greater recognition of the sexuality of people with learning disabilities (Oakes, 2003).

The law in relation to sex is fairly clear for people with profound intellectual disabilities and complex needs. It is unlawful for a person to have sex with someone who is unable to give consent (The Home Office, 2003). Holland et al. (2003) have argued that expressing sexuality is essential for well-being. It has been argued that in order to encompass the wide range of sexual needs and experiences that people have, sexuality should be seen in a broad way (Batcup and Thomas, 1994). For people with profound intellectual disabilities and complex needs, care plans might include activities to encourage bodily awareness, opportunity and support with masturbation, how clothing and appearance can be used as an expression of sexuality and sexual identity and how people should be supported through developmental changes, such as puberty, menstruation and the menopause.

Sleeping

People with profound intellectual disabilities and complex needs are dependent on others to ensure they have a safe and comfortable place to sleep. Abdul is known to be at risk of developing pressure sores on his ankles and this is thought to be caused by his positioning in bed. The physiotherapist might recommend the use of a 'sleep system' to enable carers to position Abdul in such a way that removes pressure from the areas prone to sores.

The time at which a person goes to bed and gets up should be determined by the individual's own sleep pattern. The amount of time people need to sleep varies. Lying in bed when not asleep may be boring and become uncomfortable, and not having enough sleep is thought to be detrimental to physical and psychological health and quality of life (Brostrom et al., 2004; Dogan et al.,

2005). To aid restful sleep, carers should ensure that the bedroom is quiet, neither too hot nor cold and that it is free from draughts.

Dying

Although life expectancy for people with intellectual disabilities is increasing, this group have an increased risk of early death (Hollins et al., 1998). Problems recognising and assessing symptoms of illness mean that diagnoses, and therefore access to appropriate treatment, is often delayed in this group (Tuffrey-Wijne, 2005). Pain is often the earliest indicator of illness but Donovan (2002) has found that carers can have difficulties recognising that a person with profound intellectual disabilities and complex needs is in pain, suggesting that illnesses could therefore be easily missed.

People with profound intellectual disabilities and complex needs are at greater risk of pain as a result of associated physical conditions such as cerebral palsy and gastro-oesophageal reflux (Davies and Evans, 2001). Pain management strategies, which might include the administration of analgesics and correct positioning, should be detailed in the care plan.

Tuffrey-Wijne (2005) has pointed out that an increase in life expectancy has resulted in conditions such as cardiovascular disease and cancer becoming more common in people with intellectual disabilities. When required to provide palliative care, carers should seek the support of specialist services. Some of the issues that might need to be considered at this stage of life include pain and symptom control, consent and ways of communicating about illness and death with the individual and their family, and how relatives can be supported through this difficult time (Tuffrey-Wijne, 2005). Consideration should also be given to how carers will be supported to cope with the effects of their own experience of loss and bereavement.

In a group home, people with profound intellectual disabilities and complex needs are also likely to be affected by the loss of a resident. Research on bereavement and people with intellectual disabilities has suggested that the experience of grief can be prolonged and its effects can include anxiety, depression and irritability (Oswin, 1991; Hollins and Esterhuyzen, 1997). These findings have challenged the widespread belief that people with intellectual disabilities are incapable of experiencing grief; the reader might care to refer back to Chapter 9.

One limitation of the Roper Logan Tierney model is that it does not include spirituality or relationships as activities of daily living. As both of these are thought to be equally important to the human experience they should be considered as an integral part of the care planning process.

Spirituality

Spirituality has been considered a significant dimension of well being (Narayanasamy et al., 2002). Hatton et al. (2004) have argued that meeting people's religious and spiritual needs is an essential role for services to fulfil. However, spiritual needs are probably one of the most challenging and neglected areas of care for people with profound intellectual disabilities and complex needs.

Care planning and decision making can be problematic in this area as differences in values and beliefs between different members of care staff and family members can cause tensions. Person-centred approaches offer a solution to some of these problems. By encouraging open discussion and prioritising the individual's needs above the aspirations of family and staff, decisions can be made about how to meet religious and spiritual needs.

Narayanasamy et al. (2002) have argued that a distinction must be made between religion and spirituality. They have found that services largely failed to address spiritual needs but were better at meeting religious needs which might have involved supporting individuals with religious activities and practices. Legere (1984) has defined spirituality as 'to give meaning and purpose' which might be a helpful way for carers to start to think about how to meet this area of human need.

There are some resources which might be useful for developing care plans to address religious and spiritual needs (see Hatton et al., 2004). However, these do tend to concentrate on the needs of people with mild to moderate intellectual disabilities and there is still a long way to go to understand how these needs might be met for people with profound intellectual disabilities and complex needs.

Relationships

Carers play a vital role in supporting people with profound intellectual disabilities and complex needs to maintain and develop relationships throughout their lives. Parents will have had varying experiences of parenting a child with profound intellectual disabilities and complex needs. Some may have had difficulties coming to terms with their son's or daughter's disability, and carers should be sensitive to the worries and concerns they may have about their son's or daughter's care.

The need for human touch has been well established (Montagu, 1971; Dobson et al., 2002). However, policies in human services are sometimes interpreted in a way that restricts the use of touch. This is regrettable as touch might be a person's only, or most meaningful, way of communicating and connecting with the social world. Touch can also be used to provide sensory stimulation and to offer comfort. The need for touch could be addressed through the use of massage and communication strategies.

Reader activity 13.2

Go back to the list of people who might be involved in Abdul's care. Who is likely to be involved in the direct implementation of his care plans?

> **Box 13.3 Some people who might be involved in the implementation of Abdul's care plan**
>
> - Family
> - School teacher
> - Respite care staff
> - Physiotherapist (some aspects)
> - Certain aspects of the care plan such as communication should be used by all those who come into contact with Abdul

Implementing care plans

Ultimately, the success of care planning is dependent on its implementation. Care plans should not be paper exercises whereby forms are filled out and filed away in a cabinet and retrieved only at the next date for review. They should be active documents, which should be updated on a regular basis and used by all those involved in providing care.

There is a high turnover of staff in intellectual disability services and this can have serious consequences for service quality (Felce et al., 1993; Hatton et al., 1995; Hatton et al., 2001). Care plans can be pivotal in ensuring that information is passed on to new carers when old staff leave and therefore attempt to bring about some form of continuity in someone's life.

The majority of staff who provide direct 'hands on' care do not have relevant care-related qualifications. The White Paper, *Valuing People* (Department of Health, 2001), has suggested that the lack of trained staff in intellectual disability services should be addressed by the introduction of a Learning Disabilities Awards Framework (LDAF). Service providers have a responsibility to establish and maintain a competent workforce and should ensure that all new staff enrol onto the LDAF scheme. The PMLD Network (2002) has identified the areas of accessing services and communication as priorities for staff training and these are addressed by the LDAF scheme. Professionals, such as speech and language therapists, physiotherapists and occupational therapists, can also offer valuable training to paid carers and family carers.

Hogg (1998) has acknowledged that, while we might use especially trained staff to support people with profound intellectual disabilities and complex needs, this does not mean that they always have to use special services.

Evaluating care plans

As already stated, the care plan is an active document, which should constantly evolve in response to the evaluation of current and past interventions, changes in the individual's needs and the development of new knowledge and ideas.

A lack of consensus on what constitutes quality of life (Petry et al., 2001) poses a challenge for the evaluation of care plans, as what may be a desirable outcome for one person could be entirely different for someone else. Physical outcomes are probably easier to evaluate because a comparison can be made of objective measurements (such as blood pressure or the frequency of seizures) that are taken before and after the intervention. Measuring abstract concepts, such as spiritual well-being, is more problematic. The use of communication profiles was discussed previously in this chapter. These could help carers to develop an understanding of the success of the care plan from the individual's perspective. However, for the most part, evaluation will be based on the reports and opinions of other people. Reflective practice provides an opportunity for staff to consider these different perspectives and their own contribution to care planning. The use of multiple perspectives has been commented on in the context of learning disability research by Gates and Atherton (2001):

> 'Autobiographical, participatory, oral and life history research provides evid-ence of a different nature that represents authentic accounts from people with learning disabilities concerning their experiences of disability and having to cope with professionals and caring agencies. While the reliability of such accounts may be problematic in some cases, they are clearly some of the most valid types of evidence professionals in learning disabilities presently have at their disposal. This is because the reliability of such methods is, in a sense, held ransom to the vagarious nature of human memory. Whereas human memory can be unreliable, the authenticity of such accounts repres-ents highly valid data.' (Gates and Atherton, 2001, p. 519)

Establishing long-term relationships and building and maintaining family relationships and community links are extremely valuable. Family members might be the only consistent presence in a person's life as staff members tend to come and go. Professionals should remember that a family carer is usually 'the expert' when it comes to the care of their relative.

Conclusion

This chapter has attempted to demonstrate how care can be planned and delivered for people with profound intellectual disabilities and complex needs. It has been argued that this group represents one of the most marginalised groups of people in western society. They are at risk from social exclusion and experience poorer health than the rest of the population. Care plans in this chapter have been presented as one way of ensuring that this group of people receives systematic planning and documentation of interventions by their paid carers. Such an approach should be adopted to meet an individual's daily needs for support in all aspects of their life and it has been suggested in this chapter that the use of a specific model of nursing might assist in this being undertaken in a more organised and guided way. Further, it has been suggested that care planning is particularly relevant for this group of people because of the high level of dependence they may have on others throughout their whole lives. In particular, this chapter has considered the role of the intellectual disability nurse in care planning and delivery for some of the most vulnerable people in our society.

References

American Association on Mental Retardation (1997) *Mental Retardation: Definition, Classification, and Systems of Support*, 9th edn. Washington: American Association on Mental Retardation.

Ayer, S. (1998) Use of multi-sensory rooms for children with profound and multiple intellectual disabilities. *Journal of Intellectual disabilities for Nursing, Health and Social Care* **2** (2), 89–97.

Aylott, J. (2001) The new intellectual disabilities White Paper: Did it forget something? *British Journal of Intellectual Disabilities* **10** (8), 512.

Barron, S. and Mulvany, F. (2004) *National Intellectual Disability Database Committee: Annual Report for 2004.* Dublin: Health Research Board.

Batcup, D. and Thomas, B. (1994) Mixing the genders, an ethical dilemma: how nursing theory has dealt with sexuality and gender. *Nursing Ethics* **1** (1) 43–52.

Belifore, P.J. and Toro-Zambrana, W. (1994) *Recognising Choices in Community Settings by People with Significant Disabilities.* Washington: American Association on Mental Retardation.

Bradshaw, J. (2001) Communication partnerships with people with profound and multiple intellectual disabilities. *Tizard Intellectual Disability Review* **6** (2), 6–15.

Brostrom, A., Stromberg, A., Dahlstrom, U. and Fridlund, B. (2004) Sleep difficulties, daytime sleepiness, and health-related quality of life in patients with chronic heart failure. *Journal of Cardiovascular Nursing* **19** (4), 234–2.

Caldwell, P. (1997) 'Getting in touch' with people with severe learning disabilities. *British Journal of Nursing* **6** (13), 751–6.

Cambridge, P. and Carnaby, S. (2000a) A personal touch: managing the risks of abuse during intimate and personal care. *The Journal of Adult Protection* **2** (4) 4–16.

Cambridge, P. and Carnaby, S. (2000b) *Making it Personal: Providing Intimate and Personal Care for People with Intellectual Disabilities.* Brighton: Pavilion.

Carnaby, S. (2001) Editorial. *Tizard Intellectual Disability Review* **6** (2), 2–5.

Craft, M. (1985) Classification criteria, epidemiology and causation. In: *Mental Handicap: a Multidisciplinary Approach* (Craft, M., Bicknell, J. and Hollins, S., eds.). London: Baillière Tindall.

Craig, J. and Smyth, R. (2002) *The Evidence Based Practice Manual for Nurses.* London: Churchill Livingstone.

Davies, D. and Evans, L. (2001) Assessing pain in people with profound intellectual disabilities. *British Journal of Nursing* **10** (8), 513–16.

Dealey, C. (1997) *Managing Pressure Sore Prevention.* Dinton: Quay Books.

Department of Health (1992) *Social Care for Adults with Learning Disabilities (Mental Handicap LAC (92)15).* London: Her Majesty's Stationery Office.

Department of Health (2001) *Valuing People: A New Strategy for Intellectual Disability for the 21st Century.* London: The Stationery Office.

Dobson, S., Upadhyaya, S., Conyers, I. and Raghavan, R. (2002) Touch in the care of people with profound and complex needs. *Journal of Learning Disabilities* **6** (4), 351–62.

Dogan, O., Ertekin, S. and Dogan, S. (2005) Sleep quality in hospitalized patients. *Journal of Clinical Nursing* **14** (1), 107–13.

Donovan, J. (2002) Learning disability nurses' experiences of being with clients who may be in pain. *Journal of Advanced Nursing* **38** (5), 458–66.

Emerson, E., Hatton, C., Felce, D. and Murphy, G. (2001) *Learning Disabilities: the Fundamental Facts*. London: The Foundation for People with Learning Disabilities.

Emly, M., Wilson, L. and Darby, J. (2001) Abdominal massage for adults with learning disabilities. *Nursing Times* **97** (30), 61–2.

Felce, D., Lowe, K. and Beswick, J. (1993) Staff turnover in ordinary housing services for people with severe or profound mental handicaps. *Journal of Intellectual Disability Research* **37**, 143–52.

Gates, B. and Atherton, H. (2001) The challenge of evidence based practice for learning disability professionals in health and social care. *British Journal of Nursing* **10** (8), 173–8.

Gates, B. and Wray, J. (2000) The problematic nature of evidence. In: *Behavioural Distress: Concepts and Strategies* (Gates, B., Gear, J. and Wray, J., eds.). London: Baillière Tindall.

Gibbons, G. (1996) Nurse Prescriber Supplement: skin care and incontinence. *Community Nurse* **2** (7), 37.

Goffman, E. (1961) *Asylums: Essays on the Social Situation of Mental Patients and Other Inmates*. Harmondsworth: Penguin.

Gooding, L. (2004) *Valuing People* has yet to make a real impact. *Learning Disability Practice* **7** (3), 6.

Gray, M., Ratliff, C. and Donovan, A. (2002) Tender mercies: providing skin care for an incontinent patient. *Nursing* **32** (7), 51–4.

Hatton, C., Brown, R., Caine, A. and Emerson, E. (1995) Stressors, coping strategies and stress-related outcomes among direct care staff in staffed houses for people with learning disabilities. *Mental Handicap Research* **8**, 252–71.

Hatton, C., Emerson, E., Rivers, M., Mason, H., Swarbrick, R., Mason, L., Kiernan, C., Reeves, D. and Alborz, A. (2001) Factors associated with intended staff turnover and job search behaviour in services for people with intellectual disability. *Journal of Intellectual Disability Research* **45** (3), 258–70.

Hatton, C., Turner, S., Shah, R., Rahim, N. and Stansfield, J. (2004) *Religious Expression, a Fundamental Human Right: The report of an Action Research Project on Meeting the Needs of People with Learning Disabilities*. London: The Mental Health Foundation.

Hewett, D. (2005) *How Does Intensive Interaction Work?* [online]. Available from: www.intensiveinteraction.co.uk (Accessed 6 April 2005)

Hirstwood, R. and Gray, M. (1995) *A Practical Guide to the Use of Multi-Sensory Rooms*. London: TFH Publications.

Ho, A. (2004) To be labelled, or not to be labelled: that is the question. *British Journal of Learning Disabilities* **32** (2), 86–92.

Hogg, J. (1998) Competence and quality in the lives of people with profound and multiple intellectual disabilities: some recent research. *Tizard Intellectual Disability Review* **3** (1), 6–17.

Holland, K., Jenkins, J., Solomon, J. and Whittma, S. (2003) *Applying the Roper Logan Tierney Model in Practice*. London: Churchill Livingstone.

Hollins, S. and Esterhuyzen, A. (1997) Bereavement and grief in adults with learning disabilities. *British Journal of Psychiatry* **170**, 497–501.

Hollins, S., Attard, M.T., von Fraunhofer, N., McGuigan, S. and Sedgwick, P. (1998) Mortality in people with learning disability: risks, causes and death certification findings in London. *Developmental Medicine and Child Neurology* **40** (1), 50–6.

Klotz, J. (2004) Sociocultural study of intellectual disability: moving beyond labelling and social constructionist perspectives. *British Journal of Learning Disabilities* **32**, 93–104.

Lacey, P. (1998) Meeting complex needs through collaborative multi-disciplinary team work. In: *People with Profound and Multiple Intellectual Disabilities: A Collaborative Approach to Meeting Complex Needs* (Lacey, P. and Ouvry C., eds.). London: David Foulton.

Legere, T. (1984) A spirituality for today. *Studies in Formative Spirituality* **5** (3), 375–85.

Male, D. (1996) Who goes to SLD schools? *Journal of Applied Research in Intellectual Disabilities* **9** (4), 307–23.

McConkey, R., Spollen, M. and Jamison, J. (2003) *Administrative Prevalence of Learning Disability in Northern Ireland. A Report to the Department of Health, Social Services and Public Safety*. Belfast: Department of Health, Social Services and Public Safety.

McNally, S. (2004) Plus ça change? Progress achieved in services for people with an intellectual disability in England since the publication of *Valuing People. Journal of Learning Disabilities* **8** (4), 323–9.

Mencap (2001) *No Ordinary Life: The Support Needs of Families Caring for Children and Adults with Profound and Multiple Intellectual Disabilities*. London: Mencap.

Mencap (2004) *Treat Me Right! Better Healthcare for People with a Learning Disability*. London: Mencap.

Mencap (2005) *What do we mean by Profound and Multiple Intellectual Disabilities (PMLD)?* [online] Available from: www.mencap.org.uk/html/campaigns/pmld_definition.htm (Accessed 1 February 2005)

Montagu, A. (1971) *Touching: The Human Significance of the Skin*. New York: Harper and Row.

Narayanasamy, A., Gates, B. and Swinton, J. (2002) Spirituality and intellectual disabilities: a qualitative study. *British Journal of Nursing* **11** (14), 948–57.

Nind, M. and Hewett, D. (2001) *A Practical Guide to Intensive Interaction*. Kidderminster: BILD publications.

Nursing and Midwifery Council (2004) *The NMC Code of Professional Conduct: Standards for Conduct, Performance and Ethics*. London: Nursing and Midwifery Council.

Oakes, P. (2003) Sexual and personal relationships. In: *Learning Disabilities: Toward Inclusion*, 4th edn, (Gates, B., ed.). Edinburgh: Churchill Livingstone.

Open University (1987) *Mental Handicap: Patterns for Living*. Milton Keynes: Open University Press.

Oswin, M. (1991) *Am I Allowed to Cry? A Study of Bereavement amongst People who have Learning Difficulties*. London: Human Horizons.

Oxford English Dictionary (2002) 10th edn. Revised. Oxford: Oxford University Press.

Petry, K., Maes, B. and Vlaskamp, C. (2001) Developing a procedure for evaluating quality of life for people with profound and multiple disabilities. *Tizard Learning Disability Review* **6** (2), 45–8.

Profound and Multiple Learning Disabilities Network (2002) *Valuing People with Profound and Multiple Intellectual Disabilities (PMLD)*. London: Mencap.

Roper, N., Logan, W.W. and Tierney, A. (1996) *The Elements of Nursing: A Model for Nursing Based on a Model for Living*. London: Churchill Livingstone.

Shalock, R.L. (2004) The concept of quality of life: what we know and do not know. *Journal of Intellectual Disability Research* **48** (3), 20–16.

Swinton, J. (2001) *A Space to Listen: Meeting the Spiritual Needs for People with Learning Disabilities*. The Mental Health Foundation: London.

The Home Office (2003) *The Sexual Offences Act*. London: The Home Office.

The National Society for Epilepsy (2002) *Information on Epilepsy: Epilepsy and Intellectual Disability* [online]. Available from: www.epilepsynse.org.uk/pages/info/leaflets/learning.cfm (Accessed 15 February 2005)

Tierney, A. (1998) Nursing models: extant or extinct? *Journal of Advanced Nursing* **28** (1), 77–85.

Tuffrey-Wijne, I. (2005) *Cancer, Palliative Care and Intellectual Disabilities* [online]. Available from: www.intellectualdisability.info/mental_phys_heath/cancer_id.htm (Accessed 6 April 2005)

United Kingdom Central Council for Nursing, Midwifery and Health Visiting (1998) *Guidelines for Mental Health and Learning Disabilities Nursing*. London: United Kingdom Central Council for Nursing, Midwifery and Health Visiting.

Values into Action (2001) *Demonstrating Control of Decisions by Adults with Learning Difficulties who have High Support Needs*. Joseph Rowntree Foundation: York.

Wake, E. (2003) Profound and multiple disability. In: *Learning Disabilities: Toward Inclusion*, 4th edn, (Gates, B., ed.). Edinburgh: Churchill Livingstone.

Ward, F. (1999) *Modernising the Social Care Workforce: The first National Strategy for England. Supplementary Report on Learning Disability*. Leeds: Training Organisation for the Personal Social Services.

World Health Organization (1992) *The ICD-10 Classification of Mental and Behavioural Disorders: Clinical Descriptions and Diagnostic Guidelines*. Geneva: World Health Organization.

Wolverson, M. (2003) Challenging behaviour. In: *Learning Disabilities: Toward Inclusion*, 4th edn, (Gates, B., ed.). Edinburgh: Churchill Livingstone.

Yura, H. and Walsh, M.B. (1978) *The Nursing Process*. New York: Appleton-Century-Crofts.

Further reading and resources

Chadwick, D.D., Jolliffe, J. and Goldbart, J. (2002) Carer knowledge of dysphagia management strategies. *International Journal of Language and Communication Disorders* **27** (3), 135–44.

Lacey, P. and Ouvry, C. (eds.) (1998) *People with Profound and Multiple Learning Disabilities: A Collaborative Approach to Meeting Complex Needs*. London: David Fulton.

Useful websites

General information: www.learningdisabilties.org.uk
Epilepsy: www.epilepsynse.org.uk
Cerebral palsy: www.scope.org.uk
Eating and swallowing difficulties: www.dysphagiaonline.com (free registration)
Intensive interaction: www.bild.org.uk/factsheets/intensive_interaction.htm and www.intensiveinteraction.co.uk
Learning Disabilities Award Framework: www.ldaf.org.uk

Index